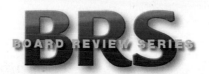

# Behavioral Science

SIXTH EDITION

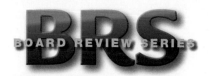

# Behavioral Science

## SIXTH EDITION

**Barbara Fadem, PhD**
Professor
Department of Psychiatry
University of Medicine and Dentistry of New Jersey
New Jersey Medical School
Newark, New Jersey

Wolters Kluwer | Lippincott Williams & Wilkins
Health
Philadelphia • Baltimore • New York • London
Buenos Aires • Hong Kong • Sydney • Tokyo

*Acquisitions Editor:* Crystal Taylor
*Product Manager:* Catherine Noonan
*Marketing Manager:* Joy Fisher-Williams
*Designer:* Holly Reid McLaughlin
*Compositor:* Aptara, Inc.

Sixth Edition

351 West Camden Street
Baltimore, MD 21201

Two Commerce Square
2001 Market Street
Philadelphia, PA 19103

Printed in China

9 8 7 6 5 4 3 2 1

**Library of Congress Cataloging-in-Publication Data**

Fadem, Barbara.
  Behavioral science / Barbara Fadem.—6th ed.
    p. ; cm.—(Board review series)
  Includes bibliographical references and index.
  ISBN 978-1-4511-3210-6
  I. Title.   II. Series: Board review series.
  [DNLM: 1. Behavioral Sciences—Examination Questions.   2. Behavioral Sciences–Outlines.
3. Behavior—Examination Questions.   4. Behavior—Outlines.   WM 18.2]
  616.890076—dc23

                              2012042579

To purchase additional copies of this book, call our customer service department at **(800) 638-3030** or fax orders to **(301) 223-2320**. International customers should call **(301) 223-2300**.

Visit Lippincott Williams & Wilkins on the Internet: http://www.lww.com. Lippincott Williams & Wilkins customer service representatives are available from 8:30 am to 6:00 pm, EST.

*I lovingly dedicate the 6th edition of this book to Daniel, Jonathan, Terri, Sarah and Joseph Fadem and Tom and Fifi Chenal*

# Preface

The function and state of the mind are of significant importance to the physical health of an individual. The United States Medical Licensing Examination (USMLE) is closely attuned to the substantial power of the mind–body relationship and extensively tests this area on all three steps of the examination. This review book was prepared as a learning tool to help the students rapidly recall information that they learned in the first two years of medical school in behavioral science, psychiatry, epidemiology, and related courses.

The sixth edition of *BRS Behavioral Science* contains 26 chapters. All chapters start with a "Typical Board Question," which serves as an example for the manner in which the subject matter of that chapter is tested on the USMLE. Each chapter has been updated to include the most current information.

A total of more than 700 USMLE-style questions (about 70 more than in the fifth edition) and answers with detailed explanations are presented after each chapter, as well as in the Comprehensive Examination. A significant number of these questions were written expressly for this sixth edition and reflect USMLE style, using clinical vignettes in the stem. Many tables are included in the book to provide quick access to essential information.

# Acknowledgments

The author wishes to thank Crystal Taylor and Catherine Noonan of Wolters Kluwer, Lippincott Williams & Wilkins, for their encouragement and practical assistance with the manuscript. As always, the author thanks with great affection and respect the caring, involved medical students with whom she has had the honor of working over the years. Special thanks to Timothy Kreider, M.D., Ph.D. for his valuable input into Chapters 25 and 26.

# Contents

## 4. GENETICS, ANATOMY, AND BIOCHEMISTRY OF BEHAVIOR — 33

I. Behavioral Genetics 33
II. Behavioral Neuroanatomy 34
III. Neurotransmission 36
IV. Biogenic Amines 37
V. Amino Acid Neurotransmitters 40
VI. Neuropeptides 40

Review Test 41

## 5. BIOLOGICAL ASSESSMENT OF PATIENTS WITH PSYCHIATRIC SYMPTOMS — 48

I. Overview 48
II. Measurement of Biogenic Amines and Psychotropic Drugs 48
III. Evaluating Endocrine Function 49
IV. Neuroimaging and Electroencephalogram Studies 49
V. Neuropsychological Tests 50
VI. Other Tests 51

Review Test 52

## 6. PSYCHOANALYTIC THEORY AND DEFENSE MECHANISMS — 56

I. Overview 56
II. Freud's Theories of the Mind 56
III. Defense Mechanisms 57
IV. Transference Reactions 57

Review Test 60

## 7. LEARNING THEORY — 64

I. Overview 64
II. Habituation and Sensitization 64
III. Classical Conditioning 65
IV. Operant Conditioning 65

Review Test 68

## 8. CLINICAL ASSESSMENT OF PATIENTS WITH BEHAVIORAL SYMPTOMS — 73

I. Overview of Psychological Testing 73
II. Intelligence Tests 73
III. Achievement Tests 74

| chapter | 1 | The Beginning of Life: Pregnancy Through Preschool |

## Typical Board Question

The mother of a 1-month-old child, her second, is concerned because the baby cries every day from 6 PM to 7 PM. She tells the doctor that, unlike her first child who was always calm, nothing she does during this hour seems to comfort this baby. Physical examination is unremarkable and the child has gained 2 pounds since birth. With respect to the mother, the physician should

- **(A)** reassure her that all children are different and that some crying is normal
- **(B)** recommend that she see a psychotherapist
- **(C)** prescribe an antidepressant
- **(D)** recommend that the father care for the child when it is crying
- **(E)** refer her to a pediatrician specializing in "difficult" infants

*(See "Answers and Explanations" at end of chapter.)*

## I. CHILDBIRTH AND THE POSTPARTUM PERIOD

A. **Birth rate and cesarean birth**
   1. About 4.3 million children are born each year in the United States; about one-third of all births are by **cesarean section**
   2. The number of cesarean births declined during the 1990s, partly in response to increasing evidence that women often undergo unnecessary surgical procedures. Since 2000, however, the rate has been increasing and is now higher than it has ever been.

B. **Premature birth**
   1. **Premature births** and **very premature births** are defined as those following a gestation of less than **37** and **32 completed weeks**, respectively.
   2. Premature birth puts a child at greater risk for dying in the first year of life and for emotional, behavioral, and learning problems; **physical disability**; and **mental retardation**.
   3. Premature births, which are associated with low income, maternal illness or malnutrition, and young maternal age, occur in almost twice as many non-Hispanic African-American infants than non-Hispanic white infants.

C. **Infant mortality**
   1. **Low socioeconomic status**, which is related in part to ethnicity, is associated with prematurity and high infant mortality (Table 1.1).
   2. In part because the United States does not have a system of health care for all citizens paid for by the government through taxes, prematurity and infant mortality rates in the United States are high as compared to the rates in other developed countries (Figure 1.1).

1

| table 1.1 | Ethnicity and Infant Mortality in the United States (2005) |
|---|---|
| **Ethnic Group** | **Infant Deaths Per 1,000 Total Live Births** |
| All ethnic groups | 6.9 |
| Asian or Pacific Islander | 4.9 |
| Mexican | 5.6 |
| White | 5.8 |
| Native American | 8.0 |
| Puerto Rican | 8.3 |
| Non-Hispanic black (African American) | 13.9 |

From Matthews TJ, MacDorman M. Infant mortality statistics from the 2005 period: Linked birth/infant death set. *Natl Vital Stat Rep.* 2007;57(2):14–17.

3. The **Apgar score (named for Dr. Virginia Apgar but useful as a mnemonic): A—appearance (color), P—pulse (heartbeat), G—grimace (reflex irritability), A—activity (muscle tone), R—respiration (breathing regularity)** quantifies physical functioning in premature and full-term newborns (Table 1.2) and can be used to predict the likelihood of immediate survival.

The infant is evaluated 1 minute and 5 (or 10) minutes after birth. Each of the five measures can have a score of 0, 1, or 2 (highest score = 10). Score >7 = no imminent survival threat; score <4 = imminent survival threat.

D. **Postpartum maternal reactions**
   1. **Baby blues**
      a. Many women experience a typical emotional reaction called "**baby blues**" or "postpartum blues" lasting up to 2 weeks after childbirth.

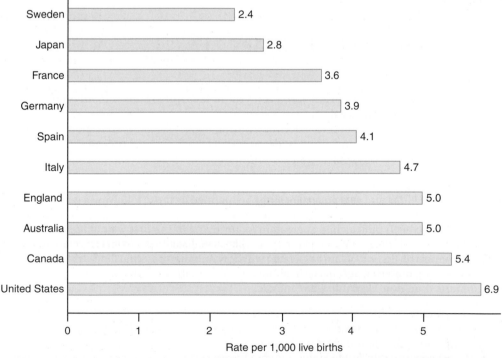

**FIGURE 1.1.** Comparison of infant mortality rates in selected countries (in alphabetical order) (Modified from CDC [2009]. Behind international rankings of infant mortality: how the United States compares with Europe. *NCHS Data Brief*, 23. Figure 1).

table **1.2** The Apgar Scoring System

| Measure | Score | | |
|---|---|---|---|
| | 0 | 1 | 2 |
| Heartbeat | Absent | Slow (<100/min) | Rapid (>100/min) |
| Respiration | Absent | Irregular, slow | Good, crying |
| Muscle tone | Flaccid, limp | Weak, inactive | Strong, active |
| Color of body and extremities | Both body and extremities pale or blue | Pink body, blue extremities | Pink body, pink extremities |
| Reflexes, e.g., heel prick or nasal tickle | No response | Grimace | Foot withdrawal, cry, sneeze, cough |

    **b.** This reaction results from **psychological factors** (e.g., the emotional stress of childbirth, the feelings of added responsibility), as well as **physiological factors** (e.g., changes in hormone levels, fatigue).

    **c.** Management involves emotional support from the physician as well as practical suggestions for child care.

  **2.** **Major depression** and **brief psychotic disorder with postpartum onset** (postpartum psychosis) are more serious reactions than postpartum blues and are treated with antidepressant and antipsychotic medications (Table 1.3) (and see Chapters 11 and 12).

    Women who have experienced these reactions once are at risk for having them after subsequent deliveries.

## II. INFANCY: BIRTH TO 15 MONTHS

**A. Bonding of the parent to the infant**

  **1.** Bonding between the caregiver and the infant is enhanced by **physical contact** between the two.

  **2.** Bonding may be adversely affected if:

    **a.** The child is of **low birth weight or ill**, leading to **separation from the mother** after delivery.

    **b.** There are problems in the mother–father relationship.

  **3.** Women who take **classes preparing them for childbirth** have shorter labors, fewer medical complications, less need for medication, and closer initial interactions with their infants.

table **1.3** Postpartum Maternal Reactions

| Maternal Reaction | Incidence | Onset of Symptoms | Duration of Symptoms | Characteristics |
|---|---|---|---|---|
| Postpartum blues ("baby blues") | 33%–50% | Within a few days after delivery | Up to 2 wks after delivery | Exaggerated emotionality and tearfulness Interacting well with friends and family Good grooming |
| Major depressive episode | 5%–10% | Within 4 wks after delivery | Up to 1 yr without treatment; 3–6 wks with treatment | Feelings of hopelessness and helplessness Lack of pleasure or interest in usual activities Poor self-care May include psychotic symptoms ("mood disorder with psychotic features"), e.g., hallucinations and delusions (see Table 11.1) Mother may harm infant |
| Brief psychotic disorder (postpartum onset) | 0.1%–0.2% | Within 4 wks after delivery | Up to 1 mo | Psychotic symptoms not better accounted for by mood disorder with psychotic features Mother may harm infant |

**B. Attachment of the infant to the parent**

1. The principal psychological task of infancy is the **formation of an intimate attachment** to the primary caregiver, usually the mother.
2. Toward the end of the first year of life, **separation from the primary caregiver** leads to initial loud protests from the infant (typical "separation anxiety").
3. With continued absence of the mother, the infant is at risk for **depression**.
   a. Infants may experience depression even when they are living with their mothers if the mother is physically and emotionally distant and insensitive to their needs.
   b. Depressed infants may exhibit **poor health** and **slowed physical growth**.
   c. The *Diagnostic and Statistical Manual of Mental Disorders, 4th Edition, Text Revision (DSM-IV-TR)* term for disturbances in otherwise typical children owing to grossly pathological care is **reactive attachment disorder of infancy or early childhood, inhibited and disinhibited type**.
      (1) **Inhibited type:** Children are withdrawn and unresponsive.
      (2) **Disinhibited type:** Children approach and attach indiscriminately to strangers as though the strangers were familiar to them.

**C. Studies of attachment**

1. **Harry Harlow** demonstrated that infant monkeys reared in relative isolation by **surrogate artificial mothers** do not develop typical mating, maternal, and social behaviors as adults.
   a. **Males** may be more affected than females by such isolation.
   b. The **length of time of isolation** is important. Young monkeys isolated for less than 6 months can be rehabilitated by playing with typical young monkeys.
2. **René Spitz** documented that children without proper mothering (e.g., those in orphanages) show severe **developmental retardation**, poor health, and higher death rates ("**hospitalism**") in spite of adequate physical care.
3. Partly because of such findings, the **foster care system** was established for young children in the United States who do not have adequate home situations. Foster families are those that have been approved and funded by the state of residence to take care of a child in their homes.

**D. Characteristics of the infant**

1. **Reflexive behavior.** At birth, the typical infant possesses simple reflexes such as the **sucking** reflex, **startle** reflex (Moro reflex), **palmar grasp** reflex, **Babinski** reflex, and **rooting** reflex. All of these reflexes disappear during the first year of life (Table 1.4).
2. **Motor, social, verbal**, and **cognitive development** (Table 1.5)
   a. Although there is a reflexive smile present at birth, the **social smile** is one of the first markers of the infant's responsiveness to another individual.
   b. Crying and withdrawing in the presence of an unfamiliar person (**stranger anxiety**) is normal and begins at about 7 months of age.
      (1) This behavior indicates that the infant has developed a specific attachment to the mother and is able to distinguish her from a stranger.

**t a b l e   1.4   Reflexes Present at Birth and the Age at which they Disappear**

| Reflex | Description | Age of Disappearance |
|---|---|---|
| Palmar grasp | The child's fingers grasp objects placed in the palm | 2 mos |
| Rooting and sucking reflexes | The child's head turns in the direction of a stroke on the cheek when seeking a nipple to suck | 3 mos |
| Startle (Moro) reflex | When the child is startled, the arms and legs extend | 4 mos |
| Babinski reflex | Dorsiflexion of the largest toe when the plantar surface of the child's foot is stroked | 12 mos |
| Tracking reflex | The child visually follows a human face | Continues |

| table **1.5** | Motor, Social, Verbal, and Cognitive Development of the Infant | | |
|---|---|---|---|
| | **Skill Area** | | |
| **Age (in Months)** | **Motor** | **Social** | **Verbal and Cognitive** |
| 1–3 | **Lifts head** when lying prone | **Smiles** in response to a human face (the "social smile") | Coos or gurgles in response to human attention |
| 4–6 | Turns over (5 mos)<br>**Sits** unassisted (6 mos)<br>Reaches for objects<br>Grasps with entire hand ("raking grasp") | Forms an attachment to primary caregiver<br>Recognizes familiar people | Babbles (repeats single sounds over and over) |
| 7–11 | **Crawls** on hands and knees<br>Pulls self up to stand<br>**Transfers** toys from hand to hand (10 mos)<br>Picks up toys and food using "pincer" (thumb and forefinger) grasp (10 mos) | Shows **stranger anxiety**<br>Plays social games such as peek-a-boo, waves "bye-bye" | Imitates sounds<br>Uses gestures<br>Responds to own name<br>Responds to simple instructions |
| 12–15 | **Walks** unassisted | Shows **separation anxiety** | Says **first words**<br>Shows **object permanence** |

**(2)** Infants exposed to many caregivers are less likely to show stranger anxiety than those exposed to few caregivers.

   **c.** At about 1 year the child can maintain the mental image of an object or of the mother without seeing it or her ("**object permanence**").

**E. Theories of development**
   **1. Chess** and **Thomas** showed that there are **endogenous differences** in the **temperaments** of infants that remain quite stable for the first 25 years of life. These differences include such characteristics as reactivity to stimuli, responsiveness to people, and attention span.
      **a. Easy children** are adaptable to change, show regular eating and sleeping patterns, and have a positive mood.
      **b. Difficult children** show traits opposite to those of easy children.
      **c. Slow-to-warm-up children** show traits of difficult children at first but then improve and adapt with increased contact with others.
   **2. Sigmund Freud** described development in terms of the parts of the body from which the most pleasure is derived at each stage of development (e.g., the "oral stage" occurs during the first year of life).
   **3. Erik Erikson** described development in terms of critical periods for the achievement of social goals; if a specific goal is not achieved at a specific age, the individual will have difficulty achieving the goal in the future. For example, in Erikson's stage of **basic trust versus mistrust**, children must learn to trust others during the first year of life or they will have trouble forming close relationships as adults.
   **4. Jean Piaget** described development in terms of learning capabilities of the child at each age.
   **5. Margaret Mahler** described early development as a sequential process of separation of the child from the mother or primary caregiver.

## III. THE TODDLER YEARS: 15 MONTHS–2½ YEARS

**A. Attachment**
   **1.** The **major theme** of the second year of life is to **separate from the mother** or primary caregiver, a process that is complete by about age 3.
   **2.** There is **no compelling evidence** that daily separation from working parents in a good day care setting has short- or long-term negative consequences for children. However, when

| table | **1.6** | Motor, Social, Verbal, and Cognitive Development of the Toddler and Preschool Child |
| --- | --- | --- |

| Age (Years) | Skill Area | | |
| --- | --- | --- | --- |
| | Motor | Social | Verbal and Cognitive |
| 1.5 | Throws a ball<br>Stacks **three blocks**<br>Climbs stairs one foot at a time<br>**Scribbles** on paper | Moves away from and then returns to the mother for reassurance **(rapprochement)** | Uses about **10** individual **words**<br>Says own name |
| 2 | Kicks a ball<br>Balances on one foot for 1 sec<br>Stacks **six blocks**<br>Feeds self with spoon | Shows negativity (e.g., the favorite word is "no")<br>Plays alongside but not with another child ("**parallel play**": 2–4 yrs of age) | Uses about **250 words**<br>Speaks in two-word sentences and uses pronouns (e.g., "me do")<br>Names body parts and objects |
| 3 | Rides a tricycle<br>Undresses and partially dresses without help<br>Climbs stairs using alternate feet<br>Stacks **nine blocks**<br>Copies a **circle** | Has a sense of self as male or female **(gender identity)**<br>Usually achieves **bowel and bladder control** (problems such as encopresis ["soiling"] and enuresis ["bedwetting"] cannot be diagnosed until 4 and 5 yrs of age, respectively)<br>Comfortably spends part of the day away from mother | Uses about **900 words** in speech<br>Understands about 3,500 words<br>Identifies some colors<br>Speaks in complete sentences (e.g., "I can do it myself")<br>Strangers can now understand her |
| 4 | Catches a ball with arms<br>Dresses independently, using buttons and zippers<br>Grooms self (e.g., brushes teeth)<br>Hops on one foot<br>Draws a person<br>Copies a **cross** | Begins to **play cooperatively** with other children<br>Engages in role playing (e.g., "I'll be the mommy, you be the daddy")<br>May have **imaginary companions**<br>Curious about sex differences (e.g., plays "doctor" with other children)<br>Has nightmares and transient phobias (e.g., of "monsters") | Shows good verbal self-expression (e.g., can tell detailed stories)<br>Comprehends and uses prepositions (e.g., under, above) |
| 5 | Catches a ball with two hands<br>Draws a person in detail (e.g., with arms, hair, eyes)<br>Skips using alternate feet<br>Copies a **square** | Has romantic feelings about the opposite sex parent (the "oedipal phase") at 4–5 yrs of age<br>Overconcerned about physical injury at 4–5 yrs of age | Shows further improvement in verbal and cognitive skills |
| 6 | Ties shoelaces<br>Rides a two-wheeled bicycle<br>Prints letters<br>Copies a **triangle** | Begins to develop an internalized moral sense of right and wrong<br>Begins to understand the finality of death | Begins to think logically (see Chapter 2)<br>Begins to **read** |

compared to children who stay at home with their mothers, those who have been in day care show more **aggressiveness**.

B. **Motor, social, verbal, and cognitive characteristics of the toddler**
See Table 1.6.

## IV. THE PRESCHOOL CHILD: 3–6 YEARS

A. **Attachment**
 1. After reaching 3 years of age a child should be able to spend a few hours away from the mother in the care of others (e.g., in day care).
 2. A child who cannot do this after age 3 is experiencing **separation anxiety disorder** (see Chapter 15).
 3. Preschool children do not yet understand that death is permanent; they typically expect that a dead relative (or pet) will come back to life.

B. **Characteristics**
   1. The child's **vocabulary increases** rapidly. The 3-year-old child can typically say about **900 words** and speaks in complete sentences.
   2. **Toilet training** typically occurs at age 3 years. Delayed toilet training is most often related to physiological immaturity due to genetic factors, for example, the father was also a "bed-wetter" as a child.
   3. The birth of a sibling or other **life stress**, such as moving or divorce, may result in a child's use of **regression**, a defense mechanism (see Chapter 6) in which the child temporarily behaves in a "baby-like" way (e.g., although he is toilet-trained, he starts wetting the bed again). Regression often occurs in typical children as a reaction to life stress.
   4. Children can distinguish fantasy from reality (e.g., they know that imaginary friends are not "real" people), although the line between them may still not be sharply drawn.
   5. Preschool children are typically active and **rarely sit still** for long.
   6. Other aspects of motor, social, verbal, and cognitive development of the preschool child can be found in Table 1.6.

C. **Changes at 6 years of age**
   1. The child begins to understand that death is final and fears that his or her parents will die and leave. It is not until about age 9, however, that the child understands that he or she also can die.
   2. At the end of the preschool years (about age 6), the child's **conscience** (the **superego** of Freud) and sense of morality begin to develop.
   3. After age 6, children can put themselves in another person's place (**empathy**) and behave in a caring and sharing way toward others.
   4. Morality and empathy increase further during the school-age years (see Chapter 2).

# Review Test

**Directions:** Each of the numbered items or incomplete statements in this section is followed by answers or by completions of the statement. Select the **one** lettered answer or completion that is **best** in each case.

**1.** The concerned parents of a 5-year-old child report that the child is still wetting the bed. The child is otherwise developing appropriately for his age and physical examination is unremarkable. The child's father was also a bedwetter until age 8 years. The most common cause of enuresis in a child of this age is

(A) emotional stress
(B) physiological immaturity
(C) sexual abuse
(D) urinary tract infection
(E) major depression

**2.** A 4-year-old boy survives a house fire in which his father was killed. He has only minor injuries. Although he has been told that his father has died, in the weeks after the fire the child continues to ask for his father. The best explanation for this boy's behavior is

(A) an acute reaction to severe stress
(B) a typical reaction for his age
(C) delayed development
(D) refusal to believe the truth
(E) an undiagnosed head injury

**3.** A 7-year-old boy has a terminal illness. His parents have told him that he is going to die. Which of the following is most likely to characterize this child's conception of death?

(A) That others can die but he cannot die
(B) That he can die but others cannot die
(C) That everyone dies at some time
(D) That people die but then come back to life

**4.** An American couple would like to adopt a 10-month-old Russian child. However, they are concerned because the child has been in an orphanage since he was separated from his birth mother 5 months ago. The orphanage is clean and well kept but has a high staff turnover ratio. Which of the following characteristics is the couple most likely to see in the child at this time?

(A) Loud crying and protests at the loss of his mother
(B) Increased responsiveness to adults
(C) Typical development of motor skills
(D) Reactive attachment disorder
(E) Typical development of social skills

**5.** When a physician conducts a well-child checkup on a typical 2-year-old girl, the child is most likely to show which of the following skills or characteristics?

(A) Speaks in two-word sentences
(B) Is toilet-trained
(C) Can comfortably spend most of the day away from her mother
(D) Can ride a tricycle
(E) Engages in cooperative play

**6.** When a physician conducts a well-child checkup on a 3-year-old boy, he finds that the child can ride a tricycle, copy a circle, engage in parallel play with other children, name some of his body parts (e.g., nose, eyes) but not others (e.g., hand, finger), and has about a 50-word vocabulary. With respect to motor, social, and cognitive/verbal skills, respectively, this child is most likely to be

(A) typical, typical, needs evaluation
(B) typical, typical, typical
(C) needs evaluation, typical, needs evaluation
(D) typical, needs evaluation, needs evaluation
(E) typical, needs evaluation, typical

**7.** A mother brings her 4-month-old child to the pediatrician for a well-baby examination. Which of the following developmental signposts can the doctor expect to be present in this infant if the child is developing typically?

**(A)** Stranger anxiety
**(B)** Social smile
**(C)** Rapprochement
**(D)** Core gender identity
**(E)** Phobias

**8.** The overall infant mortality rate in the United States in 2005 was approximately

**(A)** 1 per 1,000 live births
**(B)** 3 per 1,000 live births
**(C)** 7 per 1,000 live births
**(D)** 21 per 1,000 live births
**(E)** 40 per 1,000 live births

**9.** The most important psychological task for a child between birth and 15 months is the development of

**(A)** the ability to think logically
**(B)** speech
**(C)** stranger anxiety
**(D)** a conscience
**(E)** an intimate attachment to the mother or primary caregiver

**10.** The husband of a 28-year-old woman, who gave birth to a healthy infant 2 weeks ago, reports that he found her shaking the infant to stop it from crying. When the doctor questions the woman about the incident, she says "I did not realize it would be so much work." The patient also reports that she wakes up at 5 AM every day and cannot fall back asleep and has very little appetite. The next step in management is for the doctor to

**(A)** assess the patient for thoughts of suicide
**(B)** advise the father to hire a caregiver to assist the mother in caring for the child
**(C)** set up another appointment for the following week
**(D)** prescribe an antidepressant
**(E)** tell the father that the mother is showing evidence of the "baby blues"

**11.** A well-trained, highly qualified obstetrician has a busy practice. Which of the following is most likely to be true about postpartum reactions in this doctor's patients?

**(A)** Postpartum blues will occur in about 10% of the patients.
**(B)** Major depression will occur in about 25% of the patients.
**(C)** Brief psychotic disorder will occur in about 8% of the patients.
**(D)** Brief psychotic disorder will last about 1 year.
**(E)** Postpartum blues will usually last up to 2 weeks.

**12.** A woman in the seventh month of pregnancy with her third child tells her physician she is worried that she will experience depression after the child is born. The most important thing for the doctor to say at this time is

**(A)** "Do not worry, there are many effective medications for depression."
**(B)** "Women often become more anxious toward the end of their pregnancy."
**(C)** "Did you experience any emotional difficulties after the birth of your other children?"
**(D)** "Do you want to start taking antidepressant medication now?"
**(E)** "Most women who worry about depression never experience it."
**(F)** "Some depression is common after childbirth."

**13.** The mother of a 3-year-old child tells you that although she instructs the child to sit still at the dinner table, the child cannot seem to do so for more than 10 minutes at a time. She squirms in her seat and gets out of her chair. The child's motor and verbal skills are appropriate for her age. Which of the following best fits this picture?

**(A)** Separation anxiety disorder
**(B)** Typical behavior
**(C)** Delayed development
**(D)** Lack of basic trust
**(E)** Attention deficit/hyperactivity disorder (ADHD)

**14.** A typical 8-month-old child is brought to the pediatrician for his monthly well-baby examination. The child is the family's first and he is cared for at home by his mother. When the doctor approaches the child in his mother's arms, the child's behavior is most likely to be characterized by

**(A)** clinging to the mother
**(B)** smiling at the doctor
**(C)** indifference to the doctor
**(D)** an anticipatory posture toward the doctor (arms held out to be picked up)
**(E)** withdrawal from both the doctor and the mother

**15.** While she previously slept in her own bed, after her parents' divorce, a 5-year-old girl begs to be allowed to sleep in her mother's bed every night. She says that a "robber" is under her bed. She continues to do well in kindergarten and to play with her friends. The best description of this girl's behavior is

**(A)** separation anxiety disorder
**(B)** typical behavior with regression
**(C)** delayed development
**(D)** lack of basic trust
**(E)** ADHD

**16.** A 3-year-old girl who has been in foster care since birth is very friendly and affectionate with strangers. She puts her arms out to them to be picked up and then "cuddles up" to them. The foster mother states that the child has "behavior problems" and then notes that she has never felt "close" to the child. The most likely explanation for this child's behavior toward strangers is

**(A)** Typical behavior
**(B)** Rett's disorder
**(C)** Reactive attachment disorder, inhibited type
**(D)** Reactive attachment disorder, disinhibited type
**(E)** Asperger's disorder

**Questions 17–21**

For each developmental milestone, select the age at which it commonly first appears.

**17.** Transfers toys from one hand to the other.

**(A)** 0–3 months
**(B)** 4–6 months
**(C)** 7–11 months
**(D)** 12–15 months
**(E)** 16–30 months

**18.** Turns over.

**(A)** 0–3 months
**(B)** 4–6 months
**(C)** 7–11 months
**(D)** 12–15 months
**(E)** 16–30 months

**19.** Smiles in response to a human face.

**(A)** 0–3 months
**(B)** 4–6 months
**(C)** 7–11 months
**(D)** 12–15 months
**(E)** 16–30 months

**20.** Responds to own name.

**(A)** 0–3 months
**(B)** 4–6 months
**(C)** 7–11 months
**(D)** 12–15 months
**(E)** 16–30 months

**21.** Feeds self with a spoon.

**(A)** 0–3 months
**(B)** 4–6 months
**(C)** 7–11 months
**(D)** 12–15 months
**(E)** 16–30 months

# Answers and Explanations

**The answer is A.** The physician should reassure the mother that all children are different and that some crying is normal. The child's appropriate weight gain and negative medical findings indicate that the child is developing typically. Once the mother is reassured, it will not be necessary to recommend a psychotherapist, prescribe an antidepressant, refer her to a pediatrician specializing in "difficult" infants, or recommending that the father care for the child when it is crying.

1. **The answer is B.** Most children are toilet-trained by the age of 5 years. However, bed wetting in a 5-year-old who has never been toilet-trained and is otherwise developing appropriately is most likely to be a result of physiological immaturity, probably related to genetic factors, for example, the father was also a bedwetter. Emotional stress, sexual abuse, and depression are less likely to be the cause of bed wetting in a child who has never been toilet-trained, although they can lead to bed wetting in a previously toilet-trained child. Absence of medical findings indicates that this child is unlikely to have a urinary tract infection.

2. **The answer is B.** This 4-year-old child is showing a typical reaction for his age. Children under the age of 6 years do not understand the finality of death and fully expect dead people to come back to life. That is why, although he has been told that his father has died, this child repeatedly asks for his father. While he has been severely stressed, he is neither simply refusing to believe the truth nor showing delayed development. While it is possible that this boy has an undiagnosed head injury, a typical reaction is more likely.

3. **The answer is A.** The conception of death in a 7-year-old child is that others can die but that he cannot die. It is not until about age 9 that children begin to understand that they can also die. Children under age 6 expect that death is temporary and that people who die come back to life.

4. **The answer is D.** This child is likely to show reactive attachment disorder after this prolonged separation from his mother. Although the orphanage is well kept, it is unlikely the child has been able to form a stable attachment to another caretaker because of the high number of staff changes. Loud protests occur initially when the mother leaves the child. With her continued absence, this child experiences other serious reactions. These reactions include depression, decreased responsiveness to adults, and deficits in the development of social and motor skills.

5. **The answer is A.** Two-year-old children speak in two-word sentences (e.g., "Me go"). Toilet training or the ability to spend most of the day away from the mother does not usually occur until age 3. Children engage in cooperative play starting at about age 4 and can ride a three-wheeled bicycle at about age 3.

6. **The answer is A.** At the age of 3 years, the child can ride a tricycle, copy a circle, and engage in parallel play (play alongside but not cooperatively with other children). However, 3-year-old children such as this one should have a vocabulary of about 900 words and speak in complete sentences.

7. **The answer is B.** The social smile (smiling in response to seeing a human face) is one of the first developmental milestones to appear in the infant and is present by 1–2 months of age. Stranger anxiety (fear of unfamiliar people) appears at about 7 months of age and indicates that the infant has a specific attachment to the mother. Rapprochement (the tendency to run away from the mother and then run back for comfort and reassurance) appears at about 18 months of age. Core gender identity (the sense of self as male or female) is established between 2 and 3 years of age. Transient phobias (irrational fears) occur in typical children, appearing most commonly at 4–5 years of age.

8. **The answer is C.** In 2005, the overall infant mortality rate in the United States was 6.9 per 1,000 live births. This rate, which is closely associated with socioeconomic status, was about two times higher in African-American infants than in white infants.

9. **The answer is E.** The most important psychological task of infancy is the development of an intimate attachment to the mother or primary caregiver. Stranger anxiety, which typically appears at about 7 months of age, demonstrates that the child has developed this attachment and can distinguish its mother from others. Speech, the ability to think logically, and the development of a conscience are skills that are developed later during childhood.

10. **The answer is A.** This woman is showing evidence of a serious post-partum reaction such as major depression, not simply the "baby blues." Because she shows evidence of depression, for example, early morning awakening, lack of appetite, the next step in management is to assess her for thoughts of suicide. The child must also be protected. If she is suicidal or likely to harm the child, inpatient treatment may be indicated. Ultimately, assistance with care of the child may be helpful, but the next step is to protect the patient and the child. Just setting up another appointment for the following week or prescribing an antidepressant will not protect either.

11. **The answer is E.** Postpartum blues may occur in one-third to one-half of new mothers and can last up to 2 weeks. Intervention involves support and practical help with the child. Brief psychotic disorder is rare, occurring in less than 1% of new mothers and lasting up to 1 month after childbirth. Postpartum depression occurs in 5%–10% of new mothers and is treated primarily with antidepressant medication.

12. **The answer is C.** "Did you experience any emotional difficulties after the birth of your other children?" is an important question since a predictor of postpartum reactions is whether or not they have occurred before. This patient is probably worried because she has had previous problems. Reassuring statements such as, "Most women who worry about depression never experience it," "Do not worry, there are many effective medications for depression," "Women often become more anxious toward the end of their pregnancy," or "Some depression is common after childbirth," do not address this patient's realistic concerns.

13. **The answer is B.** It is typical for a 3-year-old child to have difficulty sitting still for any length of time. By school age, children should be able to sit still and pay attention for longer periods of time. Thus, this is not ADHD. There is also no evidence of delayed development, lack of basic trust, or separation anxiety disorder.

14. **The answer is A.** Stranger anxiety (the tendency to cry and cling to the mother in the presence of an unfamiliar person) develops in typical infants at 7–9 months of age. It does not indicate that the child is developmentally delayed, emotionally disturbed, or that the child has been abused, but rather that the child can now distinguish familiar from unfamiliar people. Stranger anxiety is more common in children who are cared for by only one person and is reduced in those exposed to many different caregivers.

15. **The answer is B.** The best description of this girl's behavior is typical. Her desire to sleep with her mother is a sign of regression, a defense mechanism that is common in typical children under stress. Because she continues to play well when away from her mother, this is not separation anxiety disorder. There is also no evidence of delayed development, lack of basic trust, or ADHD (see Chapter 15).

16. **The answer is D.** The most likely diagnosis for this child is reactive attachment disorder, disinhibited type. Children with this disorder form indiscriminate attachments to strangers because their primary attachment figure, here the foster mother, does not interact normally with the child. Autistic disorder, Asperger's disorder, and Rett's disorder are all characterized by decreased, not increased, social interaction.

17. **The answer is C.** Transferring objects from hand to hand commonly occurs at about 10 months of age.

18. **The answer is B.** Infants can usually turn over at about 5 months of age.

19. **The answer is A.** Children begin to show social smiling between 1 and 2 months of age.

20. **The answer is C.** Children begin to respond to their own names between 7 and 11 months of age.

21. **The answer is E.** Children begin to use a utensil to feed themselves at about 2 years of age.

# chapter 2

# School Age, Adolescence, Special Issues of Development, and Adulthood

**Typical Board Question**

A 15-year-old girl is brought to the doctor by her mother because she is insisting on getting a tattoo. The teenager states that she knows there is a risk of human immunodeficiency virus (HIV) infection but wants to get the tattoo anyway. What is the doctor's best next step in management?

**(A)** Say "I strongly recommend that you not get the tattoo"
**(B)** Say "Let's talk about the pros and cons of getting a tattoo"
**(C)** Ask "If you know there are risks, why do you want the tattoo?"
**(D)** Say "Tattoos are permanent and can rarely be completely removed"
**(E)** Give the teen a brochure describing the health risks of tattoos

*(See "Answers and Explanations" at end of chapter.)*

## I. TE SCHOOL AGE: 7–11 YEARS

**A. Motor development.** The typical grade-school child, 7–11 years of age, engages in complex motor tasks (e.g., plays baseball, skips rope).

**B. Social characteristics.** The school-age child:
1. Prefers to play with **children of the same sex**; typically avoids and is critical of those of the opposite sex.
2. Identifies with the parent of the same sex.
3. Has relationships with **adults other than parents** (e.g., teachers, group leaders).
4. Demonstrates little interest in psychosexual issues (sexual feelings are latent and will reappear at puberty).
5. Has internalized a **moral sense of right and wrong (conscience)** and understands how to follow rules, (e.g., playing "fair").
6. School-age children and younger children are typically interviewed and examined by the doctor with the mother present.

**C. Cognitive characteristics.** The school-age child:
1. Is **industrious** and organized (e.g., gathers collections of objects).
2. Has the capacity for **logical thought** and can determine that objects have more than one property (e.g., an object can be both red and metal).

3. Understands the concepts of **conservation and seriation**; both are necessary for certain types of learning.
   a. **Conservation** involves the understanding that a quantity of a substance remains the same regardless of the size of the container or shape it is in (e.g., two containers may contain the same amount of water even though one is a tall, thin tube and one is a short, wide bowl).
   b. **Seriation** involves the ability to arrange objects in order with respect to their sizes or other qualities.

## II. ADOLESCENCE: 11–20 YEARS

A. **Early adolescence (11–14 years of age)**
   1. **Puberty** occurs in early adolescence and is marked by:
      a. The development of **secondary sex characteristics** (Table 2.1) and increased skeletal growth.
      b. **First menstruation** (menarche) in girls, which on average occurs at 11–14 years of age.
      c. **First ejaculation** in boys, which on average occurs at 12–15 years of age.
      d. **Cognitive maturation** and **formation of the personality**.
      e. **Sex drives**, which are expressed through **physical activity** and **masturbation** (daily masturbation is typical).
   2. Early adolescents show strong sensitivity to the opinions of peers but are generally obedient and unlikely to seriously challenge parental authority.
   3. **Alterations in expected patterns of development** (e.g., acne, obesity, late breast development in girls, nipple enlargement in boys [usually temporary but may concern the boy and his parents]) may lead to psychological difficulties.

B. **Middle adolescence (15–17 years of age)**
   1. **Characteristics**
      a. There is great interest in **gender roles, body image, and popularity**.
      b. Heterosexual **crushes** (love for an unattainable person such as a rock star) are common.
      c. **Homosexual experiences** may occur. Although parents may become alarmed, such practicing is part of typical development.
      d. Efforts to **develop an identity** by adopting current teen fashion in clothing and music, and preference for spending time with peers over family are typical, but may lead to conflict with parents.
   2. **Risk-taking behavior**
      a. Readiness to challenge parental rules and feelings of **omnipotence** may result in **risk-taking behavior** (e.g., failure to use condoms, driving too fast, smoking).
      b. Education about **obvious short-term benefits** rather than references to long-term consequences of behavior is more likely to **decrease teenagers' unwanted behavior**. For example, **to discourage smoking**, telling teenagers that their teeth will stay white if they do not smoke, or that other teens find smoking disgusting, will be more helpful than telling them that they will avoid lung cancer in 30 years.

| t a b l e   **2.1**   Tanner Stages of Sexual Development | |
|---|---|
| **Stage** | **Characteristics** |
| 1 | Genitalia and associated structures are the same as in childhood; nipples (papillae) are slightly elevated in girls |
| 2 | Scant, straight pubic hair, testes enlarge, scrotum develops texture; slight elevation of breast tissue in girls |
| 3 | Pubic hair increases over the pubis and becomes curly, penis increases in length and testes enlarge |
| 4 | Penis increases in width, glans develops, scrotal skin darkens; areola rises above the rest of the breast in girls |
| 5 | Male and female genitalia are like adult; pubic hair now is also on thighs, areola is no longer elevated above the breast in girls |

C. **Late adolescence (18–20 years of age)**
   1. **Development**
      a. Older adolescents develop **morals, ethics, self-control**, and a realistic appraisal of their own abilities; they become concerned with humanitarian issues and world problems.
      b. Some adolescents, but not all, develop the ability for abstract reasoning (Piaget's **stage of formal operations**).
   2. In the effort to form one's own identity, an **identity crisis** commonly develops.
      a. If the identity crisis is not handled effectively, adolescents may experience **role confusion** in which they do not know where they belong in the world.
      b. Experiencing role confusion, the adolescent may display behavioral problems such as **criminality** or an **interest in cults**.

D. **Teenage sexuality**
   1. In the United States, **first sexual intercourse** occurs on average at **16 years** of age; by 19 years of age, most men and women have had sexual intercourse.
   2. Fewer than half of all sexually active teenagers **do not use contraceptives** for reasons that include the conviction that they will not get pregnant, lack of access to contraceptives, and lack of education about which methods are most effective.
   3. Physicians may counsel minors (persons under 18 years of age) and provide them with contraceptives without parental knowledge or consent. They may also provide to minors treatment for sexually transmitted diseases, problems associated with pregnancy, and drug and alcohol abuse (see Chapter 23).
   4. Because of their potential sensitivity, issues involving sexuality and drug abuse, as well as issues concerning physical appearance such as obesity, are typically discussed with teenagers **without the parents present.**

E. **Teenage pregnancy**
   1. Teenage pregnancy is a social problem in the United States, although the **birth rate and abortion rate** in American teenagers **has been declining**. In contrast, the birth rate among women 35–44 has been increasing (Figure 2.1).
   2. **Abortion is legal** in the United States. However, in many states, minors must obtain parental consent for abortion.
   3. Factors predisposing adolescent girls to pregnancy include depression, poor school achievement, and having divorced parents.
   4. Pregnant teenagers are at high risk for **obstetric complications** because they are less likely to get prenatal care, and because they are physically immature.

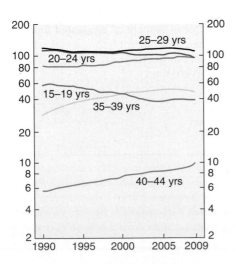

FIGURE 2.1. Birth rates in the United States by age of mother: 1990–2008 and preliminary 2009. (Reprinted from Hamilton BE, Martin JA, Ventura SJ, Division of Vital Statistics. Births: Preliminary data for 2009. *Natl Vital Stat Rep.* 2009;59(3).) Rates are plotted on a logarhithmic scale.

## III. SPECIAL ISSUES IN CHILD DEVELOPMENT

A. **Illness and death in childhood and adolescence.** A child's reaction to illness and death is closely associated with the child's developmental stage.
   1. During the **toddler years** (15 months–2½ years) hospitalized children **fear separation** from the parent more than they fear bodily harm, pain, or death.
   2. During the **preschool years** (2½–6 years) the child's greatest fear when hospitalized is of **bodily harm**.
   3. **School-age children** (7–11 years of age) cope relatively well with hospitalization. Thus, this is the **best age to perform elective surgery**.
   4. Ill **adolescents** may challenge the authority of doctors and nurses and resist being different from peers. Both of these factors can result in **lack of adherence to medical advice**.
   5. A child with an **ill sibling** or parent may respond by **acting badly** at school or home (use of the defense mechanism of "acting out" [see Chapter 6, Section II]).

B. **Adoption**
   1. An **adoptive parent** is a person who voluntarily becomes the **legal parent** of a child who is not his or her genetic offspring.
   2. Adopted children, particularly those adopted after infancy, may be at increased risk for behavioral problems in childhood and adolescence.
   3. Children **should be told** by their parents that they are adopted **at the earliest age possible** to avoid the chance of others telling them first.

C. **Mental retardation** (also referred to as intellectual and/or developmental disability)
   1. **Etiology**
      a. The most common genetic causes of mental retardation are **Down syndrome and fragile X syndrome**.
      b. Other causes include metabolic factors affecting the mother or fetus, prenatal and postnatal **infection** (e.g., rubella), and **maternal substance abuse**; many cases of mental retardation are of unknown etiology.
   2. Mildly (IQ of 50–69) and moderately (IQ of 35–49) mentally retarded children and adolescents commonly **know they are handicapped** (see Chapter 8). Because of this, they may become **frustrated and socially withdrawn**. They may have poor self-esteem because it is difficult for them to communicate and compete with peers.
   3. The **Vineland Social Maturity Scale** (see Chapter 8) can be used to evaluate social skills and skills for daily living in mentally retarded and other challenged individuals.
   4. **Avoidance of pregnancy** in adults with mental retardation can become an issue, particularly in residential social settings (e.g., summer camp). **Long-acting, reversible contraceptive methods** such as subcutaneous progesterone implants can be particularly useful to these individuals.

## IV. EARLY ADULTHOOD: 20–40 YEARS

A. **Characteristics**
   1. At about **30 years of age**, there is a **period of reappraisal** of one's life.
   2. The adult's **role in society is defined**, physical development peaks, and the adult becomes independent.

B. **Responsibilities and relationships**
   1. The development of an **intimate (e.g., close, sexual) relationship** with another person occurs.

2. According to **Erikson**, this is the stage of **intimacy versus isolation**; if the individual does not develop the ability to sustain an intimate relationship by this stage of life, he or she may experience emotional isolation in the future.
3. By 30 years of age, most Americans are in a committed relationship, e.g., marriage and have children.
4. During their middle 30s, many women alter their lifestyles by returning to work or school or by **resuming their careers**.

## V. MIDDLE ADULTHOOD: 40–65 YEARS

A. **Characteristics.** The person in middle adulthood possesses more power and authority than at other life stages.

B. **Responsibilities.** The individual either maintains a continued sense of productivity or develops a sense of emptiness (Erikson's stage of generativity versus stagnation).

C. **Relationships**
   1. Many men in their middle 40s or early 50s exhibit a **midlife crisis**. This may lead to:
      a. A change in profession or lifestyle.
      b. Infidelity, separation, or divorce.
      c. Increased use of alcohol or drugs.
      d. Depression.
   2. Midlife crisis is associated with an **awareness of one's own aging** and death and severe or unexpected lifestyle changes (e.g., death of a spouse, loss of a job, serious illness).

D. **Climacterium** is the change in physiologic function that occurs during midlife.
   1. In **men**, decreased muscle strength, physical endurance, and sexual performance (see Chapter 18) occur in midlife.
   2. In **women, menopause** occurs.
      a. The ovaries stop functioning, and menstruation stops in the **late forties or early fifties**.
      b. Absence of menstruation for 1 year defines **the end of menopause**. To avoid unwanted pregnancy, contraceptive measures should be used until at least **1 year following the last missed menstrual period**.
      c. Most women experience menopause with relatively few physical or psychological problems.
      d. Vasomotor instability, called **hot flashes or flushes**, is a common physical problem seen in women in all countries and cultural groups and may continue for years. While estrogen or estrogen/progesterone replacement therapy can relieve this symptom, use of such therapy has decreased because it is associated with increased risk of uterine and breast cancer.

# Review Test

**Directions:** Each of the numbered items or incomplete statements in this section is followed by answers or by completions of the statement. Select the **one** lettered answer or completion that is **best** in each case.

1. A mother worriedly reports that her 7-year-old son is often dirty when he comes in from playing. She notes that he digs in the dirt, wipes his face with his dirty hands, and climbs trees outside of the home. She states that she is worried that he will catch a disease or injure himself. The mother also reports that she had a meeting with the child's teacher who told her that the child is doing well in school. The next step in management is for the doctor to:

(A) Speak with the child's teacher
(B) Speak with the child
(C) Say "He must be hard to handle"
(D) Say "Tell me more about your concerns regarding your son?"
(E) Say "He is fine, do not worry"

2. A physician discovers that a 15-year-old patient is pregnant. Which of the following factors is likely to have contributed most to her risk of pregnancy?

(A) Living in a rural area
(B) Depressed mood
(C) Intact parental unit
(D) High achievement in school
(E) Having received information about contraceptive methods

3. A 50-year-old male patient comes in for an insurance physical. Which of the following developmental signposts is most likely to characterize this man?

(A) Decreased alcohol use
(B) Peak physical development
(C) Possession of power and authority
(D) Strong resistance to changes in social relationships
(E) Strong resistance to changes in work relationships

4. A 52-year-old woman in the United States has a 52-year-old female friend in Australia. Both are in good general health and neither has menstruated for about 1 year. Which of the following symptoms are both women most likely to experience at this time?

(A) Severe depression
(B) Severe anxiety
(C) Hot flashes
(D) Fatigue
(E) Lethargy

5. Increase in penis width, development of the glans, and darkening of scrotal skin characterize Tanner stage

(A) 1
(B) 2
(C) 3
(D) 4
(E) 5

6. A mother tells the physician that she is concerned about her son because he consistently engages in behavior that is dangerous and potentially life-threatening. The age of her son is most likely to be

(A) 11 years
(B) 13 years
(C) 15 years
(D) 18 years
(E) 20 years

7. A physician is conducting a school physical on a typical 10-year-old girl. When interviewing the child, the physician is most likely to find which of the following psychological characteristics?

(A) Lack of conscience formation
(B) Poor capacity for logical thought
(C) Identification with her father
(D) Relatively stronger importance of friends over family when compared to children of younger ages
(E) No preference with respect to the sex of playmates

**19**

**8.** A child's pet has recently died. The child believes that the pet will soon come back to life. This child is most likely to be of age

(A) 4 years
(B) 6 years
(C) 7 years
(D) 9 years
(E) 11 years

**9.** A 10-year-old girl with Down syndrome and an IQ of 60 is brought to the physician's office for a school physical. When the doctor interviews this girl, he is most likely to find that she

(A) has good self-esteem
(B) knows that she is handicapped
(C) communicates well with peers
(D) competes successfully with peers
(E) is socially outgoing

**10.** A 15-year-old boy tells his physician that he has been smoking cigarettes for the past year. He relates that his friends smoke and his father smokes. The most likely reason that this teenager does not attempt to stop smoking is because

(A) he is depressed
(B) his father smokes
(C) his peers smoke
(D) he does not know that smoking is harmful
(E) smoking is addictive

**11.** A formerly outgoing 10-year-old boy begins to do poorly in school after his 6-year-old brother is diagnosed with leukemia. He now prefers to watch television alone in his room and does not want to socialize with his friends. His parents are very stressed by caring for the younger child but do not ask the older child for help. The most appropriate suggestion for the doctor to make with respect to the 10-year-old is to tell the parents to

(A) insist that he take more responsibility for caring for his younger brother
(B) ignore his behavior
(C) remove the television from his room
(D) pay more attention to him
(E) tell him not to worry, everything will be fine

**12.** A woman and her 15-year-old daughter come to the physician's office together. The mother asks the physician to fit her daughter for a diaphragm. The most appropriate action for the physician to take at this time is to

(A) follow the mother's wishes
(B) ask the mother why she wants a diaphragm for her daughter
(C) recommend that the girl see a counselor
(D) ask to speak to the girl alone
(E) ask the girl if she is sexually active

**13.** A physician is asked to evaluate the development of an 11-year-old girl. Which of the following milestones is usually not acquired until after the age of 11 years?

(A) The concept of seriation
(B) The concept of conservation
(C) Parallel play
(D) The formation of a personal identity
(E) An understanding of the concept of "fair play"

**14.** A girl tells her mother that she "hates the boys because they are noisy and stupid." The age of this girl is most likely to be

(A) 4 years
(B) 6 years
(C) 9 years
(D) 13 years
(E) 15 years

**15.** At the lunch table, a child asks his mother to cut his hot dog up into three pieces so that he can have three times as much to eat. The age of this child is most likely to be

(A) 4 years
(B) 6 years
(C) 9 years
(D) 13 years
(E) 15 years

**16.** A 15-year-old overweight girl and her mother come to see the doctor for advice about diet and exercise. The mother states that she does not know why the girl is overweight because she cooks the same food for her and her slim 16-year-old brother. The doctor should first

(A) talk to the mother alone
(B) talk to both the teens with the mother present
(C) talk to the girl with the mother present
(D) talk to the mother, the brother, and the girl together
(E) talk to the girl alone

**17.** A medical student on a surgery rotation is assigned to stay with a 9-year-old girl who is waiting to have surgery to repair a cleft palate. The girl, who has recently arrived alone from Laos, does not speak English and appears anxious. The hospital administrator has requested a translator who has not yet arrived. At this time, the most appropriate action for the medical student to take is to

**(A)** sedate the child to decrease her anxiety

**(B)** give the child a toy to keep her occupied

**(C)** suggest that the nurse stay with the child so that he can review her chart

**(D)** look in the child's ears with an otoscope

**(E)** listen to the child's heart with a stethoscope and then let the child try using the stethoscope to listen to his heart

**18.** A physician is scheduled to see 8-year-old and 15-year-old sisters for routine checkups. They had consecutive appointments but when the doctor enters the examining room, they are both there with their mother. Most appropriately the doctor should

**(A)** Ask the 15-year-old to leave and talk to the 8-year-old with the mother present. Then talk to the 15-year-old alone.

**(B)** Ask both girls to leave and talk to the mother alone. Then ask the mother to leave and talk to the two girls together.

**(C)** Ask both girls to leave, talk to the mother alone, and then ask the mother to come back in and talk to all three together.

**(D)** Ask the mother to leave, talk to both girls together then talk to the mother alone

**(E)** Ask the mother and the older girl to leave, talk to the younger child alone, and then talk to the older girl alone.

# Answers and Explanations

**The answer is B.** Saying "Let's talk about the pros and cons of getting a tattoo" will encourage the girl to talk about her motivation for getting the tattoo. The current risk of getting the tattoo or problems with removal of the tattoo in the future probably are not as important at this time as why she wants it so badly. Saying "I strongly recommend that you not get the tattoo" or criticizing her by saying "If you know there are risks, why do you want the tattoo?" will not be effective. Just giving her a brochure also will not be helpful; most likely it will be ignored.

1. **The answer is D.** Although this boy is probably showing typical behavior for a 6-year-old, the doctor needs to know more about this mother's concerns regarding her son. Since he is doing well in school there is no need to speak to the teacher or the child. Simply saying "he must be hard to handle" or "he is fine, do not worry" will not address the mother's concerns.

2. **The answer is B.** Teenagers who become pregnant frequently are depressed, come from homes where the parents are divorced, have problems in school, and may not know about effective contraceptive methods. Studies have not indicated that living in a rural area is related to teenage pregnancy.

3. **The answer is C.** While midlife is associated with the possession of power and authority, physical abilities decline. This time of life is also associated with a midlife crisis, which may include increased alcohol and drug use as well as an increased likelihood of changes in social and work relationships.

4. **The answer is C.** These 52-year-old women in good general health are going through menopause. The most common symptom of menopause occurring cross-culturally is hot flashes, a purely physiological phenomenon. In most women, menopause is not characterized by psychopathology such as severe depression or anxiety or physical symptoms like fatigue and lethargy.

5. **The answer is D.** Increase in penis width, development of the glans, and darkening of scrotal skin characterize Tanner stage 4. Stage 1 is characterized by slight elevation of the papillae, and stage 2 by the presence of scant, straight pubic hair, testes enlargement, development of texture in scrotal skin, and slight elevation of breast tissue. In stage 3, pubic hair increases over the pubis and becomes curly, and the penis increases in length; in stage 5, male and female genitalia are much like those of adults.

6. **The answer is C.** The age of this woman's son is most likely to be 15 years. Middle adolescents (15–17 years) often challenge parental authority and have feelings of omnipotence (e.g., nothing bad will happen to them because they are all-powerful). Younger adolescents (11–14 years) are unlikely to challenge parental rules and authority. Older adolescents (18–20 years) have developed self-control and a more realistic picture of their own abilities.

7. **The answer is D.** When compared to younger ages, peers and nonfamilial adults become more important to the latency-age child and the family becomes less important. Children 7–11 years of age have the capacity for logical thought, have a conscience, identify with the same-sex parent, and show a strong preference for playmates of their own sex.

8. **The answer is A.** Preschool children usually cannot comprehend the meaning of death and commonly believe that the dead person or pet will come back to life. Children over the age of 6 years commonly are aware of the finality of death (see Chapter 1).

9. **The answer is B.** Mildly and moderately mentally retarded children are aware that they have a handicap. They often have low self-esteem and may become socially withdrawn. In part, these problems occur because they have difficulty communicating with and competing with peers.

10. **The answer is C.** Peer pressure has a major influence on the behavior of adolescents who tend to do what other adolescents are doing. Depression, the smoking behavior of their parents, and the addictive quality of cigarettes have less of an influence. Most teenagers have been educated with respect to the dangers of smoking.

11. **The answer is D.** The doctor should remind the parents to pay more attention to the older child. The child is likely to be frightened by his younger sibling's illness and the attitudes of his parents toward the younger child. School-age children such as this one may become withdrawn or "act out" by showing bad behavior when fearful or depressed. While he can be included in the care of his brother, it is not appropriate to insist that he take more responsibility for him. Ignoring his behavior or punishing him can increase his fear and withdrawal. False reassurance such as telling the child that everything will be fine is not appropriate.

12. **The answer is D.** As in the Typical Board Question, the most appropriate action for the physician to take at this time is to ask to speak to the girl alone. The physician can then ask the girl about her sexual activity and provide contraceptives and counseling if she wishes, without notification or consent from the mother. The mother's wishes in this circumstance are not relevant to the physician's action; the teenager is the patient.

13. **The answer is D.** The formation of a personal identity is usually achieved during the teenage years. The concepts of seriation and conservation and an understanding of the concept of "fair play" are gained during the school-age years. Parallel play is usually seen between ages 2 and 4 years.

14. **The answer is C.** Latency-age children (age 7–11 years) have little interest in those of the opposite sex and often criticize or avoid them. In contrast, younger children do not show strong gender preferences for playmates, and teenagers commonly seek the company of opposite-sex peers.

15. **The answer is A.** This child is most likely to be 4 years of age. Preschool children do not yet understand the concept of conservation (i.e., that the quantity of a substance remains the same regardless of the shape that it is in). Thus, this child believes that a hot dog cut into three pieces has more in it than when it was in only one piece. Children understand this concept better as they approach school age.

16. **The answer is E.** As in the Typical Board Question and Question 12, the physician should talk to this 15-year-old girl alone. In addition to sexual and drug abuse issues, those that involve body image such as body weight ideally should be discussed with a teenager alone, without other family members present.

17. **The answer is E.** The best thing for the medical student to do at this time is to interact with the child. Since they do not speak the same language, involving children of this age in an interactive activity such as using the stethoscope or drawing pictures together is the best choice here. Neither giving the child a toy nor looking in her ears is an interactive activity. The student, not the nurse, is responsible for the child in this instance. Sedation is inappropriate at this time; social activity is often effective in decreasing a patient's anxiety.

18. **The answer is A.** Parents should be present when a physician speaks to a younger child, but teenagers usually should be interviewed, particularly about sexual issues, without parents present. Thus, the doctor should ask the 15-year-old to leave and talk to the 8-year-old with the mother present. Then the doctor should talk to the 15-year-old alone.

# chapter 3

# Aging, Death, and Bereavement

**Typical Board Question**

An 81-year-old patient complains to his doctor that he sometimes has trouble falling asleep and would like to have "a pill to take" at those times. Physical examination is unremarkable and the patient shows no evidence of psychopathology. Of the following agents, which should be avoided in this patient?

**(A)** Diphenhydramine
**(B)** Zaleplon
**(C)** Trazodone
**(D)** Zolpidem
**(E)** Ramelteon

*(See "Answers and Explanations" at end of chapter.)*

## I. AGING

**A. Demographics**
1. By 2020, more than 15% of US population will be more than 65 years of age.
2. The fastest growing segment of the population is people over age 85.
3. Differences in life expectancies by gender and ethnicity have been decreasing over the past few years.
4. **Gerontology**, the study of aging, and **geriatrics**, the care of aging people, have become important medical fields.
    a. Geriatricians typically **manage rather than cure** the chronic illness of aging such as hypertension, cancer, and diabetes.
    b. A major aim of geriatrics is to keep elderly patients mobile and active. Because **fractures** (e.g., of the hip) are more likely than chronic illness to cause **loss of mobility** leading to disability and death in the elderly, **preventing falls** and prevention and management of **osteoporosis** are important foci in management.
    c. Prevention and management of osteoporosis includes: Increasing **weight bearing exercise**, and increasing **calcium** and **Vitamin D** in the diet. Medications which decrease bone resorption by blocking osteoclasts, for example, **alendronate sodium** (Fosamax) or increase bone formation by stimulating osteoblasts, for example, **teriparatide** (Forteo) are also useful.

**B. Somatic and neurologic changes**
1. **Strength and physical health gradually decline.** This decline shows great variability but commonly includes not only osteoporosis but also impaired vision, hearing, and

immune responses; decreased muscle mass and strength; increased fat deposits; decreased renal, pulmonary, and gastrointestinal function; reduced bladder control; and decreased responsiveness to changes in ambient temperature.

2. **Changes in the brain** occur with aging.
    a. These changes include **decreased brain weight, enlarged ventricles** and **sulci**, and **decreased cerebral blood flow**.
    b. **Amyloid (senile) plaques** and **neurofibrillary tangles** are present in the **normally aging brain** but to a lesser extent than in dementia of the Alzheimer type, hereinafter Alzheimer disease.
    c. Neurochemical changes that occur in aging include **decreased availability of neurotransmitters** such as norepinephrine, dopamine, g-aminobutyric acid, and acetylcholine; increased **availability of monoamine oxidase;** and **decreased responsiveness of neurotransmitter receptors**. These changes can be associated with psychiatric symptoms such as **depression** and **anxiety** (see below).

C. **Cognitive changes**
    1. Although learning speed may decrease, in the absence of brain disease, **intelligence remains approximately the same** throughout life.
    2. **Some memory problems** may occur in normal aging (e.g., the patient may forget the name of a new acquaintance). However, these problems **do not interfere with the patient's functioning** or ability to live independently.

D. **Psychological changes**
    1. In late adulthood there is either a sense of ego integrity (i.e., satisfaction and pride in one's past accomplishments) or a sense of despair and worthlessness (**Erikson's stage of ego integrity versus despair**). Most elderly people achieve ego integrity.
    2. Psychopathology and related problems
        a. **Depression** is the most common psychiatric disorder in the elderly. Suicide is more common in the elderly than in the general population.
            (1) Factors associated with depression in the elderly include loss of spouse, other family members, and friends; decreased social status; and decline of health.
            (2) **Depression may mimic and thus be misdiagnosed as Alzheimer disease**. This misdiagnosed disorder is referred to as **pseudodementia** because it is associated with memory loss and cognitive problems (see Chapter 14).
            (3) Depression **can be managed successfully** using supportive psychotherapy in conjunction with pharmacotherapy or electroconvulsive therapy (see Chapter 15).
        b. **Sleep patterns change**, resulting in loss of sleep, poor sleep quality, or both (see Chapter 10).
        c. **Anxiety** and fearfulness may be associated with realistic fear-inducing situations (e.g., worries about developing a physical illness or falling and breaking a bone).
        d. **Alcohol-related disorders** are often unidentified but are present in 10%–15% of the geriatric population.
        e. **Psychoactive agents** may produce different effects in the elderly than in younger patients. For example, using antihistamines such as diphenhydramine as sleep agents should be avoided because they may cause delirium (see Chapter 14) in elderly patients.
        f. For a realistic picture of the functioning level of elderly patients, the physician should ideally **evaluate patients in familiar surroundings**, such as their own homes.

E. **Life expectancy and longevity**
    1. The **average life expectancy** in the **United States** is currently about **77 years**. However, this figure varies by gender and ethnicity. Comparing the three largest ethnic groups, the **longest-lived group is Hispanic American women** and the **shortest-lived group is African American men** (Figure 3.1).
    2. Factors associated with **longevity** include:
        a. Family history of longevity.
        b. Continuation of physical and occupational activity.
        c. Advanced education.
        d. Social support systems, including marriage.

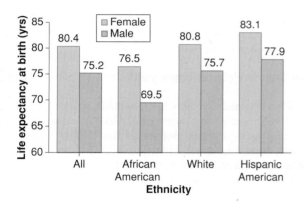

FIGURE 3.1. Life expectancy in years at birth in the United States by sex and ethnic group in 2005–2006. (Data from National Center for Health Statistics, 2008–2009.)

## II. STAGES OF DYING AND DEATH

According to **Dr. Elizabeth Kübler-Ross**, the process of dying involves **five stages: Denial, anger, bargaining, depression,** and **acceptance (DAng BaD Act).** The stages usually occur in the following order, but also may be present simultaneously or in another order.

A. **Denial.** The patient refuses to believe that he or she is dying. ("The laboratory made an error.")

B. **Anger.** The patient may become angry at the physician and hospital staff. ("It is your fault that I am dying. You should have checked on me weekly.") Physicians must learn not to take such comments personally (see Chapter 21).

C. **Bargaining.** The patient may try to strike a bargain with God or some higher being. ("I will give half of my money to charity if I can get rid of this disease.")

D. **Depression.** The patient becomes preoccupied with death and may become emotionally detached. ("I feel so distant from others and so hopeless.") Some people become "stuck" in this stage and may be diagnosed with an abnormal or complicated grief reaction (see below).

E. **Acceptance.** The patient is calm and accepts his or her fate. ("I am ready to go now.")

## III. BEREAVEMENT (NORMAL GRIEF) VERSUS DEPRESSION (ABNORMAL GRIEF OR COMPLICATED BEREAVEMENT)

After the loss of a loved one, there is a normal grief reaction. This reaction also occurs with other losses, such as loss of a body part, or, for younger people, with a miscarriage or abortion. A normal grief reaction must be distinguished from an abnormal grief reaction, which is pathologic (Table 3.1).

A. **Characteristics of normal grief (bereavement)**
   1. Grief is characterized initially by **shock** and **denial**.
   2. In normal grief, the bereaved may experience an **illusion** (see Table 11.1) that the deceased person is physically present.
   3. Normal grief generally **subsides after 1–2 years**, although some features may continue longer. Even after they have subsided, symptoms may return on holidays or special occasions (the "**anniversary reaction**").
   4. The **mortality rate** is high for close relatives (especially **widowed men**) in the first year of bereavement.

| table  **3.1** | Comparison between Normal Grief Reactions and Abnormal Grief Reactions |
|---|---|
| **Normal Grief Reaction (Bereavement)** | **Abnormal/Complicated Grief Reaction (Depression)** |
| Minor weight loss (e.g., <5 pounds) | Significant weight loss (e.g., >5% of body weight) |
| Minor sleep disturbances | Significant sleep disturbances |
| Mild guilty feelings | Intense feelings of guilt and worthlessness |
| Illusions (see Chapter 10) | Hallucinations or delusions (see Chapter 10) |
| Attempts to return to work and social activities | Resumes few, if any, work or social activities |
| Cries and expresses sadness | Considers or attempts suicide |
| Severe symptoms resolve within 2 mos | Severe symptoms persist for >2 mos |
| Moderate symptoms subside within 1 yr | Moderate symptoms persist for >1 yr |
| Management includes increased calls and visits to the physician, grief peer support groups, and short-acting sleep agents, e.g., zolpidem (Ambien) for transient problems with sleep | Management includes antidepressants, antipsychotics, electroconvulsive therapy and increased contact with the physician |

Adapted from Fadem B. *Behavioral Science in Medicine,* 2nd ed. Baltimore, MD: Lippincott Williams & Wilkins, 2012.

**B. Physician's response to death**

1. The major **responsibility of the physician** is to give support to the dying patient and the patient's family.

2. Generally, physicians **make the patient completely aware** of the diagnosis and prognosis. However, a physician should follow the patient's lead as to how much he or she wants to know about the condition. With the patient's permission, the **physician may tell the family** the diagnosis and other details of the illness (see Chapter 23).

3. Physicians often feel a **sense of failure** at not preventing the death of a patient. They may deal with this sense by becoming **emotionally detached** from the patient in order to deal with his or her imminent death. Such detachment can preclude helping the patient and family through this important transition.

# Review Test

**Directions:** Each of the numbered items or incomplete statements in this section is followed by answers or by completions of the statement. Select the **one** lettered answer or completion that is **best** in each case.

1. When questioned about her lifestyle , a 70-year-old woman tells the doctor that she eats mainly fish and chicken but enjoys an occasional steak. She also notes that she is lactose intolerant and so avoids milk products but eats almonds, beans, and canned salmon with bones daily. She also notes that she drinks one cup of coffee and one glass of wine and smokes one cigarette daily. To help prevent osteoporosis, the most important advice the physician should give this patient is to

(A) stop drinking wine
(B) stop eating steak
(C) stop drinking coffee
(D) start using dairy products despite her intolerance
(E) stop smoking

2. An 80-year-old woman is being examined by a physician for admission to a nursing home. The woman, who was brought to the doctor by her son, seems anxious and confused. The most effective action for the physician to take at this time is to

(A) arrange for immediate admission to a nursing home
(B) conduct a neuropsychological evaluation
(C) suggest immediate hospitalization
(D) ask the son if he has observed changes in the patient's behavior
(E) arrange to examine the woman in her own home

3. Each year during the first week in May, a 63-year-old woman develops chest discomfort and a feeling of foreboding. Her husband died 5 years ago during the first week in May. This woman's experience is best described as

(A) an attention-seeking device
(B) pathological grief
(C) an anniversary reaction
(D) malingering
(E) depression

4. A terminally ill patient who uses a statement such as, "It is the doctor's fault that I became ill; she didn't do an electrocardiogram when I came for my last office visit," is most likely in which stage of dying, according to Elizabeth Kübler-Ross?

(A) Denial
(B) Anger
(C) Bargaining
(D) Depression
(E) Acceptance

5. A physician conducts a physical examination on an active, independent 75-year-old woman. Which of the following findings is most likely?

(A) Increased immune response
(B) Increased muscle mass
(C) Decreased size of brain ventricles
(D) Decreased bladder control
(E) Severe memory problems

6. Ninety percent of the patients in a primary care physician's practice are over 65 years of age. When compared to the general population, these elderly patients are more likely to show which of the following psychological characteristics?

(A) Lower likelihood of suicide
(B) Less anxiety
(C) Lower intelligence
(D) Poorer sleep quality
(E) Less depression

7. The 78-year-old husband of a 70-year-old woman has just died. If this woman experiences normal bereavement, which of the following responses would be expected?

(A) Initial loss of appetite
(B) Feelings of worthlessness
(C) Threats of suicide
(D) Intense grief lasting years after the death
(E) Feelings of hopelessness

**8.** A physician has just diagnosed a case of terminal pancreatic cancer in a 68-year-old man. Which of the following statements regarding the reactions and behavior of the physician is the most true?

**(A)** She should inform the family, but not the patient, about the serious nature of the illness.

**(B)** Her involvement with the patient's family should end when he dies.

**(C)** She should provide strong sedation for family members when the patient dies until the initial shock of his death wears off.

**(D)** She will feel that she has failed when the patient dies.

**(E)** She will feel closer and closer to the patient as his death approaches.

**9.** The average difference in life expectancy between white women and African-American men is approximately

**(A)** 3 years
**(B)** 6 years
**(C)** 11 years
**(D)** 15 years
**(E)** 20 years

**10.** Six months after the death of a loved one, which of the following is most likely to indicate that a person is experiencing a complicated grief reaction?

**(A)** Longing
**(B)** Crying
**(C)** Denial that the loved one has died
**(D)** Irritability
**(E)** Illusions

**11.** An 80-year-old patient tells the doctor that she is concerned because she forgets the addresses of people she has just met and takes longer than in the past to do the Sunday crossword puzzle. She plays cards regularly with friends, is well groomed, and shops and cooks for herself. This patient is probably

**(A)** showing normal aging
**(B)** showing evidence of Alzheimer disease
**(C)** experiencing depression
**(D)** developing an anxiety disorder
**(E)** unable to live alone

**12.** A formerly well-groomed 70-year-old patient appears unshaven and disheveled since the death of his wife 8 months ago. He has lost 15 pounds, has persistent problems sleeping, and has no interest in interacting with friends and family. He also has difficulty relating what he did the previous day or what he ate for lunch today. Physical examination and laboratory tests are unremarkable. For this patient, the best recommendation of the physician is

**(A)** medication for sleep
**(B)** evaluation for major depression
**(C)** regular phone calls and visits to "check in" with the doctor
**(D)** psychotherapy
**(E)** neuropsychological evaluation for Alzheimer disease

**13.** A 50-year-old woman who is dying of cancer has a 10-year-old son. The mother does not want the child to know about her illness or prognosis. Most correctly, with respect to the mother's condition, the physician should

**(A)** talk to the mother and encourage her to tell her son
**(B)** talk to the son alone and tell him about his mother's illness
**(C)** follow the mother's wishes and do not tell the son
**(D)** talk to both the mother and son together
**(E)** insist that the mother tell her son

**14.** A 70-year-old patient whose wife died 8 months ago reports that he sometimes wakes up an hour earlier than usual and often cries when he thinks about his wife. He also tells you that on one occasion he briefly followed a woman down the street who resembled his late wife. The patient also relates that he has rejoined his bowling team and enjoys visits with his grandchildren. For this patient, the best recommendation of the physician is

**(A)** medication for sleep
**(B)** evaluation for major depression
**(C)** regular phone calls and visits to "check in" with the doctor
**(D)** psychotherapy
**(E)** neuropsychological evaluation for Alzheimer disease

**15.** An 85-year-old man and his 80-year-old wife are brought to the emergency department after an automobile accident. The man is dead on arrival. The woman is not seriously injured and is conscious and alert. The couple's son has been called and is on his way to the hospital. The woman asks the physician about her husband's condition. Most correctly, the physician should tell her

**(A)** not to worry but instead to concentrate on her own condition

**(B)** that her husband has died and then stay and offer support

**(C)** that her son is on the way and that they will discuss everything when the son arrives

**(D)** that he will check on her husband's condition after she is treated for her injuries

**(E)** what has happened to her but not what has happened to her husband

# Answers and Explanations

**The answer is A.** The antihistaminergic agent diphenhydramine (Benadryl) should be avoided in elderly patients because it is likely to cause symptoms of delirium. Unfortunately, a number of over-the-counter sleep medicines such as Tylenol PM contain diphenhydramine. Better choices for insomnia in the elderly include newer sleep agents such as zolpidem (Ambien) and ramelteon (Rozerem). Trazodone is a sedating tricyclic antidepressant which is also useful for occasional problems falling asleep in the elderly.

1. **The answer is E.** Cigarette smoking, even if moderate, is associated with the development of osteoporosis. Almonds, beans, and canned salmon with bones contain calcium and thus can help compensate for the absence of dietary dairy products. Moderate intake of steak, coffee, and alcohol as described by this patient are not associated with the development or worsening of osteoporosis.

2. **The answer is E.** The most effective action for the physician to take at this time is to examine the woman in her own home. Anxiety or depression at being in an unfamiliar situation can lead to the anxiety and confusion that this patient shows. Immediate admission to a nursing home or hospital, or interviewing the son are not appropriate until a true picture of the patient's condition has been obtained. A neuropsychological evaluation also may not be helpful while this patient is showing evidence of severe stress.

3. **The answer is C.** This woman's experience is best described as an anniversary reaction. In this reaction, the bereaved person experiences many of the feelings she experienced when her husband died at significant times in subsequent years. This is considered a normal reaction, not pathological grief, and is not associated with depression. It is also not a sign of malingering or of seeking attention.

4. **The answer is B.** During the anger stage of dying, the patient is likely to blame the physician.

5. **The answer is D.** Of the listed findings, decreased bladder control is the most likely finding in the examination of an active, independent 75-year-old woman. In aging, immune responses and muscle mass decrease and brain ventricles increase in size. While mild memory problems may occur, severe memory problems do not occur in normal aging. Severe memory problems that interfere with normal function indicate the development of a dementia such as Alzheimer disease.

6. **The answer is D.** Sleep disturbances, such as decreased delta (slow wave) sleep (see Chapter 10) commonly occur in the elderly. Suicide and depression are more common in the elderly than in the general population. Anxiety may arise easily due to fears of illness and injury. Intelligence does not decrease in typical elderly people.

7. **The answer is A.** Initial loss of appetite is common in normal bereavement. Feelings of worthlessness or hopelessness, threats of suicide, and an extended period of grief characterize depression rather than normal bereavement.

8. **The answer is D.** Physicians often feel that they have failed when a patient dies. Rather than becoming closer, this physician may become emotionally detached from the patient in order to deal with his impending death. Heavy sedation is rarely indicated as treatment for the bereaved because it may interfere with the grieving process. Generally, physicians inform patients when they have a terminal illness and provide an important source of support for the family before and after the patient's death.

9. **The answer is C.** The difference in life expectancy between white women (80.8 years) and African-American men (69.5 years) is approximately 11 years. The difference in life expectancy by age and sex is currently decreasing.

10. **The answer is C.** Six months after the death of a loved one, denying that the death has actually occurred suggests a complicated grief reaction. Normally, denial lasts up to 24 hours. Longing, crying, irritability, and illusions are all part of a normal grief reaction.

11. **The answer is A.** This 80-year-old woman is probably showing normal aging, since she can function well living alone. Minor memory loss that does not interfere with normal functioning such as she describes is typically seen in normally aging people. There is no evidence that this patient has Alzheimer disease, depression, or an anxiety disorder.

12. **The answer is B.** This patient whose wife died 8 months ago shows evidence of an abnormal grief reaction. He is showing signs of depression (e.g., poor grooming, significant weight loss, serious sleep problems, and little interest in interacting with friends and family) (see Chapter 12). Psychotherapy, while helpful, will be less useful than antidepressant medication for this patient. His sleep will improve as the depression improves. Elderly patients experiencing depression often present with memory problems that may mimic Alzheimer disease (pseudodementia). The sudden onset of memory problems (e.g., forgetting what he has been eating) with the concurrent loss of his wife indicates that the patient is likely to be experiencing depression rather than Alzheimer disease. Thus, there is no indication at this time that this patient needs a neuropsychiatric evaluation.

13. **The answer is A.** It is up to the mother to decide whether, when, and how to tell her son about her illness. However, school-age children are often aware when something serious is going on within their family and can understand the meaning of death (see Chapter 2). Therefore, while it is not appropriate for the physician to insist that the patient tell her son, the physician should talk to the mother and encourage her to talk to her son about her terminal condition. The physician can also counsel the patient on what to say to her child about her imminent death.

14. **The answer is C.** This patient, whose wife died 8 months ago, is showing a normal grief reaction. Although he sometimes wakes up an hour earlier than usual and cries when he thinks about his wife, he is attempting to return to his lifestyle by rejoining his bowling team and visiting with his family. The illusion of believing he sees and thus follows a woman who resembled his late wife is seen in a normal grief reaction. For a normal grief reaction, recommending regular phone calls and visits to "check in" with the doctor is the appropriate intervention. Sleep medication, antidepressants, psychotherapy, and a neuropsychological evaluation are not necessary for this patient at this time.

15. **The answer is B.** There is no indication that this elderly woman is impaired mentally or physically. Therefore, the physician should tell her the truth, that is, that her husband has died, and then stay and offer support. As with all adult patients, elderly patients should be told the truth. It is not necessary to wait for the son to arrive, and telling her not to worry is patronizing.

# chapter 4

# Genetics, Anatomy, and Biochemistry of Behavior

**Typical Board Question**

When a 70-year-old man who has had a stroke attempts to (a) divide a line in half, (b) turn single lines into "Xs," or (c) reproduce a clock face, he does the tasks like this (see Figure) effectively neglecting the left of the drawings. The area(s) of the brain most likely to be affected in this patient is (are) the

(A) right parietal lobe
(B) basal ganglia
(C) hippocampus
(D) reticular system
(E) amygdala
(F) left frontal lobe

*(See "Answers and Explanations" at end of chapter.)*

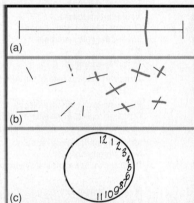

## I. BEHAVIORAL GENETICS

A. It has been difficult to link particular chromosomes with psychiatric illnesses. However, in a number of studies over years such associations have been made.
   1. **Schizophrenia** (Chapter 11) has been associated with markers on chromosomes 1, 6, 7, 8, 13, 21, and 22.
   2. **Bipolar disorder** and **major depressive disorder** (Chapter 12) recently have been associated with markers on chromosome 3, particularly 3p21.1.

B. **Specific chromosomes** have been associated with other disorders with behavioral symptoms (Table 4.1).

C. Studies for examining the genetics of behavior
   1. **Family risk studies** compare how frequently a behavioral disorder or trait occurs in the relatives of the affected individual (**proband**) with how frequently it occurs in the general population.
   2. **Twin studies**
      a. **Adoption studies** using **monozygotic twins** or **dizygotic twins** reared in the same or in different homes are used to differentiate the effects of genetic factors from environmental

| table 4.1 | Chromosomal Disorders with Behavioral Manifestations | |
|---|---|---|
| **Chromosome** | **Disorder** | **Behavioral Manifestations** |
| 1 | Alzheimer disease | Depression, anxiety, dementia (early onset) |
| 4 | Huntington disease | Erratic behavior, psychiatric symptoms (e.g., depression, psychosis), dementia |
| 5 | Sotos syndrome | Intellectual impairment, phobias, hyperphagia |
| 7 | William syndrome | Hypersociality, mental retardation, behavioral problems, hypotonia |
| 8 | Cohen syndrome | Autistic behavior, mental retardation |
| 9 | Dystonia musculorum deformans (DYT1)<br>Tuberous sclerosis | Depression, learning problems<br>Seizures, cognitive impairment, autistic behavior |
| 11 | Acute intermittent porphyria | Manic behavior, psychosis (see Chapter 5) |
| 12 | Phenylketonuria | Attention deficit/hyperactivity disorder (ADHD), mental retardation |
| 13 | Wilson disease | Depression, personality changes, psychotic symptoms |
| 14 | Alzheimer disease | Depression, anxiety, dementia (early onset) |
| 15 | Chromosome 15 inversion-duplication syndrome<br>Prader–Willi syndrome/Angelman syndrome | Seizures, autistic behavior, hypotonia<br><br>Mental retardation, rage, stubbornness, rigid thinking, and self-injury |
| 16 | Tuberous sclerosis | Seizures, cognitive impairment, autistic behavior |
| 17 | Neurofibromatosis-1<br>Charcot–Marie–Tooth disease<br>Smith–Magenis syndrome | Cognitive impairment<br>Peripheral neuropathy<br>Mental retardation, impaired expressive language, stereotyped behavior, clinging and dependency, seizures |
| 18 | Tourette syndrome | Dyscontrol of language and movements |
| 19 | Alzheimer disease (site of the APO $E_4$ gene) | Depression, anxiety, dementia (typical age of onset) |
| 21 | Progressive myoclonic epilepsy<br>Alzheimer disease (associated with Down syndrome) | Cognitive regression, aphasia, mental retardation<br>Depression, anxiety, dementia (early onset) |
| 22 | Metachromatic leukodystrophy<br>Neurofibromatosis-2<br>DiGeorge/velocardiofacial syndrome | Personality changes, psychosis, dementia<br>Hearing impairment<br>Schizophrenia, bipolar disorder, psychomotor retardation, language delay, ADHD, seizures |
| X | Fragile X syndrome<br>Kallmann syndrome<br>Lesch–Nyhan syndrome<br>Rett disorder | Autistic behavior, mental retardation<br>Anosmia, lack of sex drive, depression, anxiety, fatigue, insomnia<br>Self-mutilation and other bizarre behavior, mental retardation<br>Autistic behavior, hand-wringing, breathing abnormalities |

Adapted with permission from Fadem B, Monaco E. *High Yield Brain and Behavior.* Baltimore, MD: Lippincott Williams & Wilkins; 2007:27.

factors in the occurrence of psychiatric, substance abuse (e.g., alcoholism), and neuro-psychiatric disorders.
   **b.** If there is a genetic component to the etiology, a disorder may be expected to have a higher **concordance rate** in monozygotic twins than in dizygotic twins (i.e., if concordant, the disorder occurs in both twins).

## II. BEHAVIORAL NEUROANATOMY

The human nervous system consists of the **central nervous system (CNS)** and the **peripheral nervous system (PNS).**

**A.** The **CNS** contains the brain and spinal cord.
   **1.** The **cerebral cortex** can be divided
      **a. Anatomically** into at least four sets of lobes: Frontal, temporal, parietal, and occipital, as well as the limbic lobes (which contain medial parts of the frontal, temporal, and parietal lobes and include the hippocampus, amygdala, fornix, septum, parts of the thalamus, and cingulate gyrus and related structures).

      **b. By arrangement** of neuron layers or cytoarchitecture.

      **c. Functionally** into motor, sensory, and association areas.

  **2.** The cerebral hemispheres.

      **a.** The hemispheres are **connected** by the corpus callosum, anterior commissure, hippo-campal commissure, and habenular commissure.

      **b.** The functions of the hemispheres are **lateralized**.

         **(1)** The **right**, or **nondominant, hemisphere** is associated primarily with **perception**; it is also associated with **spatial relations, body image**, and musical and artistic ability.

         **(2)** The **left**, or **dominant, hemisphere** is associated with **language function** in about almost all right-handed people and most left-handed people.

      **c. Sex differences** in cerebral lateralization. **Women** may have a larger corpus callosum and anterior commissure and appear to have better interhemispheric communication than men. **Men** may have better-developed right hemispheres and appear to be more adept at spatial tasks than women.

  **3. Brain lesions** caused by accident, disease, surgery, or other insult are associated with particular neuropsychiatric effects (Table 4.2).

  **4. Memory systems**

      **a.** Explicit or **declarative memory** involves the knowledge of facts and is retrieved **consciously**.

      **b.** Implicit or **nondeclarative memory** involves information on how to perform an act and is recalled **unconsciously**.

      **c.** The neuroanatomy of these memory systems and clinical examples can be found in Table 4.3.

**B.** The **PNS** contains all **sensory, motor**, and **autonomic** fibers outside of the CNS, including the **spinal nerves, cranial nerves**, and **peripheral ganglia**.

  **1.** The PNS carries **sensory** information to the CNS and **motor** information away from the CNS.

---

**table 4.2** Neuropsychiatric Effects of Brain Lesions on Behavior

| Location of Lesion | Effects |
| --- | --- |
| Frontal lobes | Mood changes (e.g., depression with dominant lesions, mood elevation with nondominant lesions) <br> Difficulties with motivation, concentration, attention, orientation, and problem solving (dorsolateral convexity lesions) <br> Difficulties with judgment, inhibitions, emotions, personality changes (orbitofrontal cortex lesions) <br> Inability to speak fluently (i.e., Broca aphasia [dominant lesions]) |
| Temporal lobes | Impaired memory <br> Psychomotor seizures <br> Changes in aggressive behavior <br> Inability to understand language (i.e., Wernicke aphasia [dominant lesions]) |
| Limbic lobes <br> Hippocampus <br> Amygdala | Poor new learning; implicated specifically in Alzheimer disease <br> Klüver–Bucy syndrome (decreased aggression, increased sexual behavior, hyperorality) <br> Decreased conditioned fear response <br> Problems recognizing the meaningfulness of facial and vocal expressions of anger in others |
| Parietal lobes | Impaired processing of visual–spatial information (e.g., cannot copy a simple line drawing or neglects the numbers on the left side when drawing a clock face [right-sided lesions]) <br> Impaired processing of verbal information (e.g., cannot tell left from right, do simple math, name fingers, or write [Gerstmann syndrome; dominant lesions]) |
| Occipital lobes | Visual hallucinations and illusions <br> Inability to identify camouflaged objects <br> Blindness |
| Hypothalamus | Hunger leading to obesity (ventromedial nucleus damage); loss of appetite leading to weight loss (lateral nucleus damage) <br> Effects on sexual activity and body temperature regulation |
| Reticular system | Changes in sleep-wake mechanisms (e.g., decreased REM sleep) <br> Loss of consciousness |
| Basal ganglia | Disorders of movement (e.g., Parkinson disease [substantia nigra], Huntington disease [caudate and putamen], and Tourette syndrome [caudate]) |

| table | 4.3 | Memory Systems and Associated Neuroanatomy | | |
|---|---|---|---|---|
| **Type of System** | **Type of Memory** | **Associated Anatomy** | **Length of Recall** | **Memory Used to Remember** |
| Declarative (explicit or conscious) | Episodic | Temporal lobes (medial), anterior thalamic nuclei, fornix, hippocampus, mammillary bodies, prefrontal cortex | Long term | Personally experienced events, e.g., what you ate yesterday |
| | Semantic | Inferolateral temporal lobes | Long term | General knowledge about the world, e.g., the capital of New Jersey |
| Non-declarative (implicit or unconscious) | Procedural | Cerebellum, basal ganglia, supplementary motor area | Long term | Things you do automatically, e.g., how to tie your shoes |
| | Working | Prefrontal cortex, language and visual-association areas | Short term | Recent information, e.g., the phone number just obtained from "Information" |

2. The autonomic nervous system, which consists of **sympathetic** and **parasympathetic** divisions, innervates the internal organs.
3. The autonomic nervous system coordinates emotions with visceral responses such as heart rate, blood pressure, and peptic acid secretion.
4. Visceral responses occurring as a result of **psychological stress** are involved in the development and exacerbation of some **physical illnesses** (see Chapter 22).

# III.  NEUROTRANSMISSION

A. **Synapses and neurotransmitters**
   1. Information in the nervous system is transferred across the **synaptic cleft** (i.e., the space between the axon terminal of the presynaptic neuron and the dendrite of the postsynaptic neuron).
   2. When the presynaptic neuron is stimulated, a **neurotransmitter** is released, travels across the synaptic cleft, and acts on receptors on the postsynaptic neuron. Neurotransmitters are **excitatory** if they increase the chances that a neuron will fire and **inhibitory** if they decrease these chances.

B. **Presynaptic and postsynaptic receptors** are proteins present in the membrane of the neuron that can recognize specific neurotransmitters.
   1. The **changeability** of number or affinity of receptors for specific neurotransmitters (**neuronal plasticity**) can regulate the responsiveness of neurons.
   2. **Second messengers.** When stimulated by neurotransmitters, postsynaptic receptors may alter the metabolism of neurons by the use of second messengers, which include **cyclic adenosine monophosphate (cAMP), lipids** (e.g., diacylglycerol), **$Ca2^+$**, and **nitric oxide.**

C. **Classification of neurotransmitters. Biogenic amines** (monoamines), **amino acids**, and **peptides** are the three major classes of neurotransmitters.

D. **Regulation of neurotransmitter activity**
   1. The concentration of neurotransmitters in the synaptic cleft is closely related to mood and behavior. A number of mechanisms affect this concentration.
   2. After release by the presynaptic neuron, neurotransmitters are removed from the synaptic cleft by mechanisms including:
      a. **Reuptake** by the presynaptic neuron.
      b. **Degradation** by enzymes such as **monoamine oxidase (MAO).**

| table 4.4 | Psychiatric Conditions and Associated Neurotransmitter Activity |
|---|---|
| **Neuropsychiatric Condition** | **Neurotransmitter Activity Increased ($\uparrow$) or Decreased ($\downarrow$)** |
| Depression | Norepinephrine ($\downarrow$), serotonin ($\downarrow$), dopamine ($\downarrow$) |
| Mania | Dopamine ($\uparrow$), g-aminobutyric acid (GABA) ($\downarrow$) |
| Schizophrenia | Dopamine ($\uparrow$), serotonin ($\uparrow$), glutamate ($\uparrow$ or $\downarrow$) |
| Anxiety | GABA ($\downarrow$), serotonin ($\downarrow$), norepinephrine ($\uparrow$) |
| Alzheimer disease | Acetylcholine ($\downarrow$), glutamate ($\uparrow$) |

3. Availability of specific neurotransmitters is associated with common psychiatric conditions (Table 4.4). Normalization of neurotransmitter availability by pharmacological agents is associated with symptom improvement in some of these disorders (see Chapter 16).

# IV. BIOGENIC AMINES

## A. Overview
1. The **biogenic amines**, or **monoamines**, include catecholamines, indolamines, ethyl amines, and quaternary amines.
2. The **monoamine theory of mood disorder** hypothesizes that **lowered monoamine activity results in depression and elevated levels in mania**.
3. **Metabolites** of the monoamines are often measured in psychiatric research and diagnosis because they are more easily measured in body fluids than the actual monoamines (Table 4.5).
4. Distribution of dopaminergic, noradrenergic and serotonergic tracts in the CNS can be found in Figure 4.1.

## B. Dopamine
1. Dopamine, a catecholamine, is involved in the pathophysiology of **schizophrenia** and **other psychotic disorders, Parkinson disease, mood disorders**, the conditioned fear response (see Chapter 7), and the "rewarding" nature of drugs of abuse (see Chapter 9).
2. **Synthesis.** The amino acid tyrosine is converted to the precursor for dopamine by the enzyme **tyrosine hydroxylase**.
3. **Receptor subtypes.** At least five dopamine receptor subtypes ($D_1$–$D_5$) have been identified; the major site of action is $D_2$ for traditional antipsychotic agents and $D_1$ and $D_4$ as well as $D_2$ for the newer "atypical" antipsychotic agents (see Chapter 16).

| table 4.5 | Metabolites of Monoamines and Associated Psychopathology | |
|---|---|---|
| | **Increased ($\uparrow$) or Decreased ($\downarrow$) Concentration of Metabolite in Blood Plasma, Cerebrospinal Neurotransmitter Fluid, or Urine** | **Associated Psychopathology** |
| Dopamine | ($\uparrow$) HVA (homovanillic acid) | Schizophrenia and other conditions involving psychosis (see Chapters 9, 11, and 12) |
| | ($\downarrow$) HVA | Parkinson disease<br>Treatment with antipsychotic agents<br>Depression |
| Norepinephrine | ($\uparrow$) VMA (vanillylmandelic acid)<br>($\downarrow$) MHPG (3-methoxy-4- hydroxyphenylglycol) | Adrenal medulla tumor (pheochromocytoma)<br>Severe depression and attempted suicide |
| Serotonin | ($\downarrow$) 5-HIAA (5-hydroxyindoleacetic acid) | Severe depression<br>Attempted suicide<br>Aggressiveness and violence<br>Impulsiveness<br>Tourette syndrome<br>Alcohol abuse<br>Bulimia |

**4. Dopaminergic tracts (Figure 4.1A)**
   **a.** The **nigrostriatal tract** is involved in the regulation of muscle tone and movement.
      **(1)** This tract **degenerates in Parkinson disease**.
      **(2)** Treatment with antipsychotic drugs, which block postsynaptic dopamine receptors receiving input from the nigrostriatal tract, can result in Parkinson-like symptoms.

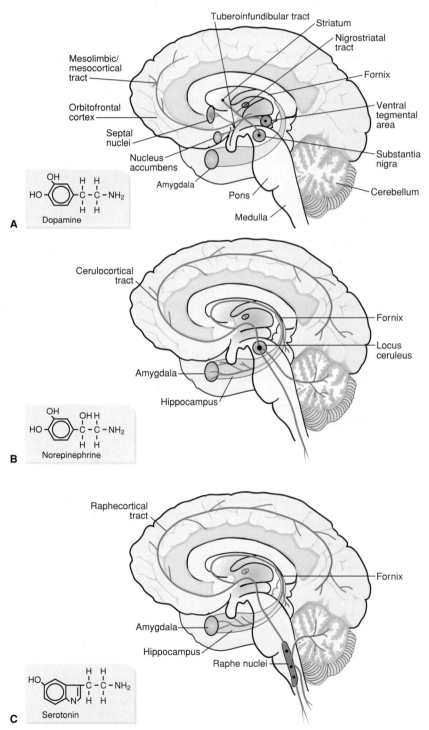

**FIGURE 4.1.** Distribution of (**A**) dopaminergic, (**B**) noradrenergic, and (**C**) serotonergic tracts in the CNS.

   **b.** Dopamine acts on the **tuberoinfundibular tract** to inhibit the secretion of prolactin from the anterior pituitary.
   
       **(1)** Blockade of dopamine receptors by antipsychotic drugs prevents the inhibition of prolactin release and results in **elevated prolactin** levels.
   
       **(2)** This elevation in turn results in symptoms such as breast enlargement, galactorrhea, and sexual dysfunction.
   
   **c.** The **mesolimbic–mesocortical tract** is associated with psychotic disorders.
   
       **(1)** This tract may have a role in the expression of **emotions** since it projects into the limbic system and prefrontal cortex.
   
       **(2)** Hyperactivity of the mesolimbic tract is associated with the positive symptoms (e.g., hallucinations) of schizophrenia; hypoactivity of the mesocortical tract is associated with the negative symptoms (e.g., apathy) of schizophrenia (see Chapter 11).

**C.** **Norepinephrine**, a catecholamine, plays a role in **mood, anxiety, arousal, learning**, and **memory**.
   1. **Synthesis**
      **a.** Like dopaminergic neurons, noradrenergic neurons synthesize dopamine.
      **b.** Dopamine b-hydroxylase, present in noradrenergic neurons, converts this dopamine to norepinephrine.
   2. **Localization.** Most noradrenergic neurons (approximately 10,000 per hemisphere in the brain) are located in the **locus ceruleus (Figure 4.1B)**.

**D.** **Serotonin**, an indolamine, plays a role in **mood, sleep, sexuality**, and **impulse control**. Elevation of serotonin is associated with improved mood and sleep but decreased sexual function (particularly delayed orgasm). Very high levels are associated with **psychotic symptoms** (see Chapter 11). Decreased serotonin is associated with poor impulse control, depression, and poor sleep.
   1. **Synthesis.** The amino acid tryptophan is converted to serotonin (also known as **5-hydroxytryptamine [5-HT]**) by the enzyme tryptophan hydroxylase as well as by an amino acid decarboxylase.
   2. **Localization.** Most serotonergic cell bodies in the brain are contained in the **dorsal raphe nucleus in the upper pons and lower midbrain (Figure 4.1C)**.
   3. **Antidepressants and serotonin.** Heterocyclic antidepressants (**HCAs**), selective serotonin reuptake inhibitors (**SSRIs**), and monoamine oxidase inhibitors (**MAOIs**) ultimately increase the presence of serotonin and norepinephrine in the synaptic cleft (Chapter 16).
      **a.** **HCAs** block reuptake of serotonin and norepinephrine, and **SSRIs** such as fluoxetine (Prozac) selectively block reuptake of serotonin by the presynaptic neuron.
      **b.** **MAOIs** prevent the degradation of serotonin and norepinephrine by MAO.

**E.** **Histamine**
   1. Histamine, an **ethylamine**, is affected by psychoactive drugs.
   2. Histamine receptor blockade with drugs such as antipsychotics and tricyclic antidepressants is associated with common side effects of these drugs such as **sedation** and **increased appetite** leading to weight gain.

**F.** **Acetylcholine (Ach)**, a quaternary amine, is the transmitter used by **nerve–skeleton–muscle junctions**.
   1. **Degeneration of cholinergic neurons** is associated with **Alzheimer disease, Down's syndrome**, and **movement and sleep disorders** (e.g., decreased REM sleep, see Chapter 10).
   2. **Cholinergic neurons** synthesize Ach from acetyl coenzyme A and choline using the enzyme **choline acetyltransferase**.
   3. The **nucleus basalis of Meynert** is a brain area involved in production of Ach.
   4. **Acetylcholinesterase** (AchE) breaks Ach down into choline and acetate.
   5. Blocking the action of **AchE** with drugs such as **donepezil** (Aricept), **rivastigmine** (Exelon), and **galantamine** (Reminyl) may delay the progression of Alzheimer disease but cannot reverse the function already lost.
   6. **Blockade of muscarinic Ach receptors** with drugs such as antipsychotics and tricyclic antidepressants results in the classic "anticholinergic" adverse effects seen with the use of

these drugs, including dry mouth, blurred vision, urinary hesitancy, and constipation. Use of these agents can also result in central anticholinergic effects such as confusion and memory problems.

**7.** Anticholinergic agents are commonly used to treat the Parkinson-like symptoms caused by antipsychotic agents (see section IV.B.4.a. above).

# V. AMINO ACID NEUROTRANSMITTERS

These neurotransmitters are involved in most synapses in the brain and include **glutamate, g-aminobutyric acid (GABA), and glycine**.

A. **Glutamate**
1. Glutamate is an excitatory neurotransmitter that contributes to the pathophysiology of **neurodegenerative illnesses** such as Alzheimer disease and schizophrenia.
   a. The mechanism of this association involves activation of the glutamate receptor **N-methyl-d-aspartate (NMDA)** by sustained elevation of glutamate.
   b. Such activation results in calcium ions entering neurons leading to nerve cell degeneration and death through **excitotoxicity**.
   c. **Memantine** (Namenda), an NMDA receptor antagonist, ultimately **blocks this influx of calcium** and is indicated for patients with moderate to severe **Alzheimer disease**.

B. **GABA**
1. GABA is the principal **inhibitory** neurotransmitter in the CNS. It is synthesized from glutamate by the enzyme glutamic acid decarboxylase, which needs vitamin B6 (pyridoxine) as a cofactor.
2. GABA is closely involved in the action of antianxiety agents such as **benzodiazepines** (e.g., diazepam [Valium]) and **barbiturates** (e.g., secobarbital [Seconal]). Benzodiazepines and barbiturates increase the affinity of GABA for its **GABA$_A$-binding site**, allowing more chloride to enter the neuron. The chloride-laden neurons become hyperpolarized and inhibited, decreasing neuronal firing and ultimately decreasing anxiety. Anticonvulsants also potentiate the activity of GABA.

C. **Glycine** is an inhibitory neurotransmitter found primarily in the spinal cord. Glycine works on its own and as a regulator of glutamate activity.

# VI. NEUROPEPTIDES

A. **Endogenous opioids such as enkephalins, endorphins, dynorphins, and endomorphins** are produced by the brain itself. They act to decrease pain and anxiety and have a role in addiction and mood.

B. **Placebo effects** (see Chapter 25) may be mediated by the endogenous opioid system. For example, prior treatment with an opioid receptor blocker such as naloxone can block placebo effects.

# Review Test

**Directions:** Each of the numbered items or incomplete statements in this section is followed by answers or by completions of the statement. Select the **one** lettered answer or completion that is **best** in each case.

**1.** A 30-year-old man who has had many negative life experiences becomes upset when he sees photographs of himself taken during these times. The brain area most likely to be activated by these photographs is the

**(A)** dorsolateral convexity of the frontal lobe
**(B)** hypothalamus
**(C)** orbitofrontal cortex
**(D)** reticular system
**(E)** amygdala
**(F)** nucleus basalis of Meynert

**2.** A 43-year-old man comes to the emergency department of a large hospital. He is very anxious and complains of abdominal cramps and diarrhea. The physician observes intense flushing of the man's skin. In this patient, a 24-hour urine study is most likely to reveal elevated levels of

**(A)** acetylcholine
**(B)** 5-hydroxyindoleacetic acid (5-HIAA)
**(C)** porphobilinogen
**(D)** vanillylmandelic acid (VMA)
**(E)** homovanillic acid (HVA)

**3.** In a clinical experiment, a 48-year-old female patient with chronic pain who, in the past, has responded to placebos is given naloxone. Shortly thereafter the patient is given an inert substance that she believes is a painkiller. After the patient receives the inert substance, her pain is most likely to

**(A)** increase
**(B)** decrease
**(C)** be unchanged
**(D)** respond to lower doses of opioids than previously
**(E)** fail to respond to opioids in the future

**4.** A 65-year-old female patient has had a stroke affecting the left hemisphere of her brain. Which of the following functions is most likely to be affected by the stroke?

**(A)** Perception
**(B)** Musical ability
**(C)** Spatial relations
**(D)** Language
**(E)** Artistic ability

**5.** Which of the following two structural entities connect the cerebral hemispheres?

**(A)** Basal ganglia and anterior commissure
**(B)** Anterior commissure and reticular system
**(C)** Reticular system and corpus callosum
**(D)** Hippocampal commissure and corpus callosum
**(E)** Amygdala and habenular commissure

**6.** A 23-year-old patient shows side effects such as sedation, increased appetite, and weight gain while being treated with antipsychotic medication. Of the following, the mechanism most closely associated with these effects is

**(A)** blockade of serotonin receptors
**(B)** blockade of dopamine receptors
**(C)** blockade of norepinephrine receptors
**(D)** blockade of histamine receptors
**(E)** decreased availability of serotonin

**7.** A 3-year-old girl who had been developing typically since birth begins to withdraw socially and then stops speaking altogether. Also, instead of purposeful hand movements, the child has begun to show repetitive hand wringing behavior. The chromosome most likely to be involved in this disorder is chromosome

**(A)** 1
**(B)** 16
**(C)** 18
**(D)** 21
**(E)** X

**8.** The major neurotransmitter implicated in **both** Alzheimer disease and schizophrenia is

**(A)** serotonin
**(B)** norepinephrine
**(C)** dopamine
**(D)** g-aminobutyric acid (GABA)
**(E)** acetylcholine (Ach)
**(F)** glutamate

**9.** The major neurotransmitter involved in the antidepressant action of fluoxetine (Prozac) is

**(A)** serotonin
**(B)** norepinephrine
**(C)** dopamine
**(D)** g-aminobutyric acid (GABA)
**(E)** acetylcholine (Ach)
**(F)** glutamate

**10.** The neurotransmitter metabolized to 5-HIAA (5-hydroxyindoleacetic acid) is

**(A)** serotonin
**(B)** norepinephrine
**(C)** dopamine
**(D)** g-aminobutyric acid (GABA)
**(E)** acetylcholine (Ach)
**(F)** glutamate

**11.** A 25-year-old male patient sustains a serious head injury in an automobile accident. He had been aggressive and assaultive, but after the accident he is placid and cooperative. He also makes inappropriate suggestive comments to the nurses and masturbates a great deal. The area(s) of the brain most likely to be affected in this patient is (are) the

**(A)** right parietal lobe
**(B)** basal ganglia
**(C)** hippocampus
**(D)** reticular system
**(E)** amygdala
**(F)** left frontal lobe

**12.** A 35-year-old female patient reports that she has difficulty sleeping ever since she sustained a concussion in a subway accident. The area(s) of the brain most likely to be affected in this patient is (are) the

**(A)** right parietal lobe
**(B)** basal ganglia
**(C)** hippocampus
**(D)** reticular system
**(E)** amygdala
**(F)** left frontal lobe

**13.** A 55-year-old woman was diagnosed with schizophrenia at the age of 22. If this diagnosis was appropriate, the volume of the hippocampus, the size of the cerebral ventricles, and glucose utilization in the frontal cortex of this patient are now most likely to be, respectively

**(A)** increased, increased, increased
**(B)** decreased, decreased, decreased
**(C)** decreased, decreased, increased
**(D)** decreased, increased, decreased
**(E)** increased, decreased, increased

**14.** An 80-year-old female patient has a resting tremor of her left hand, little expression in her face, and problems taking a first step when she has been standing still. The area(s) of the brain most likely to be affected in this patient is (are) the

**(A)** right parietal lobe
**(B)** basal ganglia
**(C)** hippocampus
**(D)** reticular system
**(E)** amygdala
**(F)** left frontal lobe

**15.** A 69-year-old former bank president cannot tell you the name of the current president and has difficulty identifying the woman sitting next to him (his wife). He began having memory problems 3 years ago. The area(s) of the brain most likely to be affected in this patient is (are) the

**(A)** right parietal lobe
**(B)** basal ganglia
**(C)** hippocampus
**(D)** reticular system
**(E)** amygdala
**(F)** left frontal lobe

**16.** A 45-year-old male patient becomes depressed following a head injury. The area(s) of the brain most likely to be affected in this patient is (are) the

**(A)** right parietal lobe
**(B)** basal ganglia
**(C)** hippocampus
**(D)** reticular system
**(E)** amygdala
**(F)** left frontal lobe

**17.** A 28-year-old male patient is brought to the emergency room after a fight in which he attacked a man who cut into his line at the supermarket checkout. In the emergency room he remains assaultive and combative. The body fluids of this patient are most likely to show

(A) increased 3-methoxy-4-hydroxyphenylg-lycol (MHPG)
(B) decreased MHPG
(C) increased 5-hydroxyindoleacetic acid (5-HIAA)
(D) decreased 5-HIAA
(E) decreased homovanillic acid (HVA)

**18.** A 30-year-old woman who is withdrawing from heroin shows intense anxiety, increased pulse, elevated blood pressure, and a hand tremor. Her symptoms improve when she is given clonidine, an alpha-2-adrenergic receptor agonist. The area(s) of the brain most likely to be involved in the improvement in this patient's symptoms is (are) the

(A) right parietal lobe
(B) basal ganglia
(C) locus ceruleus
(D) raphe nuclei
(E) amygdala
(F) substantia nigra

**19.** A very anxious 25-year-old patient is examined in the emergency room. There is no evidence of physical illness. If it could be measured, the g-aminobutyric acid (GABA) activity in the brain of this patient would most likely be

(A) increased
(B) decreased
(C) unchanged
(D) higher than the activity of serotonin
(E) higher than the activity of norepine-phrine

**20.** A 24-year-old man sustains a head injury in an automobile accident. His father relates that prior to the accident, the patient was respectful, modest, controlled, and hard working. In the hospital, the patient is rude to the nurses and aides, loses his temper with the slightest provocation, and refuses to wear a hospital gown or anything else. These behavioral changes after the accident indicate that the area of the brain most likely to have been injured in this patient is the

(A) dorsolateral convexity of the frontal lobe
(B) hypothalamus
(C) orbitofrontal cortex
(D) reticular system
(E) amygdala
(F) nucleus basalis of Meynert

**21.** Analysis of the blood plasma of a 45-year-old male patient shows increased concentration of homovanillic acid (HVA). This elevation is most likely to be associated with which of the following conditions?

(A) Parkinson disease
(B) Depression
(C) Bulimia
(D) Pheochromocytoma
(E) Schizophrenia

**22.** Remembering that school closes early before Thanksgiving Day every year is an example of which of the following types of memory?

(A) Semantic
(B) Episodic
(C) Procedural
(D) Working

**23.** A 55-year-old patient who is taking tiotropium bromide (Spiriva) for chronic obstructive pulmonary disease has memory problems due to the agent's action on which of the following receptors?

(A) Adrenergic
(B) Cholinergic
(C) Dopaminergic
(D) Histaminergic
(E) Serotonergic

**24.** A 6-year-old child shows seizures, cognitive defects, and autistic behavior. The child also shows raised discolored areas on her forehead (forehead plaques). Which of the following chromosomes is most likely to be involved in the etiology of this child's symptoms?

**(A)** 1
**(B)** 16
**(C)** 18
**(D)** 21
**(E)** X

**25.** A 72-year-old man with Alzheimer disease is being treated with memantine. What is believed to be the basis of the therapeutic action of memantine on neurons in the brain?

**(A)** To inhibit the action of acetylcholinesterase
**(B)** To block the influx of calcium
**(C)** To inhibit the action of acetylcholine
**(D)** To increase the influx of glutamate
**(E)** To facilitate the influx of calcium

# Answers and Explanations

## Typical Board Question

**The answer is A.** Damage to the right parietal lobe can result in impaired visual–spatial processing. This can lead to problems copying simple drawings and neglect of the left side as seen in this patient.

1. **The answer is E.** The amygdala is an important brain area for the evaluation of sensory stimuli with emotional significance. Thus, the brain area most likely to be activated by these photos is the amygdala.

2. **The answer is D.** A 24-hour urine study is most likely to reveal elevated levels of VMA, a metabolite of norepinephrine. Anxiety, abdominal cramps and diarrhea, and skin flushing are symptoms of pheochromocytoma, a norepinephrine-secreting adrenal tumor. This picture is not seen with elevated levels of other neurotransmitter metabolites.

3. **The answer is C.** Since the placebo response is based in part on activation of the endogenous opioid system, it will be blocked by naloxone, and this patient's pain will be unchanged. This experiment will not necessarily affect her response to opioids in the future.

4. **The answer is D.** Dominance for language in both right-handed and left-handed people is usually in the left hemisphere of the brain. Perception, musical ability, artistic ability, and spatial relations primarily are functions of the right side of the brain.

5. **The answer is D.** The corpus callosum and the hippocampal, habenular, and anterior commissures connect the two hemispheres of the brain. The basal ganglia, reticular system, and amygdala do not have this function.

6. **The answer is D.** Sedation, increased appetite, and weight gain are side effects of treatment with certain antipsychotic agents. The mechanism most closely associated with these side effects is blockade of histamine receptors since these antipsychotics are not specific for dopamine blockade. Blockade of dopamine receptors by these antipsychotic medications is associated with side effects such as Parkinsonism-like symptoms and elevated prolactin levels.

7. **The answer is E.** This 3-year-old girl is showing signs of Rett's disorder which is linked to the X chromosome. Rett's disorder is characterized by loss of social skills after a period of typical functioning as well as hand wringing and breathing abnormalities (see also Chapter 15).

8. **The answer is F.** While acetylcholine (Ach) is the major neurotransmitter implicated in Alzheimer disease, abnormalities in glutamate are seen in both Alzheimer disease and schizophrenia.

9. **The answer is A.** Blockade of serotonin reuptake by presynaptic neurons is the primary action of the antidepressant fluoxetine.

10. **The answer is A.** Serotonin is metabolized to 5-HIAA.

11. **The answer is E.** The patient is showing evidence of the Klüver–Bucy syndrome, which includes hypersexuality and docility and is associated with damage to the amygdala.

12. **The answer is D.** Sleep-arousal mechanisms are affected by damage to the reticular system.

13. **The answer is D.** Although neuroimaging cannot be used to diagnose psychiatric disorders, brains of patients with schizophrenia such as this woman are likely to show decreased volume of limbic structures such as the hippocampus; increased size of cerebral ventricles due, in part, to brain shrinkage; and decreased glucose utilization in the frontal cortex.

14. **The answer is B.** This 80-year-old female patient is showing signs of Parkinson disease (e.g., a resting tremor, little facial expression, and problems initiating movement). This disorder is associated with abnormalities of the basal ganglia.

15. **The answer is C.** This patient is showing evidence of Alzheimer disease. Of the listed brain areas, the major one implicated in Alzheimer disease is the hippocampus.

16. **The answer is F.** Of the listed brain areas, depression is most likely to be associated with damage to the left frontal lobe.

17. **The answer is D.** Assaultive, impulsive, aggressive behavior like that seen in this 28-year-old male patient is associated with decreased levels of serotonin in the brain. Levels of 5-HIAA (5-hydroxyindoleacetic acid), the major metabolite of serotonin, have been shown to be decreased in the body fluids of violent, aggressive, impulsive individuals as well as depressed individuals. MHPG (3-methoxy-4-hydroxyphenylglycol), a metabolite of norepinephrine, is decreased in severe depression, while homovanillic acid (HVA), a metabolite of dopamine, is decreased in Parkinson disease and depression.

18. **The answer is C.** The effectiveness of clonidine in treating withdrawal symptoms associated with the use of opiates and sedatives is believed to be due to its action on alpha-2-adrenergic receptors, for example, reducing the firing rate of noradrenergic neurons, most of which are located in the locus ceruleus.

19. **The answer is B.** g-Aminobutyric acid (GABA) is an inhibitory amino acid neurotransmitter in the CNS. Thus, the activity of GABA in the brain of this anxious patient is likely to be decreased. Decreased serotonin and increased norepinephrine are also involved in anxiety (Table 4.4).

20. **The answer is C.** Behavioral changes such as decreased impulse control, poor social behavior, and lack of characteristic modesty indicate that the area of the brain most likely to have been injured in this patient is the orbitofrontal cortex. Lesions of this brain area result in disinhibition, inappropriate behavior, and poor judgment. In contrast, lesions of the dorsolateral convexity of the frontal lobe result in decreased executive functioning (e.g., motivation, concentration, and attention). The hypothalamus is associated with homeostatic mechanisms and the reticular system with consciousness and sleep. Damage to the amygdala results in decreased, not increased, aggression. The nucleus basalis of Meynert is a site of Ach production; its damage could result in deficits in intellectual functioning.

21. **The answer is E.** Increased body fluid level of homovanillic acid (HVA), a major metabolite of dopamine, is seen in schizophrenia. Decreased HVA is seen in Parkinson disease, depression, and in medicated schizophrenic patients. Increased vanillylmandelic acid (VMA), a metabolite of norepinephrine, is seen in pheochromocytoma. Decreased body fluid level of 5-HIAA, a metabolite of serotonin, is seen in depression and in bulimia (Table 4.5).

22. **The answer is A.** Remembering that school closes early before Thanksgiving Day every year is an example of semantic memory. Semantic memory is a type of declarative memory which involves remembering general knowledge about the world. Episodic memory involves remembering personally experienced events, procedural memory involves remembering things one does automatically, and working memory involves remembering recent information.

23. **The answer is B.** Decreased availability of acetylcholine by blockade of muscarinic acetylcholine receptors (i.e., anticholinergic activity) in the CNS is associated with memory problems. Blockade of adrenergic, dopaminergic, histaminergic, and serotonergic receptors are not specifically associated with memory problems.

24. **The answer is B.** Chromosome 16 and chromosome 9 are both associated with tuberous sclerosis. Seizures, cognitive defects, autistic behavior, and forehead plaques in this 6-year-old child are signs of this disorder.

25. **The answer is B.** The therapeutic action of memantine is believed to be to decrease the influx of glutamate which ultimately blocks the influx of calcium which can lead to nerve cell degeneration and death. In contrast to a group of drugs also used to treat Alzheimer's, that is, the acetylcholinesterase inhibitors, memantine does not directly affect acetylcholine.

# chapter 5

# Biological Assessment of Patients with Psychiatric Symptoms

**Typical Board Question**

A 55-year-old male patient with no history of psychiatric illness is admitted to the hospital complaining of intense abdominal pain. He states that over the past few days his wife has been giving him food that is poisoned so that she can kill him and be with another man. The wife states that she loves her husband and would never harm him or leave him. When the patient's urine is collected, it appears purplish red in color. Urine testing is most likely to reveal an elevated level of

- **(A)** glucose
- **(B)** 5-hydroxyindoleacetic acid (5-HIAA)
- **(C)** porphobilinogen
- **(D)** cortisol
- **(E)** vanillylmandelic acid (VMA)

*(See "Answers and Explanations" at end of chapter.)*

## I. OVERVIEW

Biological alterations and abnormalities can underlie psychiatric symptoms and influence their occurrence. A variety of studies are used clinically to identify such alterations and abnormalities in patients.

## II. MEASUREMENT OF BIOGENIC AMINES AND PSYCHOTROPIC DRUGS

**A.** Altered levels of biogenic amines and their metabolites occur in some psychiatric conditions (see Tables 4.2 and 4.3).

**B.** Plasma levels of some antipsychotic and antidepressant agents are measured to evaluate **patient compliance** or to determine whether **therapeutic blood levels** of the agent have been reached.

**C.** Laboratory tests also are used to monitor patients for complications of pharmacotherapy.
   **1.** Patients taking certain mood stabilizers, e.g., carbamazepine (Tegretol) or antipsychotics, e.g., clozapine (Clozaril) must be observed for blood abnormalities such as **agranulocytosis** (very low, e.g., <2,000, white blood cell count or granulocyte count < 1,000).

2. **Liver function** tests are used in patients being treated with carbamazepine and valproic acid (mood stabilizers).
3. **Thyroid function** and **kidney function** tests should be used in patients who are being treated with the mood stabilizer **lithium**. Patients taking lithium can develop **hypothyroidism** and, occasionally, hyperthyroidism.
4. Lithium levels should also be monitored regularly because of the drug's **narrow therapeutic range** (see Chapter 16).

## III. EVALUATING ENDOCRINE FUNCTION

A. **Dexamethasone suppression test (DST).** In a normal patient with a normal hypothalamic–adrenal–pituitary axis, dexamethasone, a synthetic glucocorticoid, suppresses the secretion of cortisol.
   1. In contrast, approximately one-half of the patients with major depressive disorder have a positive DST (i.e., this suppression is limited or absent).
   2. Because positive findings are not specific and non-suppression is seen in conditions other than major depressive disorder, the DST has limited clinical usefulness.

B. **Thyroid** function tests are used to screen for **hypothyroidism** and **hyperthyroidism**, which can mimic depression and anxiety, respectively.
   1. Physical symptoms of hypothyroidism include fatigue, weight gain, edema, hair loss, and cold intolerance.
   2. Physical symptoms of hyperthyroidism include rapid heartbeat ("palpitations"), flushing, fever, weight loss, and diarrhea.

C. Patients with depression may have other **endocrine irregularities**, such as reduced response to a challenge with thyrotropin-releasing hormone and abnormalities in growth hormone, melatonin, and gonadotropin.

D. Psychiatric symptoms are associated with other endocrine disorders, such as **Addison disease (hypocortisolism)**, **Cushing disease (hypercortisolism)**, and enzyme disorders such as **acute intermittent porphyria**.
   1. **Addison disease**
      a. Physical signs and symptoms include **hyperpigmentation of the skin**, particularly in skin creases, low blood pressure, pain, fainting, hypoglycemia, diarrhea, and vomiting.
      b. Psychiatric symptoms include fatigue, depression, psychosis, and confusion.
   2. **Cushing's syndrome**
      a. Physical signs and symptoms include round **"moon" face**, bruising, purple striae on the skin, sweating, facial hair, hypertension, fat on the back of the neck ("buffalo hump"), and a positive DST.
      b. Psychiatric symptoms include elevated mood, psychosis, anxiety, and depression.
   3. **Acute intermittent porphyria**
      a. Physical signs and symptoms include abdominal cramps, diarrhea and vomiting, seizures, cardiac arrhythmias, flushing, and **purple/red discoloration of the urine** due to elevated **porphobilinogen**.
      b. Psychiatric symptoms include paranoid **delusions** and hallucinations as well as depression and anxiety.

## IV. NEUROIMAGING AND ELECTROENCEPHALOGRAM STUDIES

Structural brain abnormalities and EEG changes may be associated with specific behavioral disorders (Table 5.1).

| t a b l e   **5.1** | Neuroimaging and Electroencephalography in the Biological Evaluation of Psychiatric Patients |
|---|---|
| **Specific Test or Measure** | **Uses and Characteristics** |
| Computed tomography (CT) | Identifies anatomically based brain changes (e.g., enlarged brain ventricles) seen in cognitive disorders, such as Alzheimer disease, as well as in schizophrenia |
| Nuclear magnetic resonance imaging (NMRI) | Identifies demyelinating disease (e.g., multiple sclerosis)<br>Shows the biochemical condition of neural tissues without exposing the patient to ionizing radiation |
| Positron emission tomography (PET) or functional MRI (fMRI) | Localizes areas of the brain that are physiologically active during specific tasks by characterizing and measuring metabolism of glucose in neural tissue<br>Measures specific neurotransmitter receptors<br>Requires use of a cyclotron |
| Single photon emission tomography (SPECT) | Obtains similar data to PET or fMRI but is more practical for clinical use because it uses a standard gamma camera rather than a cyclotron |
| Electroencephalogram (EEG) | Measures electrical activity in the cortex<br>Is useful in diagnosing epilepsy and in differentiating delirium (abnormal EEG) from dementia (often normal EEG)<br>Shows, in patients with schizophrenia, decreased alpha waves, increased theta and delta waves, and epileptiform activity |
| Evoked EEG (evoked potentials) | Measures electrical activity in the cortex in response to tactile, auditory, sound, or visual stimulation<br>Is used to evaluate vision and hearing loss in infants and brain responses in comatose and suspected brain-dead patients |

# V. NEUROPSYCHOLOGICAL TESTS

A. Neuropsychological tests are designed to assess general intelligence, memory, reasoning, orientation, perceptuomotor performance, language function, attention, and concentration in patients with suspected neurologic problems, such as dementia and brain damage (Table 5.2).

B. In such patients, the **Folstein Mini-Mental State Examination** (Table 5.3) is designed to follow the improvement or deterioration in cognitive function and the **Glasgow Coma Scale** (Table 5.4) is designed to assess the level of consciousness by rating patient responsiveness.

| t a b l e   **5.2** | Neuropsychological Tests Used in Psychiatry |
|---|---|
| **Test** | **Used to Identify or Evaluate** |
| Halstead–Reitan battery | Brain lesion localization and effects |
| Luria–Nebraska neuropsychological battery | Cerebral dominance<br>Types of brain dysfunction, such as dyslexia |
| Bender Visual Motor Gestalt | Visual and motor ability through the reproduction of designs |
| Digit symbol substitution | Dementia, depression, and age-related cognitive decline |
| Boston naming | Dementia |
| Wisconsin card sort | Executive function |
| Stroop color-word | Directed attention |
| Folstein Mini-Mental State | Delirium and dementia (Table 5.3) |
| Glasgow Coma Scale | Level of consciousness (Table 5.4) |

| table 5.3 | Folstein Min -Mental State Examination[a] | |
|---|---|---|
| **Skill Evaluated** | **Sample Instructions to the Patient** | **Maximum Score[a]** |
| Orientation | Tell me where you are and what day it is | 10 |
| Language | Name the object that I am holding | 8 |
| Attention and concentration | Subtract 7 from 100 and then continue to subtract 7s | 5 |
| Registration | Repeat the names of these three objects | 3 |
| Recall | After 5 min, recall the names of these three objects | 3 |
| Construction | Copy this design | 1 |

[a]Maximum total score = 30; total score of 23 or higher suggests competence; total score of 18 or lower suggests incompetence (Applebaum, 2007, *N Engl J Med*, 357) (see Chapter 26).
Adapted from Fadem B. *Behavioral Science in Medicine.* 2nd ed. Lippincott Williams & Wilkins; 2012:64.

## VI. OTHER TESTS

A. **Drug-assisted interview**
   1. Administration of a **sedative**, such as amobarbital sodium ("the Amytal interview"), prior to the clinical interview may be useful in determining whether organic pathology is responsible for symptomatology in patients who exhibit certain psychiatric disorders or are **malingering** (see Chapter 14).
   2. Sedatives can **relax patients** with conditions such as **dissociative disorders, conversion disorder** (see Chapter 14), and other disorders involving high levels of anxiety and **mute psychotic states** (see Chapter 11). This will allow patients to express themselves coherently during the interview.

B. **Sodium lactate administration.** Intravenous (IV) administration of sodium lactate can **provoke panic attacks (see Chapter 13) in susceptible patients** and can thus help to identify individuals with panic disorder. Inhalation of carbon dioxide can produce the same effect.

C. **Galvanic skin response** (a component of the "**lie detector**" test)
   1. The electric resistance of skin (galvanic skin response) varies with the patient's psychological state.
   2. Higher sweat gland activity seen with **sympathetic nervous system arousal** (e.g., when lying) results in decreased skin resistance and a positive test. However, innocent but anxious people may also have positive tests (false positives) and guilty people who are not bothered by telling lies may have negative tests (false negatives).

| table 5.4 | Glasgow Coma Scale (GCS)[a] | | |
|---|---|---|---|
| **Number of Points** | **Best Eye-Opening Response (E)** | **Best Verbal Response (V)** | **Best Motor Response (M)** |
| 1 | No eye opening | No verbal response | No motor response |
| 2 | Opens eyes in response to painful stimulus | Makes incomprehensible sounds | Shows extension to painful stimulus |
| 3 | Opens eyes in response to a verbal command | Speaks using inappropriate words | Shows flexion to painful stimulus |
| 4 | Opens eyes spontaneously | Makes confused verbal response | Withdraws from painful stimulus |
| 5 | — | Is oriented and can converse | Localizes a source of pain |
| 6 | — | — | Obeys commands |

[a]Maximum total score on the GCS = 15; lowest possible score = 3; a GSC score of 13–15 indicates mild, 9–12 indicates moderate, and <9 indicates severe neurologic impairment. The reported score is commonly broken down into components (e.g., E2 V1 M3 = GCS 6).

# Review Test

**Directions:** Each of the numbered items or incomplete statements in this section is followed by answers or by completions of the statement. Select the **one** lettered answer or completion that is **best** in each case.

**1.** A 57-year-old male patient who has had a stroke cannot copy a design drawn by the examiner. The test that the examiner is most likely to be using to evaluate this patient is the
**(A)** Bender Visual Motor Gestalt Test
**(B)** Luria–Nebraska neuropsychological battery
**(C)** Halstead–Reitan battery
**(D)** dexamethasone suppression test (DST)
**(E)** electroencephalogram (EEG)

**2.** A 36-year-old female patient comes to the physician complaining of extreme fatigue and depression. Physical examination reveals a darkening of her skin, particularly in the creases of her hands as well as darkening of the buccal mucosa. The most likely cause of this picture is
**(A)** hypocortisolism
**(B)** hypercortisolism
**(C)** pheochromocytoma
**(D)** hypothyroidism
**(E)** hyperthyroidism

**3.** A physician administers sodium lactate intravenously to a 28-year-old woman. Using this technique, the physician is trying to provoke, and thus confirm, the patient's diagnosis of
**(A)** conversion disorder
**(B)** amnestic disorder
**(C)** malingering
**(D)** panic disorder
**(E)** major depression

**4.** To determine which brain area is physiologically active when a 44-year-old male patient is translating a paragraph from Spanish to English, the most appropriate diagnostic technique is
**(A)** positron emission tomography (PET)
**(B)** computed tomography (CT)
**(C)** amobarbital sodium (Amytal) interview
**(D)** electroencephalogram (EEG)
**(E)** evoked EEG
**(F)** Glasgow Coma Scale
**(G)** Folstein Mini-Mental State Examination

**5.** To determine whether a 3-month-old infant is able to hear sounds, the most appropriate diagnostic technique is
**(A)** PET
**(B)** CT
**(C)** amobarbital sodium (Amytal) interview
**(D)** EEG
**(E)** evoked EEG
**(F)** Glasgow Coma Scale
**(G)** Folstein Mini-Mental State Examination

**6.** A 27-year-old female patient shows a sudden loss of motor function below the waist that cannot be medically explained. To determine whether psychological factors are responsible for this symptom, the most appropriate diagnostic technique is
**(A)** PET
**(B)** CT
**(C)** amobarbital sodium (Amytal) interview
**(D)** EEG
**(E)** evoked EEG
**(F)** Glasgow Coma Scale
**(G)** Folstein Mini-Mental State Examination

**7.** To identify anatomical changes in the brain of an 80-year-old female patient with Alzheimer disease, the most appropriate diagnostic technique is

**(A)** PET
**(B)** CT
**(C)** amobarbital sodium (Amytal) interview
**(D)** electroencephalogram (EEG)
**(E)** evoked EEG
**(F)** Glasgow Coma Scale
**(G)** Folstein Mini-Mental State Examination

**8.** To differentiate delirium from dementia in a 75-year-old male patient, the most appropriate diagnostic technique is

**(A)** PET
**(B)** CT
**(C)** amobarbital sodium (Amytal) interview
**(D)** EEG
**(E)** evoked EEG
**(F)** Glasgow Coma Scale
**(G)** Folstein Mini-Mental State Examination

**9.** A 40-year-old woman reports that over the past 6 months she has had little appetite, sleeps poorly, and has lost interest in her normal activities. Physical exam is unremarkable. Which of the following is the most likely laboratory finding in this woman?

**(A)** Positive dexamethasone suppression test (DST)
**(B)** Normal growth hormone regulation
**(C)** Increased 5-hydroxyindoleacetic acid (5-HIAA) levels
**(D)** Normal melatonin levels
**(E)** Hyperthyroidism

**10.** A 50-year-old woman without a previous psychiatric history reports that over the past few months she has begun to experience intense anxiety and has lost 15 pounds. The patient also complains of "flushing and palpitations." Which of the following is the most likely laboratory finding in this woman?

**(A)** Positive DST
**(B)** Normal growth hormone regulation
**(C)** Increased 5-HIAA levels
**(D)** Normal melatonin levels
**(E)** Hyperthyroidism

**11.** A college-educated 72-year-old female patient has scored 15 on the Folstein Mini-Mental State Examination. From this score, the physician can conclude that this patient probably

**(A)** is normal
**(B)** cannot calculate simple sums
**(C)** is cognitively impaired
**(D)** should be placed in an assisted living facility
**(E)** has a lower-than-normal IQ

**12.** Four weeks after he begins to take a new medication, a 23-year-old male psychiatric patient develops fever and sore throat. He reports feeling tired, and blood studies reveal a white blood cell (WBC) count of less than 2,000. This patient is most likely to be taking which of the following agents?

**(A)** Amobarbital sodium
**(B)** Clozapine
**(C)** Lithium
**(D)** Dexamethasone
**(E)** Sodium lactate

# Answers and Explanations

**Typical Board Question**

**The answer is C.** This patient with abdominal pain, the false belief that his wife is trying to poison him (a delusion, see Table 11.1), and urine with a purple-red color is most likely to have porphyria, a disorder that is associated with psychiatric symptoms such as delusions. Porphyria is a metabolic disorder in which toxic porphyrins accumulate in tissue leading to high levels of porphobilinogen in urine which colors it purple-red. Purple-red urine is not seen in the serotonin syndrome (high 5-HIAA), Cushing's syndrome (high cortisol), pheochromocytoma (high VMA), or diabetes (high glucose).

1. **The answer is A.** The Bender Visual Motor Gestalt Test is used to evaluate visual and motor ability by reproduction of designs. The Luria–Nebraska neuropsychological battery is used to determine cerebral dominance and to identify specific types of brain dysfunction, while the Halstead–Reitan battery is used to detect and localize brain lesions and determine their effects. The dexamethasone suppression test is used to predict which depressed patients will respond well to treatment with antidepressant agents or electroconvulsive therapy. The electroencephalogram (EEG), which measures electrical activity in the cortex, is useful in diagnosing epilepsy and in differentiating delirium from dementia.

2. **The answer is A.** This female patient is showing evidence of hypocortisolism or Addison disease. This condition is characterized by darkening of the skin, particularly in places not exposed to the sun such as skin creases and inside the mouth. This darkening is not seen in hypercortisolism, pheochromocytoma, or hyper- or hypothyroidism. Hypercortisolism, which also may lead to depression and anxiety, is characterized by weight gain, "moon" shaped face, and skin striae. Depression, dry hair, and weight gain characterize hypothyroidism, while anxiety, fever, weight loss, and elevated heart rate characterize hyperthyroidism. Patients with pheochromocytoma show intense anxiety and elevated VMA in body fluids (see Chapter 4).

3. **The answer is D.** Intravenous administration of sodium lactate can help identify individuals with panic disorder since it can provoke a panic attack in such patients.

4. **The answer is A.** Positron emission tomography (PET) localizes physiologically active brain areas by measuring glucose metabolism. Thus, this test can be used to determine which brain area is being used during a specific task (e.g., translating a passage written in Spanish).

5. **The answer is E.** The auditory evoked EEG can be used to assess whether this child can hear. Evoked EEGs measure electrical activity in the cortex in response to sensory stimulation.

6. **The answer is C.** The amobarbital sodium (Amytal) interview is used to determine whether psychological factors are responsible for symptoms in this patient who shows a non-medically explained loss of sensory function (conversion disorder—see Chapter 14).

7. **The answer is B.** Computed tomography (CT) identifies anatomical brain changes, such as enlarged ventricles. Thus, although not diagnostic, this test can be used to identify anatomical changes in the brain, such as enlarged ventricles in a patient with suspected dementia of the Alzheimer type.

8. **The answer is D.** Electroencephalogram (EEG) measures electrical activity in the cortex and can be useful in differentiating delirium (abnormal EEG) from dementia (usually normal EEG).

9. **The answer is A.** Poor appetite, poor sleep, and lack of interest in usual activities characterize patients who have major depression (see Chapter 12). In this depressed woman, the dexamethasone suppression test is likely to be positive. A positive result is seen when the synthetic glucocorticoid dexamethasone fails to suppress the secretion of cortisol as it would in a patient with a normal mood. Also, in depression there may be abnormal growth hormone regulation and melatonin levels, and decreased 5-HIAA. Hypothyroidism may be associated with depression; hyperthyroidism is more commonly associated with the symptoms of anxiety.

10. **The answer is E.** This woman's symptoms (e.g., anxiety, fever, weight loss, and flushing) indicate that she has hyperthyroidism (also see the answer to Question 9). People commonly describe their perception of a rapid heartbeat as "palpitations."

11. **The answer is C.** Scores below 18 on the Folstein Mini-Mental State Examination indicate significant cognitive impairment. This test does not evaluate calculating ability or IQ. Although the patient is impaired, it is not clear what caused the problem or whether she needs to be placed in an assisted living facility.

12. **The answer is B.** Agranulocytosis is seen particularly in patients taking clozapine, an antipsychotic, or carbamazepine, an anticonvulsant that is used to treat bipolar disorder (see Chapter 12). Lithium, amobarbital sodium, dexamethasone, and sodium lactate are not specifically associated with agranulocytosis.

# Psychoanalytic Theory and Defense Mechanisms

## Typical Board Question

When a 27-year-old patient who had a contentious relationship with his father joins a new health insurance plan, he must change from his primary care physician, a young man, to a new physician, a middle-aged man. On his first visit to the new doctor, the patient seems annoyed with everything the doctor says and states, "You are an old man with old-fashioned ideas; you just want to control my life." This patient's behavior is most closely related to which of the following?

**(A)** Positive transference
**(B)** Negative transference
**(C)** Countertransference
**(D)** Dislike of the doctor
**(E)** Fear of the doctor

*(See "Answers and Explanations" at end of chapter.)*

## I. OVERVIEW

Psychoanalytic theory is based on Freud's concept that behavior is determined by forces derived from unconscious mental processes. Psychoanalysis and related therapies are psychotherapeutic treatments based on this concept (see Chapter 17).

## II. FREUD'S THEORIES OF THE MIND

To explain his ideas, Freud developed, early in his career, the topographic theory of the mind and, later in his career, the structural theory.

**A. Topographic theory of the mind.** In the topographic theory, the mind contains three levels: The unconscious, preconscious, and conscious.
   1. The **unconscious mind** contains repressed thoughts and feelings that are not available to the conscious mind, and uses primary process thinking.
      a. **Primary process** is a type of thinking associated with primitive drives, wish fulfillment, and pleasure seeking, and has no logic or concept of time. Primary process thinking is seen in young children and psychotic adults.
      b. **Dreams** represent gratification of unconscious instinctive impulses and wish fulfillment.

| t a b l e   **6.1**   Freud's Structural Theory of the Mind | | | |
|---|---|---|---|
| Structural Component | Topographic Level of Operation | Age at which it Develops | Characteristics |
| Id | Unconscious | Present at birth | Contains instinctive sexual and aggressive drives<br>Controlled by primary process thinking<br>Not influenced by external reality |
| Ego | Unconscious, preconscious, and conscious | Begins to develop immediately after birth | Controls the expression of the id to adapt to the requirements of the external world primarily by the use of defense mechanisms<br>Enables one to sustain satisfying interpersonal relationships<br>Through reality testing (i.e., constantly evaluating what is valid and then adapting to that reality), enables one to maintain a sense of reality about the body and the external world |
| Superego | Unconscious, preconscious, and conscious | Begins to develop by about 6 yrs of age | Associated with moral values and conscience<br>Controls the expression of the id |

2. The **preconscious mind** contains memories that, while not immediately available, can be accessed easily.
3. The **conscious mind** contains thoughts that a person is currently aware of. It operates in close conjunction with the preconscious mind but does not have access to the unconscious mind. The conscious mind uses secondary process thinking (logical, mature, time-oriented) and can delay gratification.

B. **Structural theory of the mind.** In the structural theory, the mind contains three parts: The id, the ego, and the superego (Table 6.1).

## III.  DEFENSE MECHANISMS

A. **Definition.** Defense mechanisms are **unconscious mental techniques** used by the ego to keep conflicts out of the conscious mind, thus decreasing anxiety and maintaining a person's sense of safety, equilibrium, and self-esteem. They can be useful in helping people deal with difficult life situations such as medical illness, but, when used to excess, can become a barrier to seeking care or adhering to treatment recommendations.

B. **Specific defense mechanisms (Table 6.2)**
1. Some defense mechanisms are **immature** (i.e., they are manifestations of childlike or disturbed behavior).
2. **Mature defense mechanisms** (e.g., altruism, humor, sublimation, and suppression), when used in moderation, directly help the patient or others.
3. **Repression**, pushing unacceptable emotions into the unconscious, is the **basic defense mechanism** on which all others are based.

## IV.  TRANSFERENCE REACTIONS

A. **Definition.** Transference and countertransference are **unconscious mental attitudes** based on important past personal relationships (e.g., with parents). These phenomena increase emotionality and may thus alter judgment and behavior in patients' relationships with their doctors (transference) and doctors' relationships with their patients (countertransference).

| table | 6.2 | Commonly Used Defense Mechanisms (Listed Alphabetically) |

| Defense Mechanism | Explanation | Example |
| --- | --- | --- |
| Acting out | Avoiding personally unacceptable emotions by behaving in an attention-getting, often socially inappropriate manner | A depressed 14-yr-old girl with no history of conduct disorder has sexual encounters with multiple partners after her parents' divorce |
| Altruism[a] | Assisting others to avoid negative personal feelings | A man with a poor self-image, who is a social worker during the week, donates every other weekend to charity work |
| Denial | Not accepting aspects of reality that the person finds unbearable | An alcoholic insists that he is only a social drinker |
| Displacement | Moving emotions from a personally intolerable situation to one that is personally tolerable | A surgeon with unacknowledged anger toward his sister is abrasive to the female residents on his service |
| Dissociation | Mentally separating part of one's consciousness from real life events or mentally distancing oneself from others | Although he was not injured, a teenager has no memory of a car accident in which he was driving and his girlfriend was killed |
| Humor[a] | Expressing personally uncomfortable feelings without causing emotional discomfort | A man who is concerned about his erectile problems makes jokes about Viagra (sildenafil citrate) |
| Identification (introjection) | Unconsciously patterning one's behavior after that of someone more powerful (can be either positive or negative) | A man who was terrorized by his gym teacher as a child becomes a punitive, critical gym teacher (identification with the aggressor) |
| Intellectualization | Using the mind's higher functions to avoid experiencing emotion | A sailor whose boat is about to sink calmly explains the technical aspects of the hull damage in great detail to the other crew members |
| Isolation of affect | Failing to experience the feelings associated with a stressful life event, although logically understanding the significance of the event | Without showing any emotion, a woman tells her family the results of tests that indicate her lung cancer has metastasized |
| Projection | Attributing one's own personally unacceptable feelings to others Associated with paranoid symptoms and prejudice | A man with unconscious homosexual impulses begins to believe that a male colleague is attracted to him |
| Rationalization | Distorting one's perception of an event so that its negative outcome seems reasonable | A man who loses an arm in an accident says the loss of his arm was good because it kept him from getting in trouble with the law |
| Reaction formation | Adopting opposite attitudes to avoid personally unacceptable emotions, i.e., unconscious hypocrisy | A woman who unconsciously is resentful of the responsibilities of child rearing overspends on expensive gifts and clothing for her children |
| Regression | Reverting to behavior patterns like those seen in someone of a younger age | A woman insists that her husband stay overnight in the hospital with her before surgery |
| Splitting | Categorizing people or situations into categories of either "fabulous" or "dreadful" because of intolerance of ambiguity Seen in patients with borderline personality disorder | A patient tells the doctor that while all of the doctors in the group practice are wonderful, all of the nurses and office help are unfriendly and curt |
| Sublimation[a] | Expressing a personally unacceptable feeling (e.g., rage) in a socially useful way | A man who got into fights as a teenager becomes a professional prize fighter |
| Suppression[a] | Deliberately pushing personally unacceptable emotions out of conscious awareness (the only defense mechanism that includes some aspect of consciousness) | A medical student taking a review course for the United States Medical Licensing Examination mentally changes the subject when her mind wanders to the exam during a lecture |
| Undoing | Believing that one can magically reverse past events caused by "incorrect" behavior by now adopting "correct" behavior, e.g., atonement, confession, or penance | A woman who stole money from a friend, confesses to the theft, returns the money, and then feels compelled to offer to drive the friend to and from work for a year |

[a]"Mature" defense mechanisms.
Adapted from Fadem B. *Behavioral Science in Medicine*. 2nd ed. Philadelphia, PA: Lippincott Williams & Wilkins; 2012:83.

B. Transference
1. In **positive transference**, the patient has confidence in the doctor. If intense, the patient may over-idealize the doctor or develop sexual feelings toward the doctor.
2. In **negative transference**, the patient may become resentful or angry toward the doctor if the patient's desires and expectations are not realized. This may lead to poor adherence to medical advice.

C. In **countertransference**, feelings about a patient who reminds the doctor of a close friend or relative can interfere with the doctor's medical judgment.

# Review Test

**Directions:** Each of the numbered items or incomplete statements in this section is followed by answers or by completions of the statement. Select the **one** lettered answer or completion that is **best** in each case.

**1.** A female patient who is hospitalized after making a suicide attempt because her doctor did not respond to her offer to friend him on Facebook states that all female doctors are good but all male doctors are incompetent. The best explanation for this statement by the patient is

**(A)** prejudice
**(B)** lack of basic trust
**(C)** chauvinism
**(D)** splitting
**(E)** bias

**2.** A physician becomes very angry with a patient when the patient does not take his medication. The patient reminds the doctor of her rebellious son. This physician's intense reaction to the patient's behavior is most likely to be a result of

**(A)** positive transference
**(B)** negative transference
**(C)** countertransference
**(D)** dislike of the patient
**(E)** fear of the patient

**3.** Which of the following structures of the mind work on an unconscious level?

**(A)** The id only
**(B)** The id and the ego only
**(C)** The id, ego, and superego
**(D)** The ego and superego only
**(E)** Not the id, ego, or superego

**4.** Which of the following structures of the mind are at least partly developed in a typical 4-year-old child?

**(A)** The id only
**(B)** The id and the ego only
**(C)** The id, ego, and superego
**(D)** The ego and superego only
**(E)** Not the id, ego, or superego

**5.** A primary care physician notices that many of her patients use statements like "I can't stop smoking because I'll gain weight," or "when I'm sick, I only want to eat junk food." Statements like these

**(A)** produce conflict in the conscious mind
**(B)** are conscious mental techniques
**(C)** increase anxiety
**(D)** are examples of the use of defense mechanisms
**(E)** decrease a patient's sense of self-esteem

**6.** Of the following defense mechanisms, which is considered the most mature?

**(A)** Denial
**(B)** Sublimation
**(C)** Dissociation
**(D)** Regression
**(E)** Intellectualization

**7.** When having a manic episode, a 53-year-old patient with bipolar disorder shows primary process thinking. This type of thinking

**(A)** is logical
**(B)** is closely attuned to time
**(C)** is associated with reality
**(D)** is accessible to the conscious mind
**(E)** is associated with pleasure seeking

**8.** About 1 week after her final examination for a biochemistry course, a medical student's knowledge of the details of the Krebs cycle is most likely to reside in her

**(A)** unconscious mind
**(B)** preconscious mind
**(C)** conscious mind
**(D)** superego
**(E)** ego

**9.** A 15-year-old steals from family members and friends. When no one is watching, he also tortures the family cat. Which aspect of the mind is deficient in this teenager?

**(A)** The unconscious mind
**(B)** The preconscious mind
**(C)** The conscious mind
**(D)** The superego
**(E)** The ego

**Questions 10–20**

For the individual in each of the numbered questions, choose the defense mechanism that he or she is most likely to be using. Answers can be used more than once.

**(A)** Regression
**(B)** Isolation of affect
**(C)** Denial
**(D)** Rationalization
**(E)** Projection
**(F)** Dissociation
**(G)** Reaction formation
**(H)** Intellectualization
**(I)** Sublimation
**(J)** Displacement
**(K)** Suppression
**(L)** Splitting

**10.** A 28-year-old medical resident is assigned to tell a patient that her illness is terminal. Prior to seeing the patient, the resident conducts extensive library research on the details and statistics of length of survival of people with this illness. When he speaks to the patient, he cites the journal articles that he has read, including a detailed explanation of the theories of the etiology of her condition. Later that day, the resident tells the attending physician that the patient did not seem to understand what he told her.

**11.** A 40-year-old man who is angry at his ill wife, but does not consciously acknowledge that anger, shouts at his children as soon as he returns home from work.

**12.** A 26-year-old medical student who has unconscious angry, violent feelings chooses to do a surgery residency.

**13.** A 32-year-old man who is unconsciously attracted to his wife's sister becomes extremely jealous whenever his wife speaks to another man.

**14.** A 45-year-old man who is unconsciously afraid of flying repeatedly states his love of airplanes.

**15.** A 52-year-old man receives a letter from his physician informing him that his level of prostate-specific antigen (PSA) was abnormally high during his last visit. When the man appears at his physician's office for a follow-up visit, he complains about a headache but does not mention or seem to remember receiving the letter about his PSA test.

**16.** A 34-year-old woman relates that she wakes up fully dressed at least twice a week but then is tired all day. She also notes that she frequently receives phone calls from men who say they met her in a bar but whom she does not remember meeting.

**17.** A 35-year-old lawyer scheduled for surgery the next day insists that her mother stay overnight in the hospital with her.

**18.** A woman, whose parents and teachers complained about how messy she was as a child, grows up to become a famous abstract painter. Her technique involves throwing paint and small objects at large canvases and then using her fingers to mix the colors and textures.

**19.** A man who has just received a call at work that his child has been seriously injured and is being taken to the hospital arranges for a colleague to do his work before he rushes to the child's side.

**20.** A 21-year-old woman who was physically abused by her father manages her hostility toward him by baking cookies for him.

# Answers and Explanations

**The answer is B.** The patient who becomes very angry at his new doctor is showing a negative transference reaction. This emotional demonstration is likely to be a result of re-experiencing negative feelings about his relationship with his middle-aged father in his relationship with the middle-aged male doctor. In negative transference, patients become resentful or angry toward the doctor if their desires and expectations are not realized. This may lead to noncompliance with medical advice. In positive transference, patients have a high level of confidence in the doctor. Patients may also over-idealize or develop sexual feelings toward the doctor. This patient's reaction to the new doctor is less likely to be related to dislike or fear of the doctor.

1. **The answer is D.** Dividing people or situations into categories of good and bad characterizes the defense mechanism of splitting. Splitting is commonly used by people with the borderline personality disorder (see Chapter 14).

2. **The answer is C.** The doctor who becomes very angry at her patient for not taking his medication is showing a countertransference reaction. This excessive show of emotion is a result of re-experiencing feelings about her son's behavior in her relationship with the noncompliant patient. It is important for the doctor to identify this reaction because it can interfere with her medical judgment (see also answer to the TBQ). This doctor's reaction to the patient is less likely to be related to dislike or fear of the patient.

3. **The answer is C.** In Freud's structural theory, the mind is divided into the id, ego, and superego. The id operates completely on an unconscious level, while the ego and superego operate partly on an unconscious and partly on preconscious and conscious levels.

4. **The answer is B.** The id is present at birth, the ego begins to develop immediately after birth, and the superego begins to develop at about age 6 years.

5. **The answer is D.** Statements such as "I can't stop smoking because I'll gain weight," or "when I'm sick, I only want to eat junk food" are examples of the defense mechanisms of rationalization and regression, respectively. In rationalization, a person distorts her perception of an event so that its negative outcome seems reasonable, for example, because she feels unable to stop smoking, this patient claims (and so she reasonably feels) that gaining weight is worse than smoking, a life-threatening habit. In regression, ill patients revert to behavior patterns like those seen in someone of a younger age (e.g., eating junk food, crying). Defense mechanisms such as these are unconscious mental techniques that decrease anxiety and help people to maintain a sense of equilibrium and self-esteem.

6. **The answer is B.** Sublimation, expressing an unacceptable emotion in a socially acceptable way, is classified as a mature defense mechanism. Denial, dissociation, regression, and intellectualization are all classified as less mature defense mechanisms.

7. **The answer is E.** Primary process thinking is associated with pleasure seeking, disregards logic and reality, has no concept of time, and is not accessible to the conscious mind. Secondary process thinking is logical and is associated with reality.

8. **The answer is B.** Memory of the details of the Krebs cycle, while no longer in the forefront of the medical student's mind, can be recalled relatively easily 1 week after the examination. This memory therefore resides in the preconscious mind. The unconscious mind contains repressed thoughts and feelings, which are not available to the conscious mind. The conscious mind contains thoughts that a person is currently aware of. The id contains instinctive sexual and aggressive drives and is not influenced by external reality. The ego also controls the expression of the id, sustains satisfying interpersonal relationships, and, through reality testing, maintains a sense of reality about the body and the external world (see also answer to Question 9).

9. **The answer is D.** The superego is associated with moral values and conscience, and controls impulses of the id. This teenager who steals from family members and friends and tortures the family cat is showing deficiencies in his superego. Children and adolescents under age 18 years, who have poor superego development, may be diagnosed with conduct disorder (see Chapter 15).

10. **The answer is H.** The resident's behavior in dealing with this patient reflects his use of the defense mechanism of intellectualization. The resident has used his technical knowledge to avoid experiencing the emotion associated with telling the patient that she is dying.

11. **The answer is J.** In displacement, the man's personally unacceptable angry feelings toward his wife are taken out on his children.

12. **The answer is I.** In sublimation, the surgeon reroutes his unconscious, unacceptable wish for committing a violent act to a socially acceptable route (cutting people during surgery).

13. **The answer is E.** Using projection, the husband attributes his own unconscious, unacceptable sexual feelings toward another woman to his wife.

14. **The answer is G.** In reaction formation, the man denies his unconscious fear of flying and embraces the opposite idea by stating that he loves airplanes.

15. **The answer is C.** Using denial, this patient has seemingly forgotten an aspect of external reality, that is, the letter about his problematic PSA test.

16. **The answer is F.** This patient who relates that she wakes up fully dressed at least twice a week and receives phone calls from men whom she does not remember meeting is exhibiting dissociative identity disorder (multiple personality disorder). Dissociation, separating part of one's consciousness from real life events, is the defense mechanism used by individuals with this disorder. It is likely that this patient met the men who have her phone number but does not remember meeting them because at that time she was showing another personality (see also Chapter 14).

17. **The answer is A.** Regression, going back to a less mature way of behaving, is the defense mechanism used by this woman scheduled for surgery the next day who insists that her mother stay overnight in the hospital with her.

18. **The answer is I.** The useful employment in her abstract art of this woman's "messy" tendencies is an example of the defense mechanism of sublimation.

19. **The answer is K.** This man is using the partly conscious defense mechanism of suppression during the time that he is arranging for his work to be done by someone else before going to the hospital.

20. **The answer is G.** This woman who bakes cookies for her abusive father is managing her hostility toward him by using the defense mechanism of reaction formation. In this defense mechanism, a person adopts behavior that is opposite to the way she really feels, that is, this woman feels intense anger toward her father but shows caring behavior toward him.

# 7 Learning Theory

**Typical Board Question**

A 44-year-old woman has undergone three sessions of chemotherapy in a hospital. Each session has resulted in nausea. Before the fourth session, the patient becomes nauseated when she enters the hospital lobby. This patient's reaction is a result of the type of learning best described as

- **(A)** operant conditioning
- **(B)** classical conditioning
- **(C)** modeling
- **(D)** shaping
- **(E)** extinction

*(See "Answers and Explanations" at end of chapter.)*

## I. OVERVIEW

**A.** Learning is the acquisition of new behavior patterns.

**B.** Methods of learning include simple forms, such as **habituation** and **sensitization**, and more complex types, including **classical conditioning** and **operant conditioning**.

**C.** Learning methods are the basis of **behavioral treatment techniques**, such as systematic desensitization, aversive conditioning, flooding, biofeedback, token economy, and cognitive therapy (see Chapter 17).

## II. HABITUATION AND SENSITIZATION

**A.** In **habituation** (also called desensitization), repeated stimulation results in a decreased response (e.g., a child who receives weekly allergy injections cries less and less with each injection).

**B.** In **sensitization**, repeated stimulation results in an increased response (e.g., a child who is afraid of spiders feels more anxiety each time he encounters a spider).

# III. CLASSICAL CONDITIONING

A. **Principles.** In classical conditioning, a **natural** or **reflexive response** (behavior) is elicited by a **learned stimulus** (a cue from an internal or external event). This type of learning is called **associative learning**.
1. The **hippocampus** is particularly important in associative learning.
2. The **cerebellum** participates in classical conditioning, specifically in associations involving motor skills.

B. **Elements** of classical conditioning
1. An **unconditioned stimulus** is something that automatically, without having to be learned, produces a response (e.g., the odor of food).
2. An **unconditioned response** is a natural, reflexive behavior that does not have to be learned (e.g., salivation in response to the odor of food).
3. A **conditioned stimulus** is something that produces a response following learning (e.g., the sound of the lunch bell).
4. A **conditioned response** is a behavior that is learned by an association made between a conditioned stimulus and an unconditioned stimulus (e.g., salivation in response to the lunch bell).

C. **Response acquisition, extinction, and stimulus generalization**
1. In **acquisition**, the conditioned response (e.g., salivation in response to the lunch bell) is learned.
2. In **extinction**, the conditioned response decreases if the conditioned stimulus (e.g., the sound of the lunch bell) is never again paired with the unconditioned stimulus (e.g., the odor of food).
3. In **stimulus generalization**, a new stimulus (e.g., a church bell) that resembles a conditioned stimulus (e.g., the lunch bell) causes a conditioned response (e.g., salivation).

D. **Aversive conditioning.** An unwanted behavior (e.g., setting fires) is paired with a painful or aversive stimulus (e.g., a painful electric shock). An association is created between the unwanted behavior (fire-setting) and the aversive stimulus (pain) and the fire-setting ceases.

E. **Learned helplessness**
1. An animal receives a series of painful electric shocks from which it is **unable to escape.**
2. By classical conditioning, the animal learns that there is an association between an aversive stimulus (e.g., painful electric shock) and the inability to escape.
3. Subsequently, the animal makes no attempt to escape when shocked or when faced with any new aversive stimulus; instead, the animal becomes **hopeless and apathetic.**
4. Learned helplessness in animals may be a model system for **depression** (often characterized by hopelessness and apathy) in humans.
5. Antidepressant treatment increases escape attempts in animal models.

F. **Imprinting** is the tendency of organisms to make an association with and then follow the first thing they see after birth or hatching (in birds).

# IV. OPERANT CONDITIONING

A. **Principles**
1. Behavior is determined by its consequences for the individual. The consequence (reinforcement or punishment) occurs immediately following a behavior.
2. In operant conditioning, a behavior that is **not part of the individual's natural repertoire** can be learned through reinforcement.

| t a b l e  **7.1** | Features of Operant Conditioning |

**Example: A mother would like her 8-yr-old son to stop hitting his 6-yr-old brother. She can achieve this goal by using one of the following features of operant conditioning.**

| Feature | Effect on Behavior | Example | Comments |
|---|---|---|---|
| Positive reinforcement | Behavior is increased by reward | Child increases his kind behavior toward his younger brother to get praise from his mother | Reward or reinforcement (praise) increases desired behavior (kindness toward brother)<br>A reward can be praise or attention as well as a tangible reward like money |
| Negative reinforcement | Behavior is increased by avoidance or escape | Child increases his kind behavior toward his younger brother to avoid being scolded | Active avoidance of an aversive stimulus (being scolded) increases desired behavior (kindness toward brother) |
| Punishment | Behavior is decreased by suppression | Child decreases his hitting behavior after his mother scolds him | Delivery of an aversive stimulus (scolding) decreases unwanted behavior (hitting brother) rapidly but not permanently |
| Extinction | Behavior is eliminated by non-reinforcement | Child stops his hitting behavior when the behavior is ignored | Extinction is more effective than punishment for long-term reduction in unwanted behavior<br>There may be an initial increase in hitting behavior before it disappears |

B. **Features**
   1. The likelihood that a **behavior** will occur is **increased by positive or negative reinforcement** and **decreased by punishment or extinction** (Table 7.1).
      a. Types of reinforcement include:
         (1) **Positive reinforcement** (reward) is the introduction of a positive stimulus that results in an increase in the rate of behavior.
         (2) **Negative reinforcement** (escape) is the removal of an aversive stimulus that also results in an increase in the rate of behavior.
      b. **Punishment** is the introduction of an aversive stimulus aimed at reducing the rate of an unwanted behavior.
   2. **Extinction** in operant conditioning is the gradual disappearance of a learned behavior when reinforcement (reward) is withheld.
      a. The pattern, or **schedule, of reinforcement** affects how quickly a behavior is learned and how quickly a behavior becomes extinguished when it is not rewarded (Table 7.2).

| t a b l e  **7.2** | Schedules of Reinforcement |

| Schedule | Reinforcement | Example | Effect on Behavior |
|---|---|---|---|
| Continuous | Presented after every response | A teenager receives a candy bar each time she puts a dollar into a vending machine. One time she puts a dollar in and nothing comes out. She never buys candy from the machine again | Behavior (putting in a dollar to receive candy) is rapidly learned but disappears rapidly (has little resistance to extinction) when not reinforced (no candy comes out) |
| Fixed ratio | Presented after a designated number of responses | A man is paid $10 for every five hats he makes. He makes as many hats as he can during his shift | Fast response rate (many hats are made quickly) |
| Fixed interval | Presented after a designated amount of time | A student has an anatomy quiz every Friday. He studies for 10 min on Wednesday nights, and for 2 h on Thursday nights | The response rate (studying) increases toward the end of each interval (1 wk)<br>When graphed, the response rate forms a scalloped curve |
| Variable ratio | Presented after a random and unpredictable number of responses | After a slot machine pays off $5 for a single quarter, a woman plays $50 in quarters despite the fact that she receives no further payoffs | The behavior (playing the slot machine) continues (is highly resistant to extinction) despite the fact that it is only reinforced (winning money) after a large but variable number of responses |
| Variable interval | Presented after a random and unpredictable amount of time | After 5 min of fishing in a lake, a man catches a large fish. He then spends 4 h waiting for another bite | The behavior (fishing) continues (is highly resistant to extinction) despite the fact that it is only reinforced (a fish is caught) after varying time intervals |

    **b. Resistance to extinction** is the force that prevents the behavior from disappearing when a reward is withheld.

**C. Shaping and modeling**
    **1. Shaping** involves rewarding closer and closer approximations of the wanted behavior until the correct behavior is achieved (e.g., a child learning to write is praised when she makes a letter, even though it is not formed perfectly).
    **2. Modeling** is a type of observational learning (e.g., an individual behaves in a manner similar to that of someone she admires).

# Review Test

**Directions:** Each of the numbered items or incomplete statements in this section is followed by answers or by completions of the statement. Select the **one** lettered answer or completion that is **best** in each case.

**1.** A grade school principal has 1 week to try out a new fire-alarm system for the school. He decides to test the system three times during the week. The first time the alarm is sounded, all of the students leave the school within 5 minutes. The second time, it takes the students 15 minutes to leave the school. The third time the alarm is sounded, the students ignore it. The students' response to the fire alarm the third time it is sounded is most likely to have been learned by

- **(A)** sensitization
- **(B)** habituation
- **(C)** classical conditioning
- **(D)** fixed ratio reinforcement
- **(E)** continuous reinforcement
- **(F)** variable ratio reinforcement
- **(G)** punishment

**2.** Whenever a 46-year-old man visits his physician, his blood pressure is elevated. When the patient takes his own blood pressure at home, it is usually normal. The doctor says that while other tests need to be done, the patient is probably showing "white-coat hypertension." For this scenario, the patient's blood pressure in the doctor's office represents

- **(A)** the unconditioned stimulus
- **(B)** the unconditioned response
- **(C)** the conditioned stimulus
- **(D)** the conditioned response

### Questions 3–5

For the past year, pizza has been sold from a white van outside a high school. The teenage students complain that they are often embarrassed because their stomachs begin to growl whenever they see any white vehicle, even on weekends. The principal then bans the van from selling pizza near the school and the students' stomachs stop growling at the sight of white vehicles.

**3.** For this scenario, which element represents the unconditioned response?

- **(A)** Stomach growling in response to the white van
- **(B)** Stomach growling in response to pizza
- **(C)** The white van
- **(D)** Pairing the white van with getting pizza
- **(E)** Pizza

**4.** For this scenario, which element represents the unconditioned stimulus?

- **(A)** Stomach growling in response to the white van
- **(B)** Stomach growling in response to pizza
- **(C)** The white van
- **(D)** Pairing the white van with getting pizza
- **(E)** Pizza

**5.** For this scenario, which element represents the conditioned stimulus?

- **(A)** Stomach growling in response to the white van
- **(B)** Stomach growling in response to pizza
- **(C)** The white van
- **(D)** Pairing the white van with getting pizza
- **(E)** Pizza

**6.** In the past, a child has on occasion received money for cleaning his room. Despite the fact that he has not received money for cleaning his room for the past month, the child's room-cleaning behavior continues (is resistant to extinction). This child's room-cleaning behavior was probably learned using which of the following methods?

- **(A)** Continuous reinforcement
- **(B)** Fixed ratio reinforcement
- **(C)** Fixed interval reinforcement
- **(D)** Variable ratio reinforcement
- **(E)** Punishment

**7.** A 10-year-old child who likes and looks up to her physician states that she wants to become a doctor when she grows up. This behavior by the child is an example of

**(A)** stimulus generalization
**(B)** modeling
**(C)** shaping
**(D)** imprinting
**(E)** learned helplessness

**8.** A 4-year-old child who has received beatings in the past, from which he could not escape, appears unresponsive and no longer tries to escape new beatings. This behavior by the child is an example of

**(A)** stimulus generalization
**(B)** modeling
**(C)** shaping
**(D)** imprinting
**(E)** learned helplessness

**9.** A 2-year-old child is afraid of nurses in white uniforms. When his grandmother comes to visit him wearing a white jacket, he begins to cry. This behavior by the child is an example of

**(A)** stimulus generalization
**(B)** modeling
**(C)** shaping
**(D)** imprinting
**(E)** learned helplessness

**10.** A father scolds his child when she hits the dog. The child stops hitting the dog. This change in the child's behavior is most likely to be a result of

**(A)** punishment
**(B)** negative reinforcement
**(C)** positive reinforcement
**(D)** shaping
**(E)** classical conditioning
**(F)** extinction
**(G)** sensitization
**(H)** habituation

**11.** Although a father spanks his child when she hits the dog, the child continues to hit the dog. This child's hitting behavior is most likely to be a result of

**(A)** punishment
**(B)** negative reinforcement
**(C)** positive reinforcement
**(D)** shaping
**(E)** classical conditioning
**(F)** extinction
**(G)** sensitization
**(H)** habituation

**12.** A patient with diabetes increases her time spent exercising in order to reduce the number of insulin injections she must receive. The increased exercising behavior is most likely to be a result of

**(A)** punishment
**(B)** negative reinforcement
**(C)** positive reinforcement
**(D)** shaping
**(E)** classical conditioning
**(F)** extinction
**(G)** sensitization
**(H)** habituation

**13.** A 9-year-old boy increases his television watching (when he should be doing his homework) after his father scolds him. The father then decides to ignore the boy's television-watching behavior. Within a week, the boy has stopped watching television when he should be doing homework. The father's intervention, which led to improvement in the boy's behavior, can best be described as

**(A)** punishment
**(B)** negative reinforcement
**(C)** positive reinforcement
**(D)** shaping
**(E)** classical conditioning
**(F)** extinction
**(G)** sensitization
**(H)** habituation

**14.** A 43-year-old woman is having difficulty falling asleep. Her physician advises her to listen to a 30-minute tape of ocean sounds and then go through a series of relaxation exercises every night prior to going to sleep. Two weeks later, the patient reports that she falls asleep as soon as she hears the sounds on the tape, even without doing the relaxation exercises. Falling asleep when she hears the tape is most likely to be due to which of the following

**(A)** punishment
**(B)** negative reinforcement
**(C)** positive reinforcement
**(D)** shaping
**(E)** classical conditioning
**(F)** extinction
**(G)** sensitization
**(H)** habituation

**Questions 15 and 16**

A mother picks up her 3-month-old baby each time he cries. The child cries on more and more occasions each day and the mother picks him up more frequently.

**15.** This child has learned to get picked up mainly by the process of

**(A)** punishment
**(B)** negative reinforcement
**(C)** positive reinforcement
**(D)** shaping
**(E)** classical conditioning
**(F)** extinction
**(G)** sensitization
**(H)** habituation

**16.** The mother has learned to pick up the child mainly by the process of

**(A)** punishment
**(B)** negative reinforcement
**(C)** positive reinforcement
**(D)** shaping
**(E)** classical conditioning
**(F)** extinction
**(G)** sensitization
**(H)** habituation

**Questions 17–20**

A child comes to the clinical laboratory to have a blood sample drawn for the first time and has a painful experience. The next time the child returns for this procedure, she begins to cry when she smells the odor of antiseptic in the clinic hallway. For each clinical scenario, select the definition that best describes it.

**17.** The painful blood withdrawal procedure at the child's initial visit can be called the

**(A)** unconditioned stimulus
**(B)** unconditioned response
**(C)** conditioned stimulus
**(D)** conditioned response

**18.** The antiseptic odor that leads to crying on the child's return visit to the laboratory can be called the

**(A)** unconditioned stimulus
**(B)** unconditioned response
**(C)** conditioned stimulus
**(D)** conditioned response

**19.** The child's crying upon the smell of antiseptic can be called the

**(A)** unconditioned stimulus
**(B)** unconditioned response
**(C)** conditioned stimulus
**(D)** conditioned response

**20.** The child's crying when the blood sample is drawn can be called the

**(A)** unconditioned stimulus
**(B)** unconditioned response
**(C)** conditioned stimulus
**(D)** conditioned response

# Answers and Explanations

## Typical Board Question

**The answer is B.** This common clinical phenomenon is an example of classical conditioning. In this example, a woman comes into the hospital for an intravenous (IV) chemotherapy treatment (unconditioned stimulus). The chemotherapy drug is toxic and she becomes nauseated after the treatment (unconditioned response). The following month, when she enters the hospital lobby (conditioned stimulus), she becomes nauseated (conditioned response). Thus, the hospital where the treatments took place (conditioned stimulus) has become paired with chemotherapy (the unconditioned stimulus), which elicited nausea. Now, nausea (conditioned response) can be elicited by entering the hospital lobby (conditioned stimulus), even though she has not yet received the medication. In operant conditioning, behavior is learned by its consequences. Modeling is a type of observational learning. Shaping involves rewarding closer and closer approximations of the wanted behavior until the correct behavior is achieved. Extinction is the disappearance of a learned behavior when reinforcement is withheld.

1. **The answer is B.** The students' response to the fire alarm is most likely to have been learned by habituation, that is, desensitization. In this form of learning, continued exposure to a stimulus (the fire alarm, in this example) results in a decreased response to the stimulus. Thus, while the students respond quickly to the fire alarm at first, with repeated soundings of the alarm, they ultimately fail to respond to it. If sensitization had occurred, the students would have responded more quickly with each exposure to the alarm. In classical conditioning, a natural response is elicited by a learned stimulus. In operant conditioning, reinforcement is a consequence of a behavior that alters the likelihood that the behavior will occur again. Punishment is the introduction of an aversive stimulus that reduces the rate of an unwanted behavior, while extinction is the disappearance of a learned behavior when reinforcement is withheld.

2. **The answer is D.** The patient's elevated blood pressure in the doctor's office is the conditioned (learned) response. This response results from an association that has been made by classical conditioning between the doctor and/or his white coat (conditioned stimulus) and something negative in the patient's past (unconditioned stimulus), a reaction commonly called "white-coat hypertension." The cue that this response is learned is that the patient's blood pressure is relatively normal when taken at home.

3. **The answer is B. 4. The answer is E. 5. The answer is C.** The unconditioned stimulus (pizza) produces the unconditioned response (stomach growling in response to pizza). The unconditioned response is reflexive and automatic and does not have to be learned. The unconditioned stimulus (pizza) is the only element here that by itself will elicit a natural GI reflex (stomach growling). The white van is an example of the conditioned stimulus. In this scenario, the conditioned or learned stimulus causes the same response as the unconditioned or unlearned stimulus only after it is paired with pizza (stomach growling in response to pizza).

6. **The answer is D.** This child has received money on unpredictable occasions for cleaning his room. Behavior learned in this way (i.e., by variable ratio reinforcement) is very resistant to extinction and continues even when it is not rewarded. Behavior learned by fixed schedules of reinforcement (ratio or interval) is less resistant to extinction. Behavior learned by continuous reinforcement is least resistant to extinction. Punishment is aversive and is aimed at suppressing an undesirable behavior.

7. **The answer is B.**  This behavior is an example of modeling; the child wants to become like the doctor she admires. In stimulus generalization, a new stimulus that resembles a conditioned stimulus causes a conditioned response. Modeling is a type of observational learning. Shaping involves rewarding closer and closer approximations of the wanted behavior until the correct behavior is achieved. Imprinting is the tendency of organisms to make an association with and then follow the first thing they see after birth or hatching. In learned helplessness, an association is made between an aversive stimulus and the inability to escape.

8. **The answer is E.**  This child is showing learned helplessness, in which an association is made between an aversive stimulus (beatings) and the inability to escape. After the beatings, this child makes no attempt to escape but instead becomes hopeless and apathetic when faced with another beating. Learned helplessness may be a model system for the development of depression (see also answer to Question 7).

9. **The answer is A.**  This behavior is an example of stimulus generalization. In this example, it occurs when a new conditioned stimulus (the grandmother's white jacket) that resembles the original conditioned stimulus (the nurse's white uniform) results in the conditioned response (crying when he sees his grandmother) (see also answer to Question 7).

10. **The answer is A.**  Because the behavior (hitting the dog) decreased, the scolding that this child received is probably punishment. Both negative and positive reinforcement increase behavior. Shaping involves rewarding closer and closer approximations of the wanted behavior until the correct behavior is achieved. In classical conditioning, a natural or reflexive response (behavior) is elicited by a learned stimulus (a cue from an internal or external event). (See also answers to Questions 11–16).

11. **The answer is C.**  Because the behavior (hitting the dog) is increased, the scolding that this child received is probably positive reinforcement. Both negative and positive reinforcement increase behavior. The reward or reinforcement for this hitting behavior is most likely to be increased attention from the father. Punishment decreases behavior.

12. **The answer is B.**  Because the behavior (exercise) is increased to avoid something negative (insulin injections), this is an example of negative reinforcement.

13. **The answer is F.**  The father's intervention, which led to improvement in this boy's behavior, can best be described as extinction. Initially, the child's bad behavior increased in order to gain a reward (attention, even if it was scolding). When the father stopped reinforcing the child's bad behavior and instead ignored it, the behavior ultimately disappeared (became extinct).

14. **The answer is E.**  Via classical conditioning, the patient has made an association between the sounds on the tape and sleeping, so she now falls asleep as soon as she hears the sounds.

15. **The answer is C. 16. The answer is B.**  In this example, the child's crying behavior increases as a result of positive reinforcement, being picked up by his mother each time he cries. The mother's behavior (picking up the child) increases as a result of negative reinforcement; she picks him up to avoid hearing him cry.

17. **The answer is A. 18. The answer is C. 19. The answer is D. 20. The answer is B.**  The painful blood withdrawal procedure is the unconditioned stimulus. The antiseptic odor in the clinic has become associated with the painful procedure and elicits the same response; it is therefore the conditioned stimulus. The conditioned response, crying in response to the smell of the antiseptic, has been learned. Because crying in response to the pain of an injection is automatic and does not have to be learned, it is the unconditioned response.

# chapter 8

# Clinical Assessment of Patients with Behavioral Symptoms

**Typical Board Question**

A 6-year-old child is tested and is found to have an IQ of 50. There are no significant medical findings. At this time, it can be expected that the child is able to

(A) identify some colors
(B) ride a two-wheeled bicycle
(C) understand that death is permanent
(D) copy a triangle
(E) utilize an internalized moral sense of right and wrong

*(See "Answers and Explanations" at end of chapter.)*

## I. OVERVIEW OF PSYCHOLOGICAL TESTING

A. **Types of tests**
1. Psychological tests are used to assess intelligence, achievement, personality, and psychopathology.
2. These tests are classified by functional area evaluated.

B. **Individual versus group testing**
1. Tests administered to one individual at a time allow careful observation and evaluation of that particular person; a **test battery** looks at functioning of an individual in a number of different functional areas.
2. Tests given to a group of people simultaneously have the advantages of efficient administration, grading, and statistical analysis.

## II. INTELLIGENCE TESTS

A. **Intelligence and mental age**
1. Intelligence is defined as the ability to understand abstract concepts; reason; assimilate, recall, analyze, and organize information; and meet the special needs of new situations.
2. **Mental age (MA)**, as defined by Alfred Binet, reflects a person's level of intellectual functioning. **Chronological age (CA)** is the person's actual age in years.

B. **Intelligence quotient (IQ)**
1. IQ is the ratio of MA to CA multiplied by 100: $\text{MA/CA} \times 100 = \text{IQ}$. An **IQ of 100** means that the person's mental and chronological ages are equivalent.

    **2.** The highest CA used to determine IQ is 15 years.

    **3.** IQ is determined to a large extent by genetics. However, **poor nutrition** and **illness during development** can negatively affect IQ.

    **4.** The results of IQ tests are influenced by a person's cultural background and emotional response to testing situations.

    **5.** IQ is relatively stable throughout life. In the absence of brain pathology, an individual's **IQ is essentially the same in old age as in childhood**.

**C. Normal intelligence**

    **1.** As stated above, an IQ of 100 means that the MA and CA are approximately the same. **Normal or average IQ is in the range of 90–109**.

    **2.** The standard deviation (see Chapter 26) in IQ scores is 15. A person with an IQ that is more than two standard deviations below the mean (IQ 70) is usually considered mentally retarded (see Chapter 2). **Classifications of mental retardation** (the overlap or gap in categories is related to differences in testing instruments) are:

        **a.** Mild (IQ 50–70)

        **b.** Moderate (IQ 35–55)

        **c.** Severe (IQ 20–40)

        **d.** Profound (IQ <20)

    **3.** A score between **71** and **84** indicates **borderline** intellectual functioning.

    **4.** A person with an **IQ** more than two standard deviations above the mean (IQ >130) has superior intelligence.

**D. The Wechsler intelligence tests and the Vineland Adaptive Behavior Scales**

    **1.** The Wechsler Adult Intelligence Scale-Fourth Edition (**WAIS-IV**) is the most commonly used IQ test.

    **2.** The WAIS-R has four index scores: **Verbal Comprehension Index (VCI), Working Memory Index (WMI), Perceptual Reasoning Index (PRI)**, and **Processing Speed Index (PSI)**.

        **a.** The VCI and WMI together make up the **verbal IQ**.

        **b.** The PRI and PSI together make up the **performance IQ**.

        **c.** The **Full Scale IQ** (FSIQ) is generated by all four index scores.

    **3.** The Wechsler Intelligence Scale for Children (**WISC**) is used to test intelligence in children **6–16½** years of age.

    **4.** The Wechsler Preschool and Primary Scale of Intelligence (**WPPSI**) is used to test intelligence in children **4–6½** years of age.

    **5.** The **Vineland Adaptive Behavior Scales** are used to evaluate skills for daily living (e.g., dressing, using the telephone) in people with mental retardation (see Chapter 2) and other challenges (e.g., those with impaired vision or hearing).

# III. ACHIEVEMENT TESTS

**A. Uses**

    **1.** Achievement tests evaluate how well an individual has mastered **specific subject areas,** such as reading and mathematics.

    **2.** These tests are used for evaluation and career counseling in schools and industry.

**B. Specific achievement tests**

    **1.** Achievement tests include the Scholastic Aptitude Test (**SAT**), Medical College Admission Test (**MCAT**), and United States Medical Licensing Examination (**USMLE**).

    **2.** The Wide Range Achievement Test (**WRAT**), which is often used clinically, evaluates arithmetic, reading, and spelling skills.

    **3.** Achievement tests often used by school systems include the California, Iowa, Stanford, and Peabody Achievement Tests.

| table 8.1 | Personality Tests | | |
|---|---|---|---|
| **Name of Test** | **Uses** | **Characteristics** | **Examples** |
| Minnesota Multiphasic Personality Inventory (MMPI-2) | The most commonly used objective personality test<br>Useful for primary care physicians because no training is required for administration and scoring<br>Evaluates attitude of the patient toward taking the test | Objective test<br>Patients answer 567 true (T) or false (F) questions about themselves<br>Clinical scales include depression, paranoia, schizophrenia, and hypochondriasis<br>Validity scales identify trying to look ill ("faking bad," i.e., malingering) or trying to look well ("faking good") | "I avoid most social situations" (T or F)<br>"I often feel jealous" (T or F)<br>"I like being active" (T or F) |
| Rorschach Test | The most commonly used projective personality test<br>Used to identify thought disorders and defense mechanisms | Projective test<br>Patients are asked to interpret 10 bilaterally symmetrical inkblot designs (e.g., "Describe what you see in this figure") | |
| Thematic Apperception Test (TAT) | Stories are used to evaluate unconscious emotions and conflicts | Projective test<br>Patients are asked to create verbal scenarios based on 30 drawings depicting ambiguous situations (e.g., "Using this picture, make up a story that has a beginning, a middle, and an end") | |
| Sentence Completion Test (SCT) | Used to identify worries and problems using verbal associations | Projective test<br>Patients complete sentences started by the examiner | "My mother ... "<br>"I wish ... "<br>"Most people ... " |

Original source of Rorschach illustration: Kleinmuntz B. *Essentials of Abnormal Psychology.* New York, NY: Harper & Row; 1974. Original source of TAT illustration: Phares EJ. *Clinical Psychology: Concepts, Methods, and Profession.* 2nd ed. Homewood, IL: Dorsey 1984. Both from Krebs D, Blackman R. *Psychology: A First Encounter.* Harcourt Brace Jovanovich; 1988:632. Used with permission.

## IV. PERSONALITY TESTS

A. Personality tests are used to evaluate psychopathology and personality characteristics and are categorized by whether information is gathered objectively or projectively.

B. **Objective personality tests** (e.g., the Minnesota Multiphasic Personality Inventory [MMPI] and the Million Clinical Multiaxial Inventory [MCMI]) are based on questions that are **easily scored** and statistically analyzed.

C. **Projective personality tests** (e.g., the Rorschach Test, the Thematic Apperception Test [TAT], and the Sentence Completion Test) require the subject to **interpret the questions**. Responses are assumed to be based on the subject's motivational state and defense mechanisms.

   Uses of some of these personality tests are described in Table 8.1.

## V. PSYCHIATRIC EVALUATION OF THE PATIENT WITH EMOTIONAL SYMPTOMS

A. **Psychiatric history** The patient's psychiatric history is taken as part of the medical history. The psychiatric history includes questions about mental illness, drug and alcohol use, sexual activity, current living situation, and sources of stress.

| table 8.2 | Variables Evaluated on the Mental Status Examination (MSE) |
|---|---|
| **Variable** | **Patient Example** |
| **General Presentation**<br>Appearance<br>Behavior<br>Attitude toward the interviewer<br>Level of consciousness | A 40-yr-old male patient looks older than his age but is well groomed. He seems defensive when asked about his past experiences with drugs and denies that he has ever used. He has a Glasgow Coma Scale score of 15 (see Table 5.4) |
| **Cognition**<br>Orientation, memory, attention, concentration; cognitive, spatial, and abstraction abilities; and speech (volume, speed, and articulation) | A 55-yr-old female patient is oriented to person, place, and time and shows normal memory (cognitive ability), understanding of three-dimensional space (spatial ability), and can tell you how an apple and an orange are alike (abstraction ability). However, she speaks too quickly and is difficult to understand |
| **Mood and Affect**<br>Described (mood) and demonstrated (affect) emotions<br>Match of emotions with current events | A 35-yr-old male patient describes feeling "low" and shows less external expression of mood than expected (depressed with a restricted affect) |
| **Thought**<br>Form or process of thought<br>Thought content (e.g., delusion) | A 40-yr-old female patient tells you, in excessive detail (circumstantiality: Problem in process of thought), that the Mafia is after her (a delusion: See Table 11.1) |
| **Perception**<br>Illusion (see Table 11.1)<br>Hallucination (see Table 11.1) | A 12-yr-old girl tells you that the clothes in her closet look like a person is in there (an illusion). She then describes hearing voices (a hallucination) |
| **Judgment and Insight** | A 38-yr-old woman tells you that she would open a stamped letter found on the sidewalk to see if it contained money. She also says that she knows this would be dishonest (normal, insightful response) |
| **Reliability** | A 55-yr-old patient correctly provides the details of his previous illnesses (a reliable patient) |
| **Control of Aggressive and Sexual Impulses** | A 35-yr-old man tells you that he often overreacts emotionally, although there is little provocation (poor impulse control) |

B. **The mental status examination (MSE) and related instruments**
   1. The MSE is a structured interview that is used to evaluate an individual's current state of mental functioning (Table 8.2).
   2. Objective rating scales of depression that are commonly used include the **Hamilton, Raskin, Zung,** and **Beck** scales.
      a. In the Hamilton and Raskin scales, an examiner rates the patient.
      b. In the Zung and Beck scales (Table 8.3), the patient rates himself (e.g., measures include sadness, guilt, social withdrawal, and self blame).
   3. Terms used to describe psychophysiological symptoms and mood in patients with psychiatric symptoms are listed in Table 8.4.

| table 8.3 | Items in the Beck Depression Inventory-II (BDI-II) |
|---|---|

| | |
|---|---|
| 1. Sadness | 12. Social withdrawal |
| 2. Pessimism | 13. Indecisiveness |
| 3. Sense of failure | 14. Negative body image |
| 4. Dissatisfaction | 15. Inability to work |
| 5. Guilt | 16. Insomnia |
| 6. Expectation of punishment | 17. Fatigability |
| 7. Dislike of self | 18. Loss of appetite |
| 8. Self-blame | 19. Loss of weight |
| 9. Suicidal ideation | 20. Preoccupation with health |
| 10. Episodes of crying | 21. Low level of sexual interest |
| 11. Irritability | |

Each item can be scored from 0 to 3. Total scores of 30–63 indicate severe depression; scores of 5–9 indicate little or no depression.

| table | **8.4** | Glossary of Psychophysiological States |

| Psychophysiological State | Symptom(s) |
| --- | --- |
| **Mood** | |
| Euphoric | Strong feelings of elation |
| Expansive | Feelings of self-importance and generosity |
| Irritable | Easily annoyed and quick to anger |
| Euthymic | Normal mood, with no significant depression or elevation of mood |
| Dysphoric | Subjectively unpleasant feeling |
| Anhedonic | Inability to feel pleasure |
| Labile (mood swings) | Alternates between euphoric and dysphoric moods |
| **Affect** | |
| Restricted | Decreased display of emotional responses |
| Blunted | Greatly decreased display of emotional responses |
| Flat | No display of emotional responses |
| Labile | Sudden alterations in emotional responses not related to environmental events |
| **Fear and Anxiety** | |
| Fear | Fright caused by real danger |
| Anxiety | Fright caused by imagined danger |
| Free floating anxiety | Fright not associated with any specific cause |
| **Consciousness and Attention** | |
| Normal | Alert, can follow commands, normal verbal responses |
| Clouding of consciousness | Inability to respond normally to external events |
| Somnolence | Abnormal sleepiness |
| Stupor | Responds only to shouting, shaking, or uncomfortable prodding |
| Coma | Total unresponsiveness |

**Directions:** Each of the numbered items or incomplete statements in this section is followed by answers or by completions of the statement. Select the **one** lettered answer or completion that is **best** in each case.

**1.** A 12-year-old child who is having difficulty in school is given an intelligence test. The test determines that the child is functioning mentally at the level of an 8-year-old child. What category of intellectual function best describes this child?

(A) Severely retarded
(B) Moderately retarded
(C) Mildly retarded
(D) Borderline
(E) Normal

**2.** A child is tested and found to have a mental age of 12 years. The child's chronological age is 10 years. What is the IQ of this child?

(A) 40
(B) 60
(C) 80
(D) 100
(E) 120

**3.** A 29-year-old woman tells the doctor that she often hears the voice of Abraham Lincoln speaking directly to her. This woman is showing a disorder of

(A) perception
(B) insight
(C) judgment
(D) mood
(E) affect

**4.** A child is tested and is found to have an IQ of 90. What category of intellectual function best describes this child?

(A) Severely retarded
(B) Moderately retarded
(C) Mildly retarded
(D) Borderline
(E) Normal or average

**5.** A doctor is evaluating a 20-year-old female patient. Which of the following characteristics of the patient is best evaluated using the Minnesota Multiphasic Personality Inventory-2 (MMPI-2)?

(A) Skills for daily living
(B) Depression
(C) Knowledge of general information
(D) Reading comprehension
(E) Intelligence

**6.** A physician examines a severely depressed 75-year-old woman. The woman relates that she feels so low that she cannot enjoy anything in her life, and that even winning the state lottery would not make her feel any better. The best description of this patient's mood is

(A) anhedonic
(B) dysphoric
(C) euthymic
(D) labile
(E) euphoric

**7.** For evaluating the self-care skills of a 22-year-old woman with an IQ of 60 for placement in a group home, what is the most appropriate test?

(A) Thematic Apperception Test (TAT)
(B) Minnesota Multiphasic Personality Inventory-2 (MMPI-2)
(C) Wechsler Intelligence Scale for Children-Revised (WISC-R)
(D) Rorschach Test
(E) Vineland Social Maturity Scale
(F) Wide Range Achievement Test (WRAT)
(G) Beck Depression Inventory-II (BDI-II)
(H) Raskin Depression Scale
(I) Wisconsin Card Sorting Test

**8.** For determining, using bilaterally symmetrical inkblots, which defense mechanisms are used by a 25-year-old woman, what is the most appropriate test?

**(A)** TAT
**(B)** MMPI-2
**(C)** WISC-R
**(D)** Rorschach Test
**(E)** Vineland Social Maturity Scale
**(F)** WRAT
**(G)** BDI-II
**(H)** Raskin Depression Scale
**(I)** Wisconsin Card Sorting Test

**9.** For evaluating depression in a 54-year-old male patient using a self-rating scale, what is the most appropriate test?

**(A)** TAT
**(B)** MMPI-2
**(C)** WISC-R
**(D)** Rorschach Test
**(E)** Vineland Social Maturity Scale
**(F)** WRAT
**(G)** BDI-II
**(H)** Raskin Depression Scale
**(I)** Wisconsin Card Sorting Test

**10.** For evaluating, by a primary care physician, hypochondriasis in a 54-year-old male patient using true/false questions, what is the most appropriate test?

**(A)** TAT
**(B)** MMPI-2
**(C)** WISC-R
**(D)** Rorschach Test
**(E)** Vineland Social Maturity Scale
**(F)** WRAT
**(G)** BDI-II
**(H)** Raskin Depression Scale
**(I)** Wisconsin Card Sorting Test

**11.** The most appropriate test for evaluating abstract reasoning and problem solving in a 54-year-old female patient is the

**(A)** TAT
**(B)** MMPI-2
**(C)** WISC-R
**(D)** Rorschach Test
**(E)** Vineland Social Maturity Scale
**(F)** WRAT
**(G)** BDI-II
**(H)** Raskin Depression Scale
**(I)** Wisconsin Card Sorting Test

**12.** A 24-year-old patient with schizophrenia tells the physician that the CIA is listening to his telephone conversations through his television set. This patient is describing

**(A)** a hallucination
**(B)** an illusion
**(C)** clouding of consciousness
**(D)** blunted affect
**(E)** a delusion

# Answers and Explanations

**The answer is A.** With an IQ of 50, the mental age of this 6-year-old child is 3 years. This is calculated using the IQ formula: IQ = MA/CA × 100, that is, $50 = x/6 \times 100$, $x = 3$. Children who are 3 years of age can identify some colors. However, the ability to ride a two-wheeled bicycle, understand the meaning of death, copy a triangle, or utilize an internalized moral sense of right and wrong do not develop until about the mental age of 6 years (see Chapter 1).

1. **The answer is C.** Using the IQ formula, IQ = MA/CA × 100, the IQ of this child is 8 years (mental age)/12 years (chronological age) × 100, that is, about 66 (IQ). An individual with an IQ of 66 is classified with mild mental retardation (IQ 50–70).

2. **The answer is E.** Using the IQ formula, the IQ of the child is $12/10 \times 100 = 120$.

3. **The answer is A.** This 29-year-old woman who believes that she hears the voice of Abraham Lincoln is showing an auditory hallucination, which is a disorder of perception. Disorders of judgment, insight, mood, and affect are other variables assessed on the MSE.

4. **The answer is E.** An individual with an IQ of 90 is classified as having normal or average intellectual function (IQ 90–109).

5. **The answer is B.** Clinical scales of the Minnesota Multiphasic Personality Inventory-2 (MMPI-2) evaluate depression as well as hypochondriasis, paranoia, schizophrenia, and other characteristics. Intelligence, including general information and reading comprehension, can be tested using the Wechsler Adult Intelligence Scale-Revised (WAIS-R). (See also answer to Question 7).

6. **The answer is A.** This severely depressed 75-year-old woman is showing anhedonia, the inability to feel pleasure, a characteristic of severe depression. Euphoric mood is an elated mood, while euthymic mood is a normal mood, with no significant depression or elevation. Dysphoric mood is a subjectively unpleasant feeling. Labile moods (mood swings) are alterations between elevated and dysphoric moods.

7. **The answer is E.** The Vineland Social Maturity Scale is the most appropriate test for evaluating the self-care skills of this woman with mental retardation for placement in a group home.

8. **The answer is D.** The Rorschach Test, which utilizes bilaterally symmetrical ink blots, is the most appropriate test to determine which defense mechanisms are used by this woman.

9. **The answer is G.** For evaluating depression in this patient using a self-rating scale, the most appropriate test is the Beck Depression Inventory-II (BDI-II). In the Raskin Depression Scale, the patient is rated by an examiner.

10. **The answer is B.** The Minnesota Multiphasic Personality Inventory-2 (MMPI-2) is the most appropriate test for use by a primary care physician to evaluate depression in a patient since it is an objective test and no special training is required for administration and scoring. The MMPI-2 uses true/false questions to evaluate personality characteristics and psychopathology. In contrast, interpretation of projective personality tests requires specific training.

# Substance Abuse

**Typical Board Question**

A 40-year-old woman is brought to the emergency room by a colleague. The patient initially shows clinched fists and intense tooth grinding. Shortly thereafter she begins to experience violent seizures. Her colleague states that over the past 6 months the woman has frequently been late for work and has been given warnings by the boss because her work is "not up to par." The colleague also states that the woman's mother died yesterday and that the patient had been with her mother 24 hours per day for 3 days prior to her death and came to work directly from the hospital. Of the following, which is the most likely cause of the patient's symptoms?

- **(A)** Primary seizure disorder
- **(B)** Cerebral hemorrhage
- **(C)** Malingering
- **(D)** Complicated grief reaction
- **(E)** Alcohol withdrawal

*(See "Answers and Explanations" at end of chapter.)*

## I. SUBSTANCE ABUSE, DEFINITIONS, EPIDEMIOLOGY, AND DEMOGRAPHICS

A. **Definitions**
   1. Substance use disorders include substance abuse and substance dependence.
   2. **Substance abuse** is a maladaptive pattern of substance use that leads to impairment of occupational, physical, or social functioning; it is not diagnosed if the patient meets the criteria for substance dependence.
   3. **Substance dependence** is substance abuse plus withdrawal symptoms, tolerance, or a pattern of compulsive use.
      a. **Withdrawal** is the development of physical or psychological symptoms after the reduction or cessation of intake of a substance.
      b. **Tolerance** is the need for increased amounts of the substance to achieve the same positive psychological effect.
      c. **Cross-tolerance** is the development of tolerance to one substance as the result of using another substance.

B. **Epidemiology and demographics**
   1. Alcohol, marijuana, nonmedical use of prescription agents (e.g., opioids, sedatives), cocaine, hallucinogens, inhalants, and heroin are, according to self-reports, the most commonly used substances in the United States (Table 9.1).

| t a b l e **9.1** Self-reported Substance Use in Last Month | |
|---|---|
| Substance | Number of People (in Millions) |
| Alcohol | 131.6 |
| Marijuana | 16.7 |
| Prescription agents (mainly nonmedical use of pain relievers) | 7.0 |
| Cocaine | 1.6 |
| Hallucinogen | 1.3 |
| Inhalants | 0.6 |
| Heroin | 0.2 |

Source: Substance Abuse and Mental Health Services Administration, 2010.

2. The use of illegal substances is more common among young adults (**18–25 years of age**) and is twice as **common in males**.
3. Most abused substances can be classified categorically as **stimulants, sedatives, opioids, or hallucinogens** and related agents.
4. Most abused substances can be administered by a number of routes. Routes that provide quick access to the bloodstream, and hence the brain, are often preferred by abusers (e.g., sniffing into the nose ["snorting] and smoking rather than ingesting).

## II. STIMULANTS

A. **Overview**
   1. Stimulants are **central nervous system activators** that include caffeine, nicotine, amphetamines, and cocaine.
   2. The effects of use and withdrawal of these substances can be found in Table 9.2.

B. **Caffeine** is found in coffee (125 mg/cup), tea (65 mg/cup), cola (40 mg/cup), nonprescription stimulants, and over-the-counter diet agents.

C. **Nicotine** is a toxic substance present in tobacco. Cigarette smoking decreases life expectancy more than the use of any other substance. Smoking is increasing most in teenaged girls.

D. **Amphetamines** are used clinically and also are drugs of abuse.
   1. They are medically indicated in the management of attention deficit/hyperactivity disorder (**ADHD**) (see Chapter 15) and **narcolepsy** (see Chapter 10). They are sometimes used to treat **depression** in the elderly and terminally ill, and depression and **obesity** in patients who do not respond to other treatments (see Chapter 12).
   2. The most common clinically used amphetamines are **dextroamphetamine** (Dexedrine), **methamphetamine** (Desoxyn), and a related compound, **methylphenidate** (Ritalin).
   3. "**Speed**," "**ice**" (methamphetamine), and "**ecstasy**" (methylenedioxymethamphetamine [MDMA]) are street names for amphetamine compounds.

E. **Cocaine**
   1. "**Crack**" and "**freebase**" are cheap, smokable forms of cocaine; in expensive, pure form, cocaine is **snorted.**
   2. **Hyperactivity** and **growth retardation** are seen in **newborns** of mothers who used cocaine during pregnancy.
   3. **Tactile hallucinations** of bugs crawling on the skin (i.e., **formication**) are seen with the use of cocaine ("cocaine bugs").

| t a b l e    **9.2**    Effects of Use and Withdrawal of Stimulant Agents |||
|---|---|---|
| **Substances** | **Effects of Use** | **Effects of Withdrawal** |
| | *Psychological* | |
| Caffeine, Nicotine | Increased alertness and attention span<br>Mild improvement in mood<br>Agitation and insomnia | Lethargy<br>Mild depression of mood |
| | *Physical* | |
| | Decreased appetite<br>Increased blood pressure and heart rate<br>(tachycardia)<br>Increased gastrointestinal activity | Increased appetite with slight weight gain<br>Fatigue<br>Headache |
| | *Psychological* | |
| Amphetamines, Cocaine | Significant elevation of mood (lasting only 1 h<br>with cocaine)<br>Increased alertness and attention span<br>Aggressiveness, impaired judgment<br>Psychotic symptoms (e.g., paranoid delusions<br>with amphetamines and formication with<br>cocaine)<br>Agitation and insomnia | Significant depression of mood<br>Strong psychological craving (peaking a<br>few days after the last dose)<br>Irritability |
| | *Physical* | |
| | Loss of appetite and weight<br>Pupil dilation<br>Increased energy<br>Tachycardia and other cardiovascular effects,<br>which can be life-threatening<br>Seizures (particularly with cocaine)<br>Reddening (erythema) of the nose due to<br>"snorting" cocaine<br>Hypersexuality | Hunger (particularly with amphetamines)<br>Pupil constriction<br>Fatigue |

F. **Neurotransmitter associations**
   1. Stimulant drugs work primarily by increasing the availability of **dopamine (DA)**.
   2. **Amphetamine** use causes the **release of DA. Cocaine** primarily **blocks the reuptake of DA.** Both the release of DA and the block of DA reuptake result in increased availability of this neurotransmitter in the synapse.
   3. Increased availability of DA in the synapse is apparently involved in the euphoric effects of stimulants and opioids (the "reward" system of the brain). As in schizophrenia (see Chapter 11), increased DA availability may also result in **psychotic symptoms**.

## III. SEDATIVES

A. Overview
   1. Sedatives are **central nervous system depressants** that include alcohol, barbiturates, and benzodiazepines.
   2. Sedative agents work primarily by **increasing** the activity of the inhibitory neurotransmitter g-aminobutyric acid (**GABA**).
   3. Hospitalization of patients for withdrawal from sedatives is prudent; the withdrawal syndrome may include seizures, psychotic symptoms such as hallucinations and delusions and cardiovascular symptoms that are **life threatening**. The effects of use and withdrawal of sedatives can be found in Table 9.3.

| t a b l e  **9.3**  Effects of Use and Withdrawal of Sedative Agents | | |
|---|---|---|
| Substances | Effects of Use | Effects of Withdrawal |
| | **Psychological** | |
| Alcohol, Benzodiazepines, Barbiturates | Mild elevation of mood | Mild depression of mood |
| | Decreased anxiety | Increased anxiety |
| | Somnolence | Insomnia |
| | Behavioral disinhibition | Psychotic symptoms (e.g., delusions and formication) |
| | | Disorientation |
| | **Physical** | |
| | Sedation | Tremor |
| | Poor coordination | Seizures |
| | Respiratory depression | Cardiovascular symptoms such as tachycardia and hypertension |

## B. Alcohol

**1.** Acute associated problems

   **a. Traffic accidents, homicide, suicide**, and **rape** are correlated with the concurrent use of alcohol.

   **b. Child physical** and **sexual abuse**, spouse abuse, and elder abuse are also associated with alcohol use.

**2.** Chronic associated problems

   **a. Thiamine deficiency** resulting in **Wernicke syndrome** and ultimately in **Korsakoff syndrome** (i.e., amnestic disorder: See Chapter 14) is associated with long-term use of alcohol.

   **b. Liver dysfunction**, gastrointestinal problems (e.g., ulcers), and reduced life expectancy also are seen in heavy users of alcohol.

   **c. Fetal alcohol syndrome** (including facial abnormalities, reduced height and weight, and mental retardation) is seen in the offspring of women who drink during pregnancy.

   **d.** A childhood history of problems such as **ADHD** and **conduct disorder** (see Chapter 15) correlates with alcoholism in the adult.

**3. Identification of alcoholism.** Because alcohol abusers commonly use denial as a defense mechanism (see Chapter 6), positive responses to indirect queries such as those in the **CAGE questions** can help a physician identify a person who has a problem with alcohol. The CAGE questions are: "Do you ever

   **a.** try to **C**ut down on your drinking?"

   **b.** get **A**ngry when someone comments on your drinking?"

   **c.** feel **G**uilty about your drinking?"

   **d.** take a drink as an **E**ye-opener in the morning?"

**4. Intoxication**

   **a.** Legal intoxication is defined as **0.08%–0.15% blood alcohol concentration**, depending on individual state laws.

   **b.** Coma occurs at a blood alcohol concentration of 0.40%–0.50% in nonalcoholics.

   **c.** Psychotic symptoms (e.g., hallucinations) may be seen in alcohol intoxication as well as in withdrawal (see below).

**5. Delirium tremens ("the DTs")**

   **a. Alcohol withdrawal delirium** (also called delirium tremens or "the DTs") may occur during the first week of withdrawal from alcohol (most commonly on the third day of hospitalization). It usually occurs in patients who have been drinking heavily for years.

   **b.** Delirium tremens is **life threatening**; the mortality rate is about 20%.

## C. Barbiturates

**1.** Barbiturates are used medically as **sleeping pills**, sedatives, antianxiety agents (tranquilizers), anticonvulsants, and anesthetics.

**2.** Frequently used and abused, barbiturates include amobarbital, pentobarbital, and secobarbital.

**3.** Barbiturates cause respiratory depression and have a **low safety margin**. As such they are very dangerous in overdose.

**D. Benzodiazepines**
1. Benzodiazepines are used medically as **tranquilizers**, sedatives, muscle relaxants, anticonvulsants, and anesthetics, and **to treat alcohol withdrawal** (particularly long-acting agents such as chlordiazepoxide and diazepam [see Chapter 16]).
2. Benzodiazepines have a **high safety margin** unless taken with another sedative, such as alcohol.
3. **Flumazenil** (Mazicon, Romazicon), a benzodiazepine receptor antagonist, can reverse the effects of benzodiazepines in cases of overdose.

# IV. OPIOIDS

**A. Overview**
1. Narcotics or opioid drugs include **agents used medically as analgesics** (e.g., morphine) as well as drugs of abuse (e.g., heroin). The effects of use and withdrawal of opioids can be found in Table 9.4.
2. Compared to medically used opioids such as morphine and methadone, abused opioids such as **heroin** are more potent, cross the blood–brain barrier more quickly, have a faster onset of action, and have **more euphoric action**.
3. In contrast to barbiturate withdrawal, which may be fatal, **death from withdrawal of opioids is rare** unless a serious physical illness is present.

**B. Methadone and related agents**
1. **Methadone** and **buprenorphine (Temgesic, Suboxone** [when combined with naloxone]) are **synthetic opioids** used to treat heroin addiction (see Table 9.5); they can also cause physical dependence and tolerance.
2. These legal opioids can be substituted for illegal opioids, such as heroin, to prevent withdrawal symptoms.
3. **Advantages** of methadone and buprenorphine over heroin
   a. Methadone is dispensed by **federal health authorities without charge** to registered addicts.
   b. **Buprenorphine** is an opioid receptor partial agonist-antagonist (making it unlikely to cause respiratory depression) that can block both withdrawal symptoms and, when combined with naloxone, the euphoric action of heroin. Buprenorphine can now be **prescribed by physicians in private practice** who complete a brief training program.

table **9.4** Effects of Use and Withdrawal of Opioid Agents

| Substances | Effects of Use | Effects of Withdrawal |
|---|---|---|
| | *Psychological* | |
| Heroin, Methadone, Other Opioids | Elevation of mood<br>Relaxation<br>Somnolence | Depression of mood<br>Anxiety<br>Insomnia |
| | *Physical* | |
| | Sedation<br>Analgesia<br>Respiratory depression (overdose may be fatal)<br>Constipation<br>Pupil constriction (miosis) | Sweating, muscle aches, fever<br>Rhinorrhea (running nose)<br>Piloerection (goose bumps)<br>Yawning<br>Stomach cramps and diarrhea<br>Pupil dilation (mydriasis) |

| table 9.5 | Management (in Order of Utility, Highest to Lowest) of Abuse of Sedatives, Opioids, Stimulants, and Hallucinogens and Related Agents | |
|---|---|---|
| **Category** | **Immediate Management/Detoxification** | **Extended Management/Maintenance** |
| **Minor Stimulants:** Caffeine, Nicotine | Eliminate or taper from the diet. Analgesics to control headache due to withdrawal | Peer support group (e. g., "Smokenders") Antidepressants (particularly bupropion [Zyban]) to prevent smoking Support from family members or nonsmoking physician Hypnosis to prevent smoking Nicotine-containing gum, patch, or nasal spray |
| **Stimulants:** Amphetamines, Cocaine | Benzodiazepines to decrease agitation Antipsychotics to treat psychotic symptoms Medical and psychological support | Education for initiation and maintenance of abstinence |
| **Sedatives:** Alcohol, Benzodiazepines, Barbiturates | Hospitalization Flumazenil (Mazicon) to reverse the effects of benzodiazepines Substitution of long-acting barbiturate (e.g., phenobarbital) or benzodiazepine (e.g., chlordiazepoxide [Librium] in decreasing doses; IV diazepam (Valium), lorazepam (Ativan), or phenobarbital if seizures occur Specifically for alcohol: Thiamine (vitamin B₁) and restoration of nutritional state | Education for initiation and maintenance of abstinence Specifically for alcohol: Alcoholics Anonymous (AA) or other peer support group (12-step program), disulfiram (Antabuse), psychotherapy, behavior therapy, naloxone (Narcan), naltrexone (ReVia), acamprosate (Campral), topiramate (Topamax) |
| **Opioids:** Heroin, Methadone, Opioids used medically | Hospitalization and naloxone (Narcan) for overdose Clonidine to stabilize the autonomic nervous system during withdrawal Substitution of long-acting opioid (e.g., methadone) in decreasing doses to decrease withdrawal symptoms | Methadone or buprenorphine (Temgesic) maintenance program Naltrexone or buprenorphine plus naloxone (Suboxone) used prophylactically to block the effects of abused opioids Narcotics Anonymous (NA) or other peer support program |
| **Hallucinogens and Related Agents:** Marijuana, Hashish, LSD, PCP, Psilocybin, Mescaline | Calming or "talking down" the patient Benzodiazepines to decrease agitation Antipsychotics to treat psychotic symptoms | Education for initiation and maintenance of abstinence |

PCP, phencyclidine; LSD, lysergic acid diethylamide.

c. Both agents **can be taken orally**. The intravenous method of drug use employed by many heroin addicts may involve sharing contaminated needles, thus contributing to AIDS and hepatitis B infection.

d. Both agents have a **longer duration of action**.

e. Both agents cause **less euphoria and drowsiness**, allowing people on maintenance regimens to keep their jobs and avoid the criminal activity that is necessary to maintain a costly heroin habit.

# V. HALLUCINOGENS AND RELATED AGENTS

## A. Overview

1. Hallucinogens and related agents include lysergic acid diethylamide (**LSD**), phencyclidine (**PCP** or "**angel dust**"), cannabis (tetrahydrocannabinol, marijuana, hashish), psilocybin (from mushrooms), mescaline (from cactus), and ketamine ("**Special K**").

2. Hallucinogens promote altered states of consciousness which are usually pleasurable but can also be frightening ("**bad trips**").

3. Increased availability of **serotonin** is associated with the effects of some of these agents (e.g., LSD). The effects of use and withdrawal of hallucinogens and related agents can be found in Table 9.6.

| table | **9.6** | Effects of Use and Withdrawal of Hallucinogens and Related Agents |

| Substances | Effects of Use | Effects of Withdrawal |
| --- | --- | --- |
| | *Psychological* | |
| Cannabis (marijuana, hashish), Lysergic acid diethylamide (LSD, Phencyclidine (PCP or "angel dust," Psilocybin, Mescaline | Altered perceptual states (auditory and visual hallucinations, alterations of body image, distortions of time and space)<br>Elevation of mood<br>Impairment of memory (may be long term)<br>Reduced attention span<br>"Bad trips" (frightening perceptual states)<br>"Flashbacks" (a re-experience of the sensations associated with use in the absence of the drug even months after the last dose) | Few, if any, psychological withdrawal symptoms |
| | *Physical* | |
| | Impairment of complex motor activity<br>Cardiovascular symptoms<br>Sweating<br>Tremor<br>Nystagmus (PCP) | Few, if any, physical withdrawal symptoms |

**B. Marijuana**
1. Tetrahydrocannabinol (**THC**) is the primary active compound found in marijuana.
2. In low doses, marijuana **increases appetite** and relaxation, and causes conjunctival reddening.
3. Chronic users experience **lung problems** associated with smoking and a decrease in motivation ("**the amotivational syndrome**") characterized by lack of desire to work, and increased apathy.
4. Although it is not legal in the United States, **marijuana** for medical use is permitted in some states, primarily for treating glaucoma and cancer-treatment-related nausea and vomiting.

**C. LSD and PCP**
1. **LSD is ingested** and **PCP is smoked** in a marijuana or other cigarette.
2. While LSD and PCP both cause altered perception, in contrast to LSD, **episodes of violent behavior** occur with **PCP use**.
3. Emergency department findings for **PCP** include hyperthermia and **nystagmus** (vertical or horizontal abnormal eye movements).
4. PCP binds with N-methyl-D-aspartate (NMDA) receptors of **glutamate**-gated ion channels.
5. Consumption of more than 20 mg of PCP may cause seizures, coma, and death.

# VI. CLINICAL FEATURES OF SUBSTANCE ABUSE

**A. Laboratory findings** can often confirm substance use (Table 9.7).

**B. Emergency department findings.** Changes in the pupil of the eye and presence or absence of psychotic symptoms can quickly narrow the search for the substance responsible for patients' symptoms in the emergency department (Table 9.8).

table **9.7**   Laboratory Findings for Selected Drugs of Abuse

| Category | Elevated Levels in Body Fluids (e.g., Blood, Urine) | Length of Time After Use that Substance Can Be Detected |
|---|---|---|
| Stimulants | Cotinine (nicotine metabolite)<br>Amphetamine<br>Benzoylecgonine (cocaine metabolite) | 1–2 days<br>1–2 days<br>1–3 days in occasional users; 7–12 days in heavy users |
| Sedatives | Alcohol<br>g-Glutamyltransferase (GGT)<br>Specific barbiturate or benzodiazepine or its metabolite | 7–12 h<br>7–12 h<br>1–3 days |
| Opioids | Heroin<br>Methadone | 1–3 days<br>2–3 days |
| Hallucinogens and related agents | Cannabinoid metabolites<br>Phencyclidine (PCP)<br>Serum glutamic oxaloacetic transaminase (SGOT) (also called aspartate transaminase [AST] or aspartate aminotransferase [ASAT/AAT]) or creatine phosphokinase (CPK) (with PCP use) | 3–28 days<br>7–14 days in heavy users<br>More than 7 days |

## VII. MANAGEMENT

A. **Management of substance abuse** ranges from abstinence and peer support groups to drugs that block physical and psychological withdrawal symptoms.

B. Management of withdrawal symptoms includes immediate treatment or **detoxification** ("detox") and extended management aimed at preventing relapse ("**maintenance**") (Table 9.5).

C. **Dual diagnosis** or mentally ill–chemically addicted (**MICA**) patients require treatment for both substance abuse and the comorbid psychiatric illness (e.g., major depression), often in a special unit in the hospital.

table **9.8**   Quick Emergency Department Identification of the Abused Substance

| Emergency Department Observation | Seen with Use of | Seen with Withdrawal from |
|---|---|---|
| Pupil dilation | Stimulants<br>Hallucinogens (e.g., LSD) | Opioids<br>Alcohol and other sedatives |
| Pupil constriction | Opioids | Stimulants |
| Psychotic symptoms (e.g., hallucinations, delusions) | Stimulants<br>Alcohol<br>Hallucinogens | Alcohol and other sedatives |
| Cardiovascular symptoms | Stimulants | Alcohol and other sedatives |

LSD, lysergic acid diethylamide.

# Review Test

**Directions:** Each of the numbered items or incomplete statements in this section is followed by answers or by completions of the statement. Select the **one** lettered answer or completion that is **best** in each case.

**Questions 1 and 2**

A 29-year-old man comes to the emergency department complaining of stomach cramps, agitation, severe muscle aches, and diarrhea. Physical examination reveals that the patient is sweating, has dilated pupils, a fever, and a runny nose, and shows goose bumps on his skin.

**1.** Of the following, the most likely cause of this picture is

(A) alcohol use
(B) alcohol withdrawal
(C) heroin use
(D) heroin withdrawal
(E) amphetamine withdrawal

**2.** Of the following, the most effective immediate treatment for relief of this patient's symptoms is

(A) naloxone
(B) naltrexone
(C) an antipsychotic
(D) a stimulant
(E) clonidine

**3.** Which of the following drugs is (are), by self-report, the most frequently used in the United States?

(A) Hallucinogens
(B) Inhalants
(C) Cocaine
(D) Heroin
(E) Marijuana

**4.** A physician is doing an employment physical on a 40-year-old male patient. The physician suspects that the patient has a problem with alcohol. The next step that the physician should take is to

(A) check his liver function
(B) ask him if he has a problem with alcohol
(C) call his previous employer for information
(D) ask him the CAGE questions
(E) check for the stigmata of alcoholism (e.g., stria, broken blood vessels on the nose)

**5.** A 20-year-old female patient tells the doctor that she has little interest in going back to school or in getting a job. She also reports that she often craves snack food and has gained over 10 pounds in the past 4 months. What substance is this patient most likely to be using?

(A) Phencyclidine (PCP)
(B) Lysergic acid diethylamide (LSD)
(C) Marijuana
(D) Cocaine
(E) Heroin

**6.** A 22-year-old student tells the doctor that he has been using "speed" nightly. Which of the following effects of the drug is the student most likely to experience when he is using?

(A) Increased fatigue
(B) Decreased pain threshold
(C) Increased appetite
(D) Decreased appetite
(E) Decreased libido

**7.** A patient has been using heroin for the past year. Which of the following is most likely to characterize this patient?

(A) Age 48 years
(B) Female gender
(C) Insomnia when using the drug
(D) Anxious mood when using the drug
(E) Elevated mood when using the drug

**8.** A person who uses illegal drugs is most likely to be in which of the following age groups?

(A) 10–15 years
(B) 15–18 years
(C) 18–25 years
(D) 25–35 years
(E) 35–45 years

**9.** A 60-year-old man is brought to the hospital after a fall outside of a neighborhood bar. Radiologic studies indicate that the patient has a fractured hip and surgery is performed immediately. Two days later, the patient begins to show an intense hand tremor and tachycardia. He tells the doctor that he has been "shaky" ever since his admission and that the shakiness is getting worse. The patient states that while he feels frightened, he is comforted by the fact that the nurse is an old friend (he has never met the nurse before). He also reports that he has started to see spiders crawling on the walls and can feel them crawling on his arms. The doctor notes that the patient's speech seems to be drifting from one subject to another. Of the following, what is the most likely cause of this picture?

(A) Alcohol use
(B) Alcohol withdrawal
(C) Heroin use
(D) Heroin withdrawal
(E) Amphetamine withdrawal

**10.** A physician discovers that his 28-year-old female patient is abusing cocaine. Which of the following can the doctor expect to see in this patient?

(A) Severe physical signs of withdrawal
(B) Little psychological craving in withdrawal
(C) Euphoria lasting 3–4 days
(D) Delusions
(E) Sedation with use

**11.** A 20-year-old man who has been drinking eight cups of coffee a day for the past week comes in for a physical examination. At this time, this man is most likely to show

(A) tachycardia
(B) decreased peristalsis
(C) weight gain
(D) fatigue
(E) headache

**12.** A 40-year-old female patient who has been taking a benzodiazepine daily in moderate doses over the past 5 years abruptly stops taking the drug. When a physician sees her 2 days after her last dose, she is most likely to show

(A) hypersomnia
(B) tremor
(C) lethargy
(D) respiratory depression
(E) sedation

**13.** A 24-year-old patient is experiencing intense hunger as well as tiredness and headache. This patient is most likely to be withdrawing from which of the following substances?

(A) Alcohol
(B) Amphetamines
(C) Benzodiazepines
(D) Phencyclidine (PCP)
(E) Heroin

**14.** In the United States, the group in which smoking currently shows the largest increase is

(A) teenaged males
(B) middle-aged males
(C) teenaged females
(D) middle-aged females
(E) elderly females

**15.** What is the major mechanism of action of cocaine on neurotransmitter systems in the brain?

(A) Blocks reuptake of dopamine
(B) Blocks release of dopamine
(C) Blocks reuptake of serotonin
(D) Blocks release of serotonin
(E) Blocks release of norepinephrine

**16.** After 20 years of smoking, a 45-year-old female patient has decided to quit. Of the following, what physical effect is most likely to be seen as a result of this patient's withdrawal from nicotine?

**(A)** Weight gain
**(B)** Euphoria
**(C)** Excitability
**(D)** Delirium tremens
**(E)** Long-term abstinence

**17.** A 43-year-old man with a 5-year history of HIV tells his physician that he has been smoking marijuana a few times a day to treat his symptoms of nausea and lack of appetite. To obtain the marijuana, the patient notes that he grows it in his backyard. The doctor's best response to this patient's revelation is

**(A)** "I am sorry but growing or using marijuana is illegal and I must notify the police"
**(B)** "I have read about other patients growing marijuana"
**(C)** "Are you aware that marijuana can cause respiratory problems?"
**(D)** "There are a number of medications that I can prescribe to help alleviate your nausea and lack of appetite in place of marijuana"
**(E)** "Do you think that using marijuana has negative long-term effects?"

**18.** A 35-year-old man is brought to the emergency department confused and anxious. The man reports that someone is trying to kill him but he does not know who the person is. Initial physical examination reveals elevated heart and respiration rates. While in the emergency room the patient has a seizure and then develops life-threatening cardiovascular symptoms. The drug that this patient is most likely to be withdrawing from is

**(A)** phencyclidine (PCP)
**(B)** lysergic acid diethylamide (LSD)
**(C)** heroin
**(D)** secobarbital
**(E)** marijuana

**Questions 19–23**

For the patient in each numbered question, select the lettered drug he or she is most likely to be using.

**(A)** Alcohol
**(B)** Secobarbital
**(C)** Cocaine
**(D)** Methylphenidate
**(E)** Caffeine
**(F)** Diazepam
**(G)** Heroin
**(H)** Marijuana
**(I)** Nicotine
**(J)** Phencyclidine (PCP)
**(K)** Lysergic acid diethylamide (LSD)

**19.** A 32-year-old man is brought to a New York City hospital. He appears sedated, but shows an elevated mood. A blood test reveals the presence of HIV.

**20.** A 25-year-old man is brought to the hospital after being involved in an automobile accident in which he was driving and the other driver was killed.

**21.** When a physician examines a 17-year-old high school student, she notes that he has erythema of the nose. During the interview, the student seems withdrawn and sad.

**22.** A 28-year-old man is hospitalized after trying to jump from the roof of one apartment building to another. His friends relate that prior to the jump, the man angrily threatened them because they would not jump with him.

**23.** A 22-year-old woman is brought to the emergency room at 8 AM by her friend, who states that the woman has been acting strangely since the previous evening. While lying on the examining table the patient states that she feels like she is floating in the air and the sun is big and glaring above her.

# Answers and Explanations

**The answer is E.** The violent seizures in this 40-year-old woman are most likely to be a sign of alcohol withdrawal. Her lateness and poor performance at work over the past 6 months are evidence that she has been impaired by alcohol. She has probably become physically dependent on alcohol and, because she been with her dying mother for at least 3 days, has not had the opportunity to drink and now is in withdrawal from alcohol. It is much less likely that the seizures are due to a primary seizure disorder or cerebral hemorrhage. There is no reason for this woman to be feigning her symptoms as would be the case in malingering (see Chapter 13), and the physical findings suggest an organic cause rather than a complicated grief reaction (see Chapter 3).

1. **The answer is D. 2. The answer is E.** The most likely cause of this patient's symptoms of sweating, muscle aches, stomach cramps, diarrhea, fever, runny nose, goose bumps, yawning, and dilated pupils is heroin withdrawal. While alcohol withdrawal may be associated with pupil dilation, alcohol use and withdrawal and amphetamine withdrawal are less likely to cause this constellation of symptoms. Of the choices given, the most effective immediate treatment for heroin withdrawal is clonidine to stabilize the autonomic nervous system. Psychotic symptoms are uncommon in opioid withdrawal and this patient does not need an antipsychotic. Naloxone and naltrexone as well as stimulants will worsen rather than ameliorate the patient's withdrawal symptoms.

3. **The answer is E.** Almost 17 million Americans report that they use marijuana. In contrast, 1.6 million, 1.3 million, 0.6 million, and 0.2 million report that they use cocaine, hallucinogens, inhalants, and heroin, respectively.

4. **The answer is D.** The next step in management is for the physician to ask this patient the CAGE questions. Positive answers to any two of these questions or to the last one alone indicate that he has a problem with alcohol. Patients with such problems typically use denial as a defense mechanism and so rarely believe or admit that they have a problem with alcohol. Liver function problems or presence of the stigmata of alcoholism (e.g., stria, broken blood vessels on the nose) do not necessarily indicate the patient currently has a problem with alcohol. It is inappropriate for the doctor to call the previous employer for information.

5. **The answer is C.** The amotivational syndrome (e.g., lack of interest in getting a job or going to school) and increased appetite, particularly for snack foods, are characteristically seen in chronic users of marijuana. Use of cocaine, heroin, phencyclidine (PCP), or lysergic acid diethylamide (LSD) may cause work-related problems, but are less likely to increase appetite.

6. **The answer is D.** Like other stimulant drugs, amphetamines like "speed" reduce appetite; use can thus result in decreased body weight. Amphetamines also decrease fatigue, increase pain threshold, and increase libido.

7. **The answer is E.** Heroin users show an elevated, relaxed mood and somnolence. Users are most likely to be young adult males.

8. **The answer is C.** Illegal drug use is most common in people 18–25 years of age.

9. **The answer is B.** The most likely cause of tremor, tachycardia, illusions (e.g., believing the nurse is an old friend), and visual and tactile hallucinations (e.g., formication—the feeling of insects crawling on the skin) in this patient is alcohol withdrawal, since the use of alcohol during the past few days of hospitalization is unlikely (see also the TBQ). His fractured hip may have been sustained in the fall while he was intoxicated. Heroin use and heroin and amphetamine withdrawal generally are not associated with psychotic symptoms.

10. **The answer is D.** Delusions and other symptoms of psychosis are seen with the use of cocaine. The intense euphoria produced by cocaine lasts only about 1 hour. Severe psychological craving for the drug peaks 2–4 days after the last dose, although there may be few physiologic signs of withdrawal. Cocaine intoxication is characterized by agitation and irritability, not sedation.

11. **The answer is A.** Tachycardia, increased peristalsis, increased energy, and decreased appetite are physical effects of stimulants like caffeine. Headaches are more likely to result from withdrawal rather than use of stimulant drugs.

12. **The answer is B.** Withdrawal from benzodiazepines is associated with tremor, insomnia, and anxiety. Respiratory depression and sedation are associated with the use of, not withdrawal from, sedative drugs.

13. **The answer is B.** Tiredness and headache are seen with withdrawal from stimulants. While increased appetite can be seen in withdrawal from all stimulants, the most intense hunger is seen with withdrawal from amphetamines.

14. **The answer is C.** In the United States, the group in which smoking currently shows the largest increase is teenaged females.

15. **The answer is A.** The major mechanism of action of cocaine on neural systems is to block the reuptake of dopamine, thereby increasing its availability in the synapse. Increased availability of dopamine is involved in the "reward" system of the brain and the euphoric effects of stimulants.

16. **The answer is A.** Weight gain commonly occurs following withdrawal from stimulants such as nicotine. Mild depression of mood and lethargy are also seen. Long-term abstinence is uncommon in smokers; most smokers who quit relapse within 2 years. Delirium tremens occur with withdrawal from sedatives such as alcohol.

17. **The answer is D.** The best response to this patient's revelation about growing and using marijuana is to recommend effective but safer substitutes, for example, prescription medications to treat his nausea and lack of appetite. It is neither appropriate nor necessary for a physician to report the patient's actions to the police. Also, this HIV-positive patient is likely to be more concerned about feeling ill in the short-term than long-term consequences of marijuana use such as respiratory problems.

18. **The answer is D.** This 35-year-old patient is most likely to be withdrawing from secobarbital, a barbiturate. Barbiturate withdrawal symptoms appear about 12–20 hours after the last dose and include anxiety, elevated heart and respiration rates, psychotic symptoms (e.g., the belief that someone is trying to kill him), confusion, and seizures, and can be associated with life-threatening cardiovascular symptoms. There are few physical withdrawal symptoms associated with marijuana, phencyclidine (PCP), or lysergic acid diethylamide (LSD), and those associated with heroin are uncomfortable but rarely physically dangerous.

19. **The answer is G.** The presence of HIV as well as signs of sedation and euphoria indicate that this patient is an intravenous heroin user.

20. **The answer is A.** Alcohol use is commonly associated with automobile accidents.

21. **The answer is C.** Erythema of the nose is a result of snorting cocaine, and depressed mood is seen in withdrawal from the drug.

22. **The answer is J.** Aggressiveness and psychotic behavior (jumping from one rooftop to another) indicate that this patient has used PCP.

23. **The answer is K.** This woman, who has been acting strangely over a number of hours and is experiencing out-of-body experiences (e.g., feelings of floating in the air) and illusions (e.g., mistaking the overhead light for the sun), has probably taken LSD. The patient's lack of aggression or agitation indicates that the hallucinogen she has used is less likely to have been PCP.

# chapter 10

# Normal Sleep and Sleep Disorders

**Typical Board Question**

The wife of a 62-year-old man tells the doctor that for the past year, her husband has punched and kicked her repeatedly during the night. When she wakes him during these episodes, her husband relates that he has been having a dream in which he is trying to escape from or fighting with a frightening attacker. Over the next few years, this man is at increased risk to develop

(A) Kleine–Levin syndrome
(B) sleep terror disorder
(C) nocturnal myoclonus
(D) Alzheimer disease
(E) Lewy body dementia

*(See "Answers and Explanations" at end of chapter.)*

## I. NORMAL AWAKE AND SLEEP STATES

A. **Circadian cycle.** In the absence of outside information about light and dark periods (i.e., zeitgebers), humans show a circadian cycle, including awake and sleeping states closer to **25 hours** than to 24 hours in length.

B. **Awake state.** Beta and alpha waves characterize the electroencephalogram (EEG) of the awake individual (Table 10.1).
   1. **Beta waves** over the frontal lobes are commonly seen with **active mental concentration**.
   2. **Alpha waves** over the occipital and parietal lobes are seen when a person **relaxes** with **closed eyes**.
   3. **Sleep latency** (period of time from going to bed to falling asleep) is typically less than 10 minutes.

C. **Sleep state.** During sleep, brain waves show distinctive changes (Table 10.1).
   1. Sleep is divided into rapid eye movement (**REM**) sleep and **non-REM** sleep. Non-REM sleep consists of **stages 1, 2, 3, and 4**.
   2. Mapping the transitions from one stage of sleep to another during the night produces a structure known as **sleep architecture** (Figure 10.1).
      a. Sleep architecture changes with age. The elderly often have poor sleep quality because aging is associated with **reduced REM sleep and delta sleep** (stages 3–4, or slow wave) and increased nighttime awakenings, leading to **poor sleep efficiency** (percent of time actually spent sleeping per percent of time trying to sleep) (Table 10.2).

| table 10.1 | Electroencephalographic Tracings and Characteristics of the Awake State and Sleep Stages | | |
|---|---|---|---|
| **Sleep Stage** | **Associated EEG Pattern** | **% Sleep Time in Young Adults** | **Characteristics** |
| Awake | Beta waves | — | Active mental concentration |
| | Alpha waves | — | Relaxed with eyes closed |
| Stage 1 | Theta waves | 5% | Lightest stage of sleep characterized by peacefulness, slowed pulse and respiration, decreased blood pressure, and episodic body movements |
| Stage 2 | Sleep spindle and K-complex | 45% | Largest percentage of sleep time; bruxism (tooth grinding) |
| Stages 3 and 4 | Delta (slow-wave sleep) waves | 25% (decreases with age) | Deepest, most relaxed stage of sleep; sleep disorders, such as night terrors, sleepwalking (somnambulism), and bed-wetting (enuresis) may occur |
| Rapid eye movement (REM) sleep | "Sawtooth," beta, alpha, and theta waves | 25% (decreases with age) | Dreaming; penile and clitoral erection; increased pulse, respiration, and blood pressure; absence of skeletal muscle movement |

b. **Sedative agents**, such as alcohol, barbiturates, and benzodiazepines, also are associated with **reduced REM sleep and delta sleep**.

c. Most **delta sleep** occurs during the **first half of the sleep cycle**.

d. **Longest REM periods** occur during the **second half of the sleep cycle**.

3. **During REM sleep, high levels of brain activity occur.**

   a. Average time to the first REM period after falling asleep **(REM latency) is 90 minutes**.

   b. REM periods of 10–40 minutes each occur about **every 90 minutes** throughout the night.

   c. A person who is deprived of REM sleep one night (e.g., because of inadequate sleep, repeated awakenings, or sedative use) has increased REM sleep the next night (**REM rebound**).

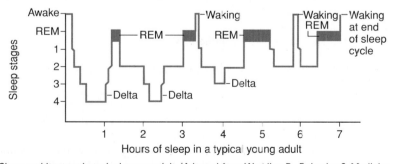

**FIGURE 10.1.** Sleep architecture in typical young adult. (Adapted from Wedding D. *Behavior & Medicine*. St. Louis, MO: Mosby Year Book, 1995:416.)

| table 10.2 | Summary of Characteristics of Sleep in Typical, Depressed, and Elderly People | | |
|---|---|---|---|
| Sleep Measure | Typical Young Adult | Depressed Young Adult | Typical Elderly Adult |
| Sleep latency | About 10 min | >10 min | >10 min |
| REM latency | About 90 min | About 45 min | About 90 min |
| Sleep efficiency | About 100% | <100% | <100% |
| Percentage delta | About 25% | <25% | <25% |
| Percentage REM | About 25% | >25% | <25% |

REM, rapid eye movement.

      **d.** Extended REM deprivation or total sleep deprivation may also result in the transient display of **psychopathology**, usually anxiety or psychotic symptoms.

**D. Neurotransmitters** are involved in the production of sleep.
    **1. Increased** levels of **acetylcholine (ACh)** in the reticular formation **increase both sleep efficiency and REM sleep**.
      **a.** ACh levels, sleep efficiency, and REM sleep decrease in typical aging as well as in Alzheimer disease.
      **b.** Patients taking anticholinergic agents show decreased REM sleep while patients taking cholinomimetic agents (e.g., physostigmine) show increased REM sleep.
    **2. Increased** levels of **dopamine decrease sleep efficiency.** Treatment with antipsychotics, which block dopamine receptors, may improve sleep in patients with psychotic symptoms.
    **3. Increased** levels of **norepinephrine decrease both sleep efficiency and REM sleep**.
    **4. Increased** levels of **serotonin increase both sleep efficiency and delta sleep**. Damage to the dorsal raphe nuclei, which produce serotonin, decreases both of these measures. Treatment with antidepressants, which increase serotonin availability, can improve sleep efficiency in depressed patients.

## II. CLASSIFICATION OF SLEEP DISORDERS

The *Diagnostic and Statistical Manual of Mental Disorders, 4th Edition Text Revision (DSM-IV-TR)* classifies sleep disorders into two major categories.

**A. Dyssomnias** are characterized by problems in the timing, quality, or amount of sleep. They include **insomnia, breathing-related sleep disorder (sleep apnea)**, and **narcolepsy**, as well as **circadian rhythm sleep disorder, nocturnal myoclonus, restless legs syndrome**, and **the primary hypersomnias (e.g., Kleine–Levin syndrome** and **menstrual-associated syndrome)**.

**B. Parasomnias** are characterized by abnormalities in physiology or in behavior associated with sleep. They include **bruxism** (tooth grinding) and **sleepwalking**, as well as **sleep terror, REM sleep behavior**, and **nightmare disorders**.

**C.** These sleep disorders are described in **Table 10.3**.

**D.** Insomnia, breathing-related sleep disorder, and narcolepsy are described below.

## III. INSOMNIA

**A.** Insomnia is **difficulty falling asleep or staying asleep** that lasts **for at least 1 month**, and leads to sleepiness during the day or causes problems fulfilling social or occupational obligations. It is present in at least 30% of the population.

| t a b l e  **10.3**  Other Sleep Disorders and Their Characteristics | |
|---|---|
| **Sleep Disorder** | **Characteristics** |
| Sleep terror disorder | Repetitive experiences of fright in which a person screams in fear during sleep (usually normal in children) The person cannot be awakened The person has no memory of having a dream Occurs during delta sleep Onset in adolescence may indicate temporal lobe epilepsy |
| Nightmare disorder | Repetitive, frightening dreams that cause nighttime awakenings The person usually can recall the nightmare Occurs during REM sleep |
| Sleepwalking disorder | Repetitive walking around during sleep No memory of the episode on awakening Begins in childhood (usually 4–8 yrs of age) Occurs during delta sleep |
| Circadian rhythm sleep disorder | Inability to sleep at appropriate times Delayed sleep phase type involves falling asleep and waking later than wanted Jet lag type lasts 2–7 days after a change in time zones Shift work type (e.g., in physician training) can result in work errors |
| Nocturnal myoclonus | Repetitive, abrupt muscular contractions in the legs from toes to hips Causes nighttime awakenings Treat with benzodiazepine, quinine, or antiparkinsonian, i.e., dopaminergic agent (e.g., levodopa, ropinirole [Requip]) |
| Restless legs syndrome | Uncomfortable sensation in the legs necessitating frequent motion Repetitive limb jerking during sleep Causes difficulty falling asleep and nighttime awakenings More common with aging, Parkinson disease, pregnancy, and kidney disease Treat with antiparkinsonian agent, iron supplements, or magnesium supplements |
| Primary hypersomnias (Kleine–Levin syndrome and menstrual-associated syndrome [symptoms only in the pre-menstruum]) | Recurrent periods of excessive sleepiness occurring almost daily for weeks to months Sleepiness is not relieved by daytime naps Often accompanied by hyperphagia (overeating) Kleine–Levin syndrome is more common in adolescent males |
| Sleep drunkenness | Difficulty awakening fully after adequate sleep Rare, must be differentiated from substance abuse or other sleep disorder Associated with genetic factors |
| Bruxism | Tooth grinding during sleep (stage 2) Can lead to tooth damage and jaw pain Treat with dental appliance worn at night or corrective orthodontia |
| REM sleep behavior disorder | REM sleep without the typical skeletal muscle paralysis While dreaming, patients can injure themselves or their sleeping partners Associated with Parkinson disease and Lewy body dementia Treat with antiparkinsonian agent, REM suppressor (e.g., benzodiazepines) or anticonvulsant (e.g., carbamazepine) |

B. **Psychological causes** of insomnia include the mood and anxiety disorders.
   1. **Major depressive disorder** (see Chapter 12).
      a. Characteristics of the **sleep pattern** in depression (Table 10.2):
         (1) Long sleep latency.
         (2) Repeated nighttime awakenings leading to poor sleep efficiency.
         (3) **Waking too early** in the morning (terminal insomnia) is the most common sleep characteristic of depressed patients.
      b. Characteristics of the **sleep stages** in depression (Table 10.2):
         (1) **Short REM latency** (appearance of REM within about 45 minutes of falling asleep).
         (2) **Increased REM early in the sleep cycle** and decreased REM later in the sleep cycle (e.g., in the early morning hours).
         (3) Long first REM period and **increased total REM**.
         (4) **Reduced delta** sleep.

2. **Bipolar disorder. Manic or hypomanic** patients have trouble falling asleep and sleep fewer hours.
3. **Anxious** patients often have trouble falling asleep.

C. **Physical causes** of insomnia:
1. **Use of central nervous system (CNS) stimulants** (e.g., caffeine) is the most common cause of insomnia.
2. **Withdrawal of agents with sedating action** (e.g., alcohol, benzodiazepines) can result in wakefulness.
3. **Medical conditions** causing pain also result in insomnia, as do endocrine and metabolic disorders.

## IV. BREATHING-RELATED SLEEP DISORDER (SLEEP APNEA)

A. Patients with sleep apnea **stop breathing** for brief intervals. Low oxygen or high carbon dioxide level in the blood **repeatedly awakens the patient** during the night, resulting in **daytime sleepiness** and **respiratory acidosis** (blood pH<7.35).
1. In patients with **central sleep apnea** (more common in the elderly), little or no respiratory effort occurs, resulting in less air reaching the lungs.
2. In patients with **obstructive sleep apnea**, respiratory effort occurs, but an airway obstruction prevents air from reaching the lungs. Obstructive sleep apnea occurs most often in people 40–60 years of age, and is more common in men (8:1 male-to-female ratio) and in the obese. Patients often **snore**.
3. **Pickwickian syndrome** is a related condition in which airway obstruction results in daytime sleepiness.

B. Sleep apnea occurs in **1%–10% of the population** and is related to depression, morning headaches, and **pulmonary hypertension**. It may also result in **sudden death** during sleep in the elderly and in infants.

## V. NARCOLEPSY

A. Patients with narcolepsy have **sleep attacks** (i.e., fall asleep suddenly during the day) despite having a normal amount of sleep at night. While typical in amount, their nighttime sleep is characterized by **decreased sleep latency, very short REM latency (<10 minutes), less total REM**, and **interrupted REM** (sleep fragmentation).

B. Decreased REM sleep at night leads to the intrusion of characteristics of REM sleep (e.g., paralysis, nightmares) while the patient is awake resulting in:
1. **Hypnagogic or hypnopompic hallucinations.** These are strange perceptual experiences that occur just as the patient falls asleep or wakes up, respectively, and occur in 20%–40% of patients.
2. **Cataplexy.** This is a sudden physical collapse caused by the loss of all muscle tone after a strong emotional stimulus (e.g., laughter, fear) and occurs in 30%–70% of patients.
3. **Sleep paralysis.** This is the inability to move the body for a few seconds after waking.

C. Narcolepsy is uncommon.
1. It occurs most frequently in **adolescents and young adults**.
2. There may be a **genetic component**.
3. **Daytime naps** allow the patient to make up some lost REM sleep and, as such, leave the patient feeling refreshed.

| table | **10.4** | Management of the Major Sleep Disorders |

| Disorder | Management (in Order of Highest to Lowest Utility) |
|---|---|
| Insomnia | Avoidance of caffeine, especially before bedtime<br>Development of a series of behaviors associated with bedtime (i.e., "a sleep ritual" or "sleep hygiene")<br>Maintaining a fixed sleeping and waking schedule<br>Daily exercise (but not just before sleep)<br>Relaxation techniques<br>Psychoactive agents (i.e., limited use of sleep agents to establish an effective sleep pattern and antide-pressants or antipsychotics, if appropriate) (see Table 16.3) |
| Breathing-related sleep disorder (obstructive sleep apnea) | Weight loss (if overweight)<br>Continuous positive airway pressure (CPAP) (a device applied to the face at night to gently move air into the lungs)<br>Breathing stimulant, e.g. medroxyprogesterone acetate, protriptyline (Vivactil), fluoxetine (Prozac)<br>Surgery to enlarge the airway, e.g., uvulopalatoplasty<br>Tracheostomy (as a last resort) |
| Narcolepsy | Stimulant agents (e.g., methylphenidate [Ritalin], modafinil [Provigil]; if cataplexy is present, sodium oxybate [Xyrem] or an antidepressant may be added)<br>Scheduled daytime naps |

# VI. MANAGEMENT OF SLEEP DISORDERS

The management of insomnia, breathing-related sleep disorder, and narcolepsy are described in Table 10.4.

# Review Test

**Directions:** Each of the numbered items or incomplete statements in this section is followed by answers or by completions of the statement. Select the **one** lettered answer or completion that is **best** in each case.

**1.** The parents of a 5-year-old boy report that the child often screams during the night. They are particularly concerned because during these disturbances the child sits up, opens his eyes, and "looks right through them," and they are unable to awaken him. The child has no memory of these experiences in the morning. Physical examination is unremarkable and the child is doing well in kindergarten. During these disturbances the child's electroencephalogram is most likely to be primarily characterized by

(A) sawtooth waves
(B) theta waves
(C) K complexes
(D) delta waves
(E) alpha waves

**2.** During a sleep study a physician discovers that a patient shows too little REM sleep during the night. Theoretically, to increase REM sleep the physician should give the patient a medication aimed at increasing circulating levels of

(A) serotonin
(B) norepinephrine
(C) acetylcholine
(D) dopamine
(E) histamine

**3.** During a sleep study a male patient's electroencephalogram (EEG) shows primarily sawtooth waves. Which of the following is most likely to characterize this patient at this time?

(A) Penile erection
(B) Movement of skeletal muscles
(C) Decreased blood pressure
(D) Decreased brain oxygen use
(E) Decreased pulse

**4.** During a sleep study a female patient's EEG shows primarily delta waves. Which of the following is most likely to characterize this patient at this time?

(A) Clitoral erection
(B) Paralysis of skeletal muscles
(C) Sleepwalking (somnambulism)
(D) Nightmares
(E) Increased brain oxygen use

**5.** An 85-year-old patient reports that he sleeps poorly. Sleep in this patient is most likely to be characterized by increased

(A) sleep efficiency
(B) REM sleep
(C) nighttime awakenings
(D) stage 3 sleep
(E) stage 4 sleep

**6.** A woman reports that most nights during the last year she has lain awake in bed for more than 2 hours before she falls asleep. After these nights, she is tired and forgetful and makes mistakes at work. Of the following, the most effective long-term treatment for this woman is

(A) continuous positive airway pressure (CPAP)
(B) an antipsychotic agent
(C) a sedative agent
(D) a stimulant agent
(E) development of a "sleep ritual"

### Questions 7 and 8

A 22-year-old medical student who goes to sleep at 11 PM and wakes at 7 AM falls asleep in laboratory every day. He tells the doctor that he sees strange images as he is falling asleep and sometimes just as he wakes up. He has had a few minor car accidents that occurred because he fell asleep while driving.

**7.** Of the following the best first step in management of this student is

**(A)** continuous positive airway pressure (CPAP)
**(B)** an antipsychotic agent
**(C)** a sedative agent
**(D)** a stimulant agent
**(E)** development of a "sleep ritual"

**8.** Which of the following is this student most likely to experience?

**(A)** Long REM latency
**(B)** Auditory hallucinations
**(C)** Tactile hallucinations
**(D)** Delusions
**(E)** Cataplexy

**Questions 9 and 10**

A patient reports that he is sleepy all day despite having 8 hours of sleep each night. His wife reports that his loud snoring keeps her awake.

**9.** Of the following, the best first step in the management of this patient is

**(A)** continuous positive airway pressure (CPAP)
**(B)** an antipsychotic agent
**(C)** a sedative agent
**(D)** a stimulant agent
**(E)** development of a "sleep ritual"

**10.** Of the following, this patient is most likely to be

**(A)** depressed
**(B)** aged 25 years
**(C)** overweight
**(D)** using a stimulant agent
**(E)** withdrawing from a sedative agent

**11.** Sawtooth waves are most characteristic of what sleep stage?

**(A)** Stage 1
**(B)** Stage 2
**(C)** Stages 3 and 4
**(D)** REM sleep

**12.** Sleep spindles, K complexes, and bruxism are most characteristic of what sleep stage?

**(A)** Stage 1
**(B)** Stage 2
**(C)** Stages 3 and 4
**(D)** REM sleep

**13.** Theta waves are most characteristic of what sleep stage?

**(A)** Stage 1
**(B)** Stage 2
**(C)** Stages 3 and 4
**(D)** REM sleep

**14.** What sleep stage takes up the largest percentage of sleep time in young adults?

**(A)** Stage 1
**(B)** Stage 2
**(C)** Stages 3 and 4
**(D)** REM sleep

**15.** Bed-wetting is characteristic of what sleep stage?

**(A)** Stage 1
**(B)** Stage 2
**(C)** Stages 3 and 4
**(D)** REM sleep

**16.** A 22-year-old student in the middle of finals week tells her doctor that for the last 2 weeks she has been studying late into the night and has started to have trouble falling asleep. What is the doctor's most appropriate recommendation?

**(A)** Exercise before bedtime
**(B)** A large meal before bedtime
**(C)** A glass of milk before bedtime
**(D)** A fixed wake-up and bedtime schedule
**(E)** A short-acting benzodiazepine at bedtime

**17.** A 45-year-old female patient reports that over the last 3 months she has lost her appetite and interest in her usual activities, and often feels that life is not worth living. Compared with typical sleep, in this patient the percentage of REM sleep, percentage of delta sleep, and sleep latency, respectively, are most likely to

**(A)** increase, decrease, decrease
**(B)** increase, decrease, increase
**(C)** decrease, stay the same, increase
**(D)** decrease, decrease, increase
**(E)** increase, increase, increase

**18.** In a sleep laboratory, a woman shows 10% of sleep time in stage 1 sleep, 75% of sleep time in stage 2 sleep, 15% of sleep time in REM sleep, no delta sleep, and six night-time awakenings. This sleep pattern indicates that this woman

(A) has narcolepsy
(B) has depressive illness
(C) is elderly
(D) has an anxiety disorder
(E) has nocturnal myoclonus

**19.** A 5-year-old child often wakes during the night, crying and fearful. When his parents come to him, he relates details of dreams involving frightening creatures and situations. Which of the following sleep disorders best matches this picture?

(A) Kleine–Levin syndrome
(B) Nightmare disorder
(C) Sleep terror disorder
(D) Sleep drunkenness
(E) Circadian rhythm sleep disorder
(F) Nocturnal myoclonus
(G) Restless legs syndrome
(H) Bruxism

**20.** The mother of a 13-year-old boy reports that he has "bouts" of overeating and of oversleeping, each lasting a few days to a few weeks. Which of the following sleep disorders best matches this picture?

(A) Kleine–Levin syndrome
(B) Nightmare disorder
(C) Sleep terror disorder
(D) Sleep drunkenness
(E) Circadian rhythm sleep disorder
(F) Nocturnal myoclonus
(G) Restless legs syndrome
(H) Bruxism

**21.** A 32-year-old man has a 9 to 5 job in a law office. Sunday night through Thursday night the man goes to bed at 10 PM, but is unable to fall asleep until about 2 AM. His alarm wakens him at 6 AM and he feels tired all day. On Friday and Saturday nights, the man goes to bed at 2 AM, falls asleep quickly, sleeps until 10 AM, and wakes feeling refreshed. Which of the following sleep disorders best matches this picture?

(A) Kleine–Levin syndrome
(B) Nightmare disorder
(C) Sleep terror disorder
(D) Sleep drunkenness
(E) Circadian rhythm sleep disorder
(F) Nocturnal myoclonus
(G) Restless legs syndrome
(H) Bruxism

**22.** A 70-year-old man cannot fall asleep because of crawling feelings and aching in his calves and thighs. He can suppress the urge to move his legs for a short period but then must move them. Which of the following best fits this clinical picture?

(A) Kleine–Levin syndrome
(B) Nightmare disorder
(C) Sleep terror disorder
(D) Sleep drunkenness
(E) Circadian rhythm sleep disorder
(F) Nocturnal myoclonus
(G) Restless legs syndrome
(H) Bruxism

**23.** The sleep of a patient who begins taking a moderate dose of diazepam (Valium) daily is most likely to be characterized by which of the following changes?

(A) Increased stage 1 and increased stage 2
(B) Increased stage 1 and decreased delta
(C) Decreased REM and decreased delta
(D) Decreased REM and increased delta
(E) Increased REM and decreased delta

**24.** A 21-year-old student who is part of a study of circadian rhythms, sleeps in a cave for 1 month with no access to clocks or watches. At the end of the month, the length of her circadian cycle is likely to be closest to

**(A)** 21 hours
**(B)** 22 hours
**(C)** 23 hours
**(D)** 24 hours
**(E)** 25 hours

**25.** A 52-year-old overweight man reports that he often wakes up with a headache. He also notes that he is tired all the time and repeatedly falls asleep during the day. Evaluation of the arterial blood of this patient is most likely to reveal

**(A)** respiratory acidosis
**(B)** respiratory alkalosis
**(C)** metabolic alkalosis
**(D)** increased $PaO_2$
**(E)** decreased $PaCO_2$

**26.** A 33-year-old man with myasthenia gravis is taking physostigmine for symptom relief. The effect of this agent on sleep architecture in this patient is most likely to be increased

**(A)** stage 1 sleep
**(B)** stage 2 sleep
**(C)** stage 3 sleep
**(D)** stage 4 sleep
**(E)** REM sleep

# Answers and Explanations

**The answer is E.** Dreaming typically occurs during REM sleep. Because typically there is muscle atonia during REM sleep, this man who is moving while dreaming is showing signs of REM sleep behavior disorder. This disorder is associated with an increased risk for Parkinson disease and Lewy body dementia. Kleine–Levin syndrome, sleep terror disorder, nocturnal myoclonus, and Alzheimer disease are not specifically associated with REM sleep behavior disorder (see also answer to Question 19).

1. **The answer is D.** This child demonstrates sleep terror disorder, which is characterized by repetitive occurrences of screaming during the night and the inability to be awakened or to remember those experiences in the morning. Sleep terrors typically occur during delta sleep. If the child were having nightmares, which occur in REM sleep, the child would awaken and relate the nature of his frightening dreams (see also answer to Question 19).

2. **The answer is C.** Acetylcholine (Ach) is involved in both increasing REM sleep and increasing sleep efficiency. Increased levels of dopamine decrease sleep efficiency. Increased levels of norepinephrine decrease both sleep efficiency and REM sleep while increased levels of serotonin increase both sleep efficiency and delta (slow-wave) sleep.

3. **The answer is A.** Sawtooth waves characterize REM sleep, which is also associated with penile erection; dreaming; increased pulse, respiration, and blood pressure; and paralysis of skeletal muscles.

4. **The answer is C.** Delta waves characterize sleep stages 3 and 4 (slow-wave sleep), which is also associated with somnambulism, night terrors, episodic body movements, and enuresis. Delta sleep is the deepest, most relaxed stage of sleep. Clitoral erection, paralysis of skeletal muscles, nightmares, and increased brain oxygen use occur during REM sleep.

5. **The answer is C.** Sleep in the elderly is characterized by increased nighttime awakenings, decreased REM sleep, decreased delta sleep, and decreased sleep efficiency.

6. **The answer is E.** The most effective long-term management for this woman with insomnia is the development of a series of behaviors associated with bedtime (i.e., a "sleep ritual"). By the process of classical conditioning (see Chapter 7) the sleep ritual then becomes associated with going to sleep. Sleep rituals can include things like taking a warm bath, pulling down the blinds, and listening to soothing music. Continuous positive airway pressure is used to treat sleep apnea; stimulant agents are used to treat narcolepsy; and antipsychotics are used to treat psychotic symptoms. Sedative agents have a high abuse potential and, because they tend to reduce REM and delta sleep, their use may result in sleep of poorer quality.

7. **The answer is D. 8. The answer is E.** This medical student who falls asleep in laboratory every day despite a normal amount of sleep at night probably has narcolepsy. Of the listed choices, the most effective management for narcolepsy is the administration of stimulant agents such as modafinil. Sedative agents are not useful for narcolepsy. In narcolepsy, short REM latency, sleep paralysis, and cataplexy occur. The student's strange perceptual experiences as he is falling asleep and waking up are hypnagogic and hypnopompic hallucinations, respectively.

9. **The answer is A. 10. The answer is C.** This man who snores and reports that he is sleepy all day despite having 8 hours of sleep each night probably has obstructive sleep apnea. Of the listed choices, the best first step in management of this patient is continuous positive airway pressure (CPAP). Since obesity is associated with obstructive sleep apnea, other suggestions for this patient would include weight loss. Use of stimulants and withdrawal from sedatives are associated with wakefulness rather than the daytime sleepiness seen here. Also, most sleep apnea patients are middle aged (age 40–60 years). Although depression and anxiety are associated with sleep problems, this man's snoring indicates that his sleep problem is more likely to have a physical basis.

11. **The answer is D.** Sawtooth waves are primarily seen in REM sleep.

12. **The answer is B.** Sleep spindles, K complexes, and bruxism are primarily seen in stage 2 sleep.

13. **The answer is A.** Theta waves are primarily seen in stage 1 sleep.

14. **The answer is B.** In young adults, 45% of total sleep time is spent in stage 2 sleep. Five percent is spent in stage 1, 25% in REM, and 25% in delta sleep.

15. **The answer is C.** Bed-wetting occurs primarily in stages 3–4 (delta) sleep.

16. **The answer is D.** The most appropriate first step in management of this 22-year-old student who is having temporary problems with sleep during finals week is to recommend a fixed wake-up and bedtime schedule. Benzodiazepines are not appropriate because of their high abuse potential and possibility of causing daytime sedation in this student during examinations. These agents also decrease sleep quality by reducing REM and delta sleep. Exercise should be done early in the day; if done before bedtime it can be stimulating and cause wakefulness. A large meal before bedtime is more likely to interfere with sleep than to help sleep. While many people believe that milk helps induce sleep, this effect has never been shown empirically.

17. **The answer is B.** This woman's symptoms indicate that she is likely to be experiencing a major depressive episode (see Chapter 12). Sleep in major depression is associated with increased REM sleep, reduced delta sleep, and increased sleep latency.

18. **The answer is C.** This sleep pattern indicates that this woman is elderly. Sleep in elderly patients is characterized by increased stage 1 and stage 2 sleep, increased nighttime awakenings, decreased REM sleep, and much reduced or absent delta sleep.

19. **The answer is B.** This child is experiencing nightmare disorder, which occurs during REM sleep. In contrast to the child with sleep terror disorder (see also answer to Question 1), this child wakes up and can relate the nature of his frightening dreams. Kleine–Levin syndrome is usually seen in adolescents and involves recurrent periods of hypersomnia and hyperphagia, each lasting days to weeks. In sleep drunkenness a patient cannot come fully awake after sleep, and in circadian rhythm sleep disorder the individual sleeps and wakes at inappropriate times. Nocturnal myoclonus (muscular contractions involving the legs) and restless legs syndrome (uncomfortable sensation in the legs) occur more commonly in middle-aged and elderly people. Bruxism is tooth grinding during sleep.

20. **The answer is A.** The fact that this patient is an adolescent, as well as the recurrent periods of hypersomnia and hyperphagia each lasting for weeks to months, indicate that this patient has Kleine–Levin syndrome (and see also answer to Question 19).

21. **The answer is E.** Circadian rhythm sleep disorder involves the inability to sleep at appropriate times. This man shows the delayed sleep phase type of this disorder, which is characterized by falling asleep and waking later than wanted. When the man is able to follow his preferred sleep schedule (e.g., on weekends), he sleeps well and wakes refreshed (see also answer to Question 19).

22. **The answer is G.** In restless legs syndrome, there are crawling, aching feelings in the legs making it necessary for the patient to move them and causing difficulty in falling asleep (see also answer to Question 19).

23. **The answer is C.** Decreased REM sleep and decreased delta sleep characterize the sleep of patients such as this one, who are taking sedatives such as diazepam (a benzodiazepine), barbiturates, or alcohol.

24. **The answer is E.** At the end of the month, the length of this student's circadian cycle in the absence of cues from the outside world is likely to be close to 25 hours.

25. **The answer is A.** This overweight middle-aged male patient is likely to have sleep apnea. Like other patients with pulmonary disorders leading to depressed breathing, patients with sleep apnea typically show chronic respiratory acidosis (increased partial pressure of carbon dioxide [$PaCO_2$]). Respiratory alkalosis (decreased $PaCO_2$) results from hyperventilation as a result of anxiety, high fever, or stimulant abuse. Metabolic alkalosis typically results from excessive vomiting and resulting hypokalemia (see also answers to Questions 9 and 10).

26. **The answer is E.** Physostigmine is a cholinomimetic agent used to treat myasthenia gravis. The increase in acetylcholine resulting from treatment with this agent is most likely to result in increased REM sleep in this patient.

# Schizophrenia and Other Psychotic Disorders

## Typical Board Question

A 40-year-old attorney is convinced that his wife is trying to kill him. When he locks himself in the basement and refuses to come out, the police are called and he is taken to the emergency room of the local hospital. The wife, who denies her husband's charge, notes that the patient has been showing increasingly strange behavior over the past 9 months. An abnormal gait is observed on physical examination. The history reveals that the patient's mother and uncle, who had shown similar psychiatric and physical symptoms, died in their early 50s after being institutionalized in long-term care facilities for many years. What is the most appropriate diagnosis for this patient?

**(A)** Schizophrenia
**(B)** Schizoaffective disorder
**(C)** Schizophreniform disorder
**(D)** Brief psychotic disorder
**(E)** Delusional disorder
**(F)** Shared psychotic disorder
**(G)** Psychosis due to a general medical condition

*(See "Answers and Explanations" at end of chapter.)*

# I. SCHIZOPHRENIA

### A. Overview

1. Schizophrenia is a **chronic, debilitating** mental disorder characterized by periods of loss of touch with reality (psychosis); persistent disturbances of thought, behavior, appearance, and speech; abnormal affect; and social withdrawal.
2. Peak **age of onset** of schizophrenia is **15–25 years for men and 25–35 years for women**.
3. Schizophrenia occurs **equally in men and women, all cultures, and all ethnic groups** studied.

### B. Symptoms of schizophrenia can be classified as **positive** or **negative**.

1. **Positive symptoms** are things **additional to expected behavior** and include delusions, hallucinations, agitation, and talkativeness.
2. **Negative symptoms** are things **missing from expected behavior** and include lack of motivation, social withdrawal, flattened affect, cognitive disturbances, poor grooming, and poor (i.e., impoverished) speech content.
3. These classifications can be useful in predicting the effects of antipsychotic medication.
   a. **Positive symptoms** respond well to most **traditional** and **atypical antipsychotic agents**.
   b. **Negative symptoms** respond better to **atypical** than to traditional antipsychotics (see Chapter 16).

| t a b l e  **11.1** | Symptoms of Schizophrenia: Disorders of Perception, Thought Content, Thought Process, and Form of Thought | | |
|---|---|---|---|
| Disorder of | Symptom | Definition | Example |
| Perception | Illusions | Misperception of real external stimuli | Interpreting the appearance of a coat in a dark closet as a man |
| | Hallucinations | False sensory perception | Hearing voices when alone in a room |
| Thought content | Delusions | False belief not shared by others | The idea of being followed by the FBI |
| | Ideas of reference | False belief of being referred to by others | The feeling of being discussed by someone on television |
| Thought processes | Impaired abstraction ability | Problems discerning the essential qualities of objects or relationships | When asked what brought her to the emergency room, the patient says, "An ambulance" |
| | Magical thinking | Belief that thoughts affect the course of events | Knocking on wood to prevent something bad from happening |
| Form of thought | Circumstantiality | Inclusion of too much detail | When asked about her health, the patient explains everything that she did since getting up that day before getting to the subject of her health |
| | Loose associations | Shift of ideas from one subject to another in an unrelated way | The patient begins to answer a question about her health and then shifts to a statement about baseball |
| | Neologisms | Inventing new words | The patient refers to her doctor as a "medocrat" |
| | Perseveration | Repeating words or phrases | The patient says, "I'm evil, I'm evil, I'm evil" |
| | Tangentiality | Getting further away from the point as speaking continues | The patient begins to answer a question about her health and ends up talking about her sister's abortion; she never gets back to the subject of her health |

4. Patients with predominantly negative symptoms have more **neuroanatomic** (see below) and **metabolic abnormalities** (e.g., decreased cerebral metabolism of glucose) than those with predominantly positive symptoms.

C. **Course.** Schizophrenia has three **phases:** Prodromal, active, (i.e., psychotic and residual).
   1. **Prodromal** signs and symptoms occur prior to the first psychotic episode and include avoidance of social activities; physical complaints; and new interest in religion, the occult, or philosophy.
   2. In the **active phase**, the patient loses touch with reality. Disorders of perception, thought content, thought processes, and form of thought (Table 11.1) occur during an acute psychotic episode.
   3. In the **residual phase** (time period between psychotic episodes), the patient is in touch with reality but does not behave normally.
      a. This phase is characterized by **negative symptoms**.
      b. In this phase the patient typically shows intact memory capacity; **is oriented** to person, place, and time; and has a **normal level of consciousness** (e.g., is alert).

D. **Prognosis**
   1. Schizophrenia usually involves repeated psychotic episodes and a **chronic, downhill course** over years. The illness often stabilizes in midlife.
   2. **Suicide is common** in patients with schizophrenia. More than 50% attempt suicide (often during post-psychotic depression or when having hallucinations "commanding" them to harm themselves), and 10% of those die in the attempt.
   3. The **prognosis is better** and the suicide risk is lower if the patient is older at onset of illness, is married, has social relationships, is female, has a good employment history, has mood symptoms, has few negative symptoms, and has few relapses.

| t a b l e   **11.2**   The Genetics of Schizophrenia | |
|---|---|
| Group | Approximate Occurrence |
| The general population | 1% |
| Person who has one parent or sibling (or dizygotic twin) with schizophrenia | 10% |
| Person who has two parents with schizophrenia | 40% |
| Monozygotic twin of a person with schizophrenia | 50% |

E. **Etiology.** While the etiology of schizophrenia is not known, certain factors have been implicated in its development.
   1. **Genetic factors**
      a. Schizophrenia occurs in **1% of the population.** Persons with a close genetic relationship to a patient with schizophrenia are more likely than those with a more distant relationship to develop the disorder (Table 11.2).
      b. Markers on **chromosomes** 1, 6, 7, 8, 13, 21, and 22 have been associated with schizophrenia.
   2. **Other factors**
      a. The **season of birth** is related to the incidence of schizophrenia. More people with schizophrenia are **born during cold weather months** (i.e., January to April in the northern hemisphere, and July to September in the southern hemisphere). One possible explanation for this finding is **viral infection of the mother** during pregnancy, since such infections occur seasonally.
      b. **No social or environmental factor causes schizophrenia.** However, because patients with schizophrenia tend to drift down the socioeconomic scale as a result of their social deficits (the **"downward drift" hypothesis**), they are often found in lower socioeconomic groups (e.g., homeless people).

F. **Neural pathology**
   1. **Anatomy**
      a. **Abnormalities of the frontal lobes,** as evidenced by decreased use of glucose in the frontal lobes on positron emission tomography (PET) scans are seen in the brains of people with schizophrenia.
      b. **Lateral and third ventricle enlargement,** abnormal cerebral symmetry, and changes in brain density also may be present.
      c. **Decreased volume of limbic structures** (e.g., amygdala, hippocampus) is also seen.
   2. **Neurotransmitter abnormalities** (see also Table 4.3)
      a. The **dopamine hypothesis** of schizophrenia states that the positive symptoms result from excessive dopaminergic activity (e.g., an excessive number of dopamine receptors, excessive concentration of dopamine, hypersensitivity of receptors to dopamine) in the limbic system. As evidence for this hypothesis, stimulant drugs that increase dopamine availability (e.g., amphetamines and cocaine) can cause psychotic symptoms (see Chapter 9). Also, laboratory tests may show **elevated levels of homovanillic acid (HVA),** a metabolite of dopamine, in the body fluids of patients with schizophrenia. The negative symptoms of schizophrenia are believed to result from reduced dopaminergic activity in the frontal cortex (see Chapter 4).
      b. **Serotonin hyperactivity** is implicated in schizophrenia because hallucinogens that increase serotonin concentrations cause psychotic symptoms, and because some effective antipsychotics, such as clozapine (see Chapter 16), have anti-serotonergic-2 (5-HT$_2$) activity.
      c. **Glutamate** is implicated in schizophrenia; N-methyl-d-aspartate (NMDA) antagonists (e.g., memantine) are useful in treating some of the neurodegenerative symptoms (e.g., loss of cognitive abilities) in patients with schizophrenia.

G. **Subtypes.** The **_Diagnostic and Statistical Manual of Mental Disorders, Fourth Edition, Text Revision (DSM-IV-TR)_** lists five subtypes of schizophrenia (Table 11.3).

| table **11.3** | *DSM-IV-TR* Subtypes of Schizophrenia |
|---|---|
| **Subtype** | **Characteristics** |
| Catatonic | Stupor or agitation, lack of coherent speech<br>Bizarre posturing (waxy flexibility)<br>Rarely seen since the introduction of antipsychotic agents |
| Disorganized | Poor grooming and disheveled personal appearance<br>Inappropriate emotional responses (e.g., silliness)<br>Facial grimacing, mirror gazing<br>Onset before the age of 25 yrs |
| Paranoid | Delusions of persecution<br>Better functioning and older age at onset than other subtypes |
| Residual | At least one previous psychotic episode<br>Subsequent residual symptoms but no current frank psychotic symptoms |
| Undifferentiated | Characteristics of more than one subtype |

H. **Differential Diagnosis**

1. **Medical illnesses** that can cause psychotic symptoms, and thus mimic schizophrenia (i.e., psychotic disorder caused by a general medical condition), include neurologic infection, neoplasm, trauma, disease (e.g., Huntington disease, multiple sclerosis), temporal lobe epilepsy, and endocrine disorders (e.g., Cushing syndrome, acute intermittent porphyria).

2. **Medications** that can cause psychotic symptoms include analgesics, antibiotics, anticholinergics, antihistamines, antineoplastics, cardiac glycosides (e.g., digitalis), and steroid hormones.

3. **Psychiatric illnesses** other than schizophrenia that may be associated with psychotic symptoms include:
   a. Other psychotic disorders (see below).
   b. Mood disorders (e.g., the manic phase of bipolar disorder, major depression [see Chapter 12]).
   c. Cognitive disorders (e.g., delirium, dementia, and amnestic disorder [see Chapter 14]).
   d. Substance-related disorders (see Chapter 9).

4. **Schizotypal, paranoid**, and **borderline personality disorders** (see Chapter 14) are not characterized by frank psychotic symptoms but have other characteristics of schizophrenia (e.g., odd behavior, avoidance of social relationships).

I. **Management**

1. **Pharmacologic management** of schizophrenia includes traditional antipsychotics (dopamine-2 [$D_2$]-receptor antagonists) and atypical antipsychotic agents (see Chapter 16). Because of their better side-effect profiles, the atypical agents are now first-line treatments. Long-acting injectable "depot" forms (e.g., haloperidol decanoate) of antipsychotics are useful options in patients whose symptoms lead to noncompliance with medication.

2. **Psychological management**, including individual, family, and group psychotherapy (see Chapter 17), is useful to **provide long-term support** and to foster adherence to the drug regimen.

## II. OTHER PSYCHOTIC DISORDERS

A. **Overview.** Psychotic disorders are all characterized at some point during their course by a loss of touch with reality. However, the other psychotic disorders do **not include all of the criteria** required for the diagnosis of schizophrenia.

| t a b l e **11.4** | Schizophrenia and Other Psychotic Disorders | |
|---|---|---|
| **Disorder** | **Characteristics** | **Prognosis** |
| Schizophrenia | Psychotic and residual symptoms lasting at least 6 mos | Lifelong social and occupational impairment |
| Brief psychotic disorder | Psychotic symptoms lasting >1 day but <1 mo; often precipitating psychosocial factors | 50%–80% recover completely |
| Schizophreniform disorder | Psychotic and residual symptoms lasting 1–6 mos | 33% recover completely |
| Schizoaffective disorder | Symptoms of both a mood disorder and schizophrenia; presence of psychotic symptoms for at least 2 wks without mood symptoms | Lifelong social and occupational impairment (somewhat higher overall level of functioning than in schizophrenia) |
| Delusional disorder | Fixed, persistent, non-bizarre delusional system (paranoid in the persecutory type and romantic [often with a famous person] in the erotomanic type); few, if any, other thought disorders | 50% recover completely; many have relatively normal social and occupational functioning |
| Shared psychotic disorder (folie à deux) | Development of delusions in a person in a close relationship (e.g., spouse, child) with someone with delusional disorder (the inducer) | 10%–40% recover completely when separated from the inducer |

B. Other psychotic disorders include (Table 11.4):
   1. Brief psychotic disorder
   2. Schizophreniform disorder
   3. Schizoaffective disorder
   4. Delusional disorder
   5. Shared psychotic disorder (folie à deux)

# Review Test

**Directions:** Each of the numbered items or incomplete statements in this section is followed by answers or by completions of the statement. Select the **one** lettered answer or completion that is **best** in each case.

**Questions 1–3**

A 26-year-old medical student is brought to the emergency department by her husband. The husband tells the doctor that his wife has shown odd behavior ever since failing an exam 2 weeks ago. In particular, she tells him that people are trying to poison her. The woman has no prior psychiatric history, and physical examination and laboratory results are unremarkable.

**1.** What is the most appropriate diagnosis for this patient at this time?

**(A)** Schizophrenia
**(B)** Schizoaffective disorder
**(C)** Schizophreniform disorder
**(D)** Brief psychotic disorder
**(E)** Delusional disorder
**(F)** Shared psychotic disorder
**(G)** Psychosis due to a general medical condition

**2.** The patient's belief that people are trying to poison her is an example of

**(A)** an illusion
**(B)** a neologism
**(C)** a hallucination
**(D)** a delusion
**(E)** an idea of reference

**3.** Analysis of neurotransmitter availability in the brain of this patient is most likely to reveal

**(A)** increased dopamine
**(B)** decreased dopamine
**(C)** increased acetylcholine
**(D)** decreased histamine
**(E)** decreased serotonin

**4.** A 27-year-old patient with schizophrenia shows extreme psychomotor agitation to the point of physical exhaustion. At times, he holds unusual, uncomfortable-looking body positions. This patient is most likely to have which of the following subtypes of schizophrenia?

**(A)** Catatonic
**(B)** Disorganized
**(C)** Paranoid
**(D)** Residual
**(E)** Undifferentiated

**Questions 5 and 6**

A 36-year-old patient with schizophrenia tells the physician that the government has been listening in on all of his phone conversations for the past year.

**5.** This symptom indicates that the patient is most likely to have which of the following types of schizophrenia?

**(A)** Catatonic
**(B)** Disorganized
**(C)** Paranoid
**(D)** Residual
**(E)** Undifferentiated

**6.** The patient's false belief about the government is an example of a disorder of

**(A)** thought processes
**(B)** thought content
**(C)** form of thought
**(D)** perception
**(E)** affect

**7.** Which of the following symptoms of schizophrenia is likely to respond best to antipsychotic medication?

**(A)** Delusions
**(B)** Flattening of affect
**(C)** Poor speech content
**(D)** Lack of motivation
**(E)** Social withdrawal

**8.** When compared to traditional antipsychotic medication, atypical antipsychotic medication is more likely to be helpful for which of the following symptoms?

**(A)** Hallucinations
**(B)** Delusions
**(C)** Agitation
**(D)** Over-talkativeness
**(E)** Social withdrawal

**9.** A 20-year-old woman tells the physician that sometimes she becomes frightened when her room is dark because her computer looks like a lion lurking in the corner. This is an example of

**(A)** an illusion
**(B)** a neologism
**(C)** a hallucination
**(D)** a delusion
**(E)** an idea of reference

**10.** A 53-year-old hospitalized patient with schizophrenia tells the physician that a newscaster was talking about her when he said on television, "A woman was found shoplifting today." This patient's statement is an example of

**(A)** an illusion
**(B)** a neologism
**(C)** a hallucination
**(D)** a delusion
**(E)** an idea of reference

**11.** A 35-year-old man who lives in a group home says that his roommates are spying on him by listening to him through the electrical outlets. For this reason, he has changed roommates a number of times over the last 5 years. He dresses strangely, is dirty with unkempt hair, and seems preoccupied. He reports that he has trouble paying attention to the doctor's questions because "I am listening to my leader giving me instructions in my head." Neuropsychological evaluation of this patient when he is not hearing voices is most likely to reveal

**(A)** memory impairment
**(B)** inability to state his name
**(C)** mental retardation
**(D)** frontal lobe dysfunction
**(E)** lack of orientation to place

**12.** A 20-year-old man reports that he just found out that his mother (whom he believed had died when he was a child) has been in an institution for the past 15 years with schizophrenia. He asks what the chances are that he will develop schizophrenia over the course of his life. The most correct answer is approximately

**(A)** 1%
**(B)** 5%
**(C)** 10%
**(D)** 50%
**(E)** 80%

**13.** A patient reports that his 19-year-old identical twin brother has just been diagnosed with schizophrenia and wants to know what the likelihood is that he will develop this disorder. The most correct answer is approximately

**(A)** 1%
**(B)** 5%
**(C)** 10%
**(D)** 50%
**(E)** 80%

**14.** The percentage of patients with schizophrenia who attempt suicide is approximately

**(A)** 1%
**(B)** 5%
**(C)** 12%
**(D)** 50%
**(E)** 80%

**15.** Which of the following is most closely associated with a good prognosis in schizophrenia?

**(A)** Younger age of onset
**(B)** Catatonic symptoms
**(C)** Negative symptoms
**(D)** Many relapses
**(E)** Mood symptoms

**16.** The most common type of hallucination seen in schizophrenia is

**(A)** visual
**(B)** gustatory
**(C)** auditory
**(D)** olfactory
**(E)** hypnagogic

**17.** A 45-year-old man with a 20-year history of severe depression and psychotic symptoms has held different jobs, but none of them for more than 6 months. He is successfully treated for his severe depressive symptoms, but he remains withdrawn and odd and expresses the belief that he has been "chosen" for a special mission on earth. What is the most appropriate diagnosis for this patient?

**(A)** Schizophrenia
**(B)** Schizoaffective disorder
**(C)** Schizophreniform disorder
**(D)** Brief psychotic disorder
**(E)** Delusional disorder
**(F)** Shared psychotic disorder
**(G)** Psychosis due to a general medical condition

**18.** A 68-year-old patient tells the physician that for the last 7 years his neighbor has been trying to get him evicted from his apartment by telling lies about him to the landlord. The patient is married and is working full time in a job, which he has held for over 30 years. What is the most appropriate diagnosis for this patient?

**(A)** Schizophrenia
**(B)** Schizoaffective disorder
**(C)** Schizophreniform disorder
**(D)** Brief psychotic disorder
**(E)** Delusional disorder
**(F)** Shared psychotic disorder
**(G)** Psychosis due to a general medical condition

**19.** A 60-year-old woman whose husband believes (in the absence of any evidence) that their house is filled with radioactive dust worries about her ability to clear the house of the dust when he is hospitalized. What is the most appropriate diagnosis for this woman?

**(A)** Schizophrenia
**(B)** Schizoaffective disorder
**(C)** Schizophreniform disorder
**(D)** Brief psychotic disorder
**(E)** Delusional disorder
**(F)** Shared psychotic disorder
**(G)** Psychosis due to a general medical condition

**20.** In a 50-year-old patient with schizophrenia, the size of the cerebral ventricles, glucose utilization in the frontal lobes, and size of limbic structures are most likely to be, respectively

**(A)** increased, decreased, decreased
**(B)** increased, decreased, increased
**(C)** increased, increased, decreased
**(D)** decreased, decreased, decreased
**(E)** decreased, increased, decreased
**(F)** decreased, increased, increased

# Answers and Explanations

**Typical Board Question**

**The answer is G.** This patient is showing evidence of psychosis due to a general medical condition. The abnormal gait, age of the patient, and family history strongly suggest Huntington disease, which often presents with psychiatric symptoms such as psychosis and depression (see also answer to Question 1).

1. **The answer is D.** This patient is showing evidence of brief psychotic disorder. This disorder is characterized by psychotic symptoms lasting >1 day, but <1 month; she has had symptoms for the past 2 weeks. Also, the stress of failing the exam is likely to be a precipitating psychosocial factor in this patient. Schizoaffective disorder is characterized by symptoms of both a mood disorder and schizophrenia, as well as psychotic symptoms that occur even in the absence of mood symptoms, and lifelong social and occupational impairment. In schizophrenia, psychotic and residual symptoms last 6 months, and there is lifelong social and occupational impairment. Schizophreniform disorder is characterized by psychotic and residual symptoms lasting 1–6 months. In delusional disorder, which often lasts for years, there is a fixed, non-bizarre delusional system; few, if any, other thought disorders; and relatively normal social and occupational functioning. In shared psychotic disorder, a person develops the same delusion as a person with delusional disorder with whom they are in a close relationship. Psychosis due to a general medical condition involves psychotic symptoms occurring as a result of physical illness (see the TBQ).

2. **The answer is D.** Believing that you are being poisoned is a delusion, that is, a false belief. A hallucination is a false perception; an illusion is a misperception of real external stimuli; an idea of reference is the false belief of being referred to by others; and a neologism is a new, invented word. All of these phenomena can be seen in patients exhibiting psychotic symptoms no matter what the cause.

3. **The answer is A.** Analysis of neurotransmitter availability in the brain of this patient with a positive psychotic symptom (e.g., a delusion) is most likely to reveal increased levels of dopamine or serotonin. Acetylcholine and histamine are not so closely involved in the pathophysiology of psychotic symptoms.

4. **The answer is A.** This patient who shows extreme psychomotor agitation and unusual uncomfortable-looking body positions is most likely to have catatonic schizophrenia. Disorganized schizophrenia is characterized by disinhibition, poor grooming, poor personal appearance, and inappropriate emotional responses. Paranoid schizophrenia is characterized by delusions of persecution; undifferentiated schizophrenia has the characteristics of more than one subtype. In residual schizophrenia, there is one previous psychotic episode and residual symptoms, but no current psychotic symptoms.

5. **The answer is C.** This patient is most likely to have paranoid schizophrenia, which is characterized by delusions of persecution (see also answer to Question 4).

6. **The answer is B.** This paranoid belief is a delusion, an example of a disorder of thought content. An idea of reference is also an example of a disorder of thought content. Illusions and hallucinations are disorders of perception, and loose associations and tangentiality are disorders of form of thought. Problems with affect are more characteristic of the mood disorders (see Chapter 12) but also are seen in schizoaffective disorder.

7. **The answer is A.** When compared to negative symptoms (e.g., flattening of affect, poor speech content, lack of motivation, and social withdrawal), positive symptoms such as delusions respond better to antipsychotic medication.

8. **The answer is E.** Social withdrawal is a negative symptom of schizophrenia. Negative symptoms respond better to atypical antipsychotic medication than to traditional antipsychotics. Hallucinations, delusions, agitation, and over-talkativeness are positive symptoms of schizophrenia.

9. **The answer is A.** An illusion is a misperception of a real external stimulus (e.g., a computer looking like a lion lurking in the corner in a darkened room). A hallucination is a false sensory perception, and a delusion is a false belief not shared by others. An idea of reference is the false belief of being referred to by others, and a neologism is a new word invented by a psychotic person.

10. **The answer is E.** An idea of reference is the false belief of being referred to by others (e.g., a newscaster talking about the patient on television) (see also answer to Question 9).

11. **The answer is D.** This man, who dresses strangely, shows poor grooming, and has paranoid delusions and auditory hallucinations over a prolonged period, is most likely to have schizophrenia. Neuropsychological evaluation of a patient with schizophrenia is most likely to reveal frontal lobe dysfunction. People with schizophrenia usually show intact memory; orientation to person, place, and time; and normal intelligence.

12. **The answer is C.** The chance that the son (or other first-degree relative) of a person with schizophrenia will develop the disorder over the course of his life is approximately 10%.

13. **The answer is D.** The chance that the identical twin of a person with schizophrenia will develop the disorder over the course of his or her life is approximately 50%.

14. **The answer is D.** Approximately 50% of patients with schizophrenia attempt suicide at some point in their lives.

15. **The answer is E.** Mood symptoms are associated with a good prognosis in schizophrenia. A good prognosis is also associated with older age of onset, positive symptoms, and few relapses. Catatonic symptoms are associated with a poor prognosis.

16. **The answer is C.** Auditory hallucinations are the most common type of hallucinations seen in schizophrenia.

17. **The answer is B.** This patient is showing evidence of schizoaffective disorder. This disorder is characterized by symptoms of a mood disorder, as well as psychotic symptoms (the delusion that he has been "chosen") as well as and lifelong social and occupational impairment (see also answer to Question 1). Schizoaffective disorder is distinguished from a mood disorder in that the psychotic symptoms persist in the absence of mood symptoms.

18. **The answer is E.** This patient is showing evidence of delusional disorder, persecutory type. In this disorder, there is a fixed, non-bizarre delusional system (paranoid in the persecutory type); few, if any, other thought disorders; and relatively normal social and occupational functioning (e.g., this patient is married and has held a job for over 30 years) (see also answer to Question 1).

19. **The answer is F.** This patient is showing evidence of shared psychotic disorder. She has developed the same delusion that her husband has (i.e., their house is filled with radioactive dust). If separated for a period of time from her husband (the inducer), her psychotic symptoms are likely to remit (see also answer to Question 1).

20. **The answer is A.** In patients with schizophrenia, the size of cerebral ventricles, glucose utilization in the frontal lobes, and size of limbic structures are most likely to be increased, decreased, and decreased, respectively.

# chapter 12 Mood Disorders

**Typical Board Question**

A 43-year-old school teacher relates that over the past year he has often felt that life is not worth living. He also notes that during this time he has noticed a gradual slowing of cognition, and the development of a gravelly voice, constipation, and hair loss. Physical examination is normal, except for noticeable dryness of the skin and a lag in the relaxation phase of the ankle jerk reflex. At this time, the most likely diagnosis for this patient is

**(A)** major depressive disorder
**(B)** bipolar I disorder
**(C)** bipolar II disorder
**(D)** dysthymic disorder
**(E)** cyclothymic disorder
**(F)** substance-induced mood disorder
**(G)** mood disorder due to a general medical condition

*(See "Answers and Explanations" at end of chapter.)*

## I. OVERVIEW

### A. Definitions

1. The mood or affective disorders are characterized by a primary **disturbance** in **internal emotional state**, causing subjective distress and problems in social and occupational functioning.

2. **Given the patient's current social and occupational situation** he or she emotionally feels
   a. somewhat worse than would be expected (**dysthymia**)
   b. very much worse than would be expected (**depression**)
   c. somewhat better than would be expected (**hypomania**)
   d. very much better than would be expected (**mania**)

3. The *Diagnostic and Statistical Manual of Mental Disorders, Fourth edition, Text Revision (DSM-IV-TR)* **categories** of primary mood disorders are
   a. **Major depressive disorder:** Recurrent episodes of depression, each continuing for at least **2 weeks**.
   b. **Bipolar disorder:** Episodes of both mania (continuing for at least **1 week**) and depression (**bipolar I disorder**) or both hypomania (continuing for at least **4 days**) and depression (**bipolar II disorder**).
   c. **Dysthymic disorder:** Dysthymia continuing over a **2-year** period (1 year in children) with no discrete episodes of illness.

   **d. Cyclothymic disorder:** Hypomania and dysthymia occurring over a **2-year** period (1 year in children) with no discrete episodes of illness.
   **e. Mood disorder due to a general medical condition and substance-induced mood disorder** are secondary mood disorders.

## B. Epidemiology
   1. There are **no differences** in the occurrence of mood disorders associated with ethnicity, education, marital status, or income.
   2. The **lifetime prevalence** of mood disorders is
      **a.** Major depressive disorder: 5%–12% for men; 10%–20% for women.
      **b.** Bipolar disorder: 1% overall; no sex difference.
      **c.** Dysthymic disorder: 6% overall; up to three times more common in women.
      **d.** Cyclothymic disorder: Less than 1% overall; no sex difference.

# II. CLASSIFICATION OF MOOD DISORDERS

## A. Major depressive disorder
   ### 1. Characteristics
      **a. SWAG** is a mnemonic device that can quickly identify depression and differentiate it from normal sadness. If one of the following symptoms is present, it is most likely that the patient is depressed:
      **(1) S** – Suicidality (having a plan or a means of self-destruction).
      **(2) W** – Weight loss (>5% of body weight).
      **(3) A** – Anhedonia (loss of pleasure or interest in usually pleasurable activities).
      **(4) G** – Guilt (feelings of responsibility for negative life events when little or none exists).
      **b. These and other symptoms** of depression are listed and described in Table 12.1.

table **12.1** Signs and Symptoms of Depression and Mania

| Depression | Likelihood of Occurrence |
| --- | --- |
| SWAG (suicidality, weight loss, anhedonia, guilt) symptom | ++++ |
| Sadness, hopelessness, helplessness, low self-esteem | ++++ |
| Reduced energy and motivation | ++++ |
| Anxiety (is apprehensive about imagined dangers) | ++++ |
| Sleep problems (wakes frequently at night and too early in the morning) | ++++ |
| Cognitive problems (has difficulty with memory and concentration) | +++ |
| Change in physical activity (psychomotor retardation or agitation) | +++ |
| Decreased or increased (in atypical depression) appetite for food and sex | +++ |
| Poor grooming | ++ |
| Diurnal variation in symptoms (worse in the morning, better in the evening) | ++ |
| Suicidal ideation (has thoughts of killing oneself) | ++ |
| Suicide (takes one's own life) | + |
| Psychotic symptoms (has delusions of destruction and fatal illness) | + |
| **Mania** | **Likelihood of Occurrence** |
| Elevated mood (has strong feelings of happiness and physical well-being) | ++++ |
| Grandiosity and expansiveness (has feelings of self-importance) | ++++ |
| Irritability and impulsivity (is easily bothered and quick to anger) | ++++ |
| Disinhibition (shows uncharacteristic lack of modesty in dress or behavior) | ++++ |
| Assaultiveness (cannot control aggressive impulses; causes legal problems) | ++++ |
| Distractibility (cannot concentrate on relevant stimuli) | ++++ |
| Flight of ideas (thoughts move rapidly from one to the other) | ++++ |
| Pressured speech (seems compelled to speak quickly) | ++++ |
| Impaired judgment (provides unusual responses to hypothetical questions, [e.g., says she would buy a blood bank if she inherited money]) | ++++ |
| Psychotic symptoms (has delusions of power and influence) | +++ |

Approximate percentage of patients in which the sign or symptom is seen: + <25%; ++ 50%; +++ 70%; ++++ >70%.

2. **Masked depression**
   a. As many as 50% of depressed patients seem unaware of or deny depression and thus are said to have "**masked depression**."
   b. Patients with masked depression often visit primary care doctors complaining of **vague physical symptoms**.
   c. In contrast to patients who have somatoform disorders (physical symptoms resulting from psychological factors; see Chapter 14) depressed patients show at least one SWAG symptom in addition to their physical complaints.
3. **Seasonal affective disorder (SAD)**
   a. SAD is a subtype of major depressive disorder associated with the winter season and short days.
   b. SAD is characterized by **atypical symptoms** of depression (e.g., oversleeping and over-eating) and a heavy feeling in the limbs ("leaden paralysis").
   c. Many SAD patients improve in response to full-spectrum **light exposure**.
4. **Suicide risk**
   a. Patients with mood disorders are at increased **risk for suicide**.
   b. Certain demographic, psychosocial, and physical factors affect this risk (Table 12.2).
   c. The top five risk factors for suicide from higher to lower risk are
      (1) serious prior suicide attempt
      (2) age older than 45 years
      (3) alcohol dependence
      (4) history of rage and violent behavior
      (5) male sex.

B. **Bipolar disorder**
   1. In bipolar disorder, there are episodes of **both mania and depression (bipolar I disorder)** or **both hypomania and depression (bipolar II disorder)**.
   2. There is no simple manic disorder because depressive symptoms eventually occur. Therefore, **one episode of symptoms of mania** (Table 12.1) alone or hypomania plus one episode of major depression defines bipolar disorder.
   3. **Psychotic symptoms**, such as delusions, can occur in depression (depression with psychotic features) as well as in mania.
      a. In some patients (e.g., poor patients with low access to health care), a mood disorder with psychotic symptoms can become severe enough to be **misdiagnosed as schizophrenia**.
      b. In contrast to schizophrenia and schizoaffective disorder, in which patients are chronically impaired, in mood disorders the patient's mood and functioning usually **return to normal** between episodes.

C. **Dysthymic disorder and cyclothymic disorder.** In contrast to major depressive disorder and bipolar disorder, respectively, dysthymic disorder and cyclothymic disorder are
   1. less severe
   2. nonepisodic
   3. chronic
   4. not associated with psychosis or suicide.

## III. ETIOLOGY

A. The **biologic** etiology of mood disorders includes
   1. **Altered neurotransmitter activity** (see Chapter 4).
   2. A **genetic component**, strongest in bipolar disorder (Table 12.3).
   3. **Physical illness** and related factors (Table 12.4).
   4. Abnormalities of the limbic–hypothalamic–pituitary–adrenal axis (see Chapter 5).

| t a b l e  **12.2**  Risk Factors for Suicide | | | |
|---|---|---|---|
| Category | Factor | Increased Risk | Decreased Risk |
| History | Personal history | Serious suicide attempt (about 30% of people who attempt suicide try again and 10% succeed) | Suicidal gesture, but not a serious attempt |
| | | <3 mos since previous attempt | >3 mos since previous attempt |
| | | Possibility of rescue was remote | Rescue was very likely |
| | Family history | Parent committed suicide | No family history of suicide |
| | | Early loss of a parent through divorce or death | Intact family throughout childhood |
| Current, social, psychological, and physical factors | Psychiatric symptoms | Depression | Dysthymia or no depressive symptoms |
| | | Psychotic symptoms | No psychotic symptoms |
| | | Hopelessness | Some hopefulness |
| | | Impulsiveness | Thinks things out |
| | Depth of depression | Initial stages of recovery from deep depression; recovering patients may have enough energy to commit suicide | The depth of severe depression; patients rarely have the clarity of thought or energy needed to plan and commit suicide |
| | Substance use | Alcohol and drug dependence | Little or no substance use |
| | | Current intoxication | |
| | Physical health | Serious medical illness (e.g., cancer, AIDS) | Good health |
| | | Perception of serious illness (most patients have visited a physician in the 6 mos prior to suicide) | No recent visit to a physician |
| | Social relationships | Divorced (particularly men) | Married |
| | | Widowed | Strong social support |
| | | Single, never married | Has children |
| | | Lives alone | Lives with others |
| Demographic factors | Age | Elderly (persons age 65 and older, especially men) | Children (up to age 15 yrs) |
| | | Middle-aged (over age 55 yrs in women and age 45 yrs in men) | Young adults (age 25–40 yrs) |
| | | Adolescents (suicide is the third leading cause of death in those 15–24 yrs of age; rates increase after neighborhood suicide of a teen or when media depict teenage suicide) | |
| | Sex | Male sex (men successfully commit suicide three times more often than women) | Female sex (although women attempt suicide three times more often than men) |
| | Occupation | Professionals | Non-professionals |
| | Specific occupation | Physicians (especially women and psychiatrists) | |
| | | Dentists and veterinarians | |
| | | Police officers | |
| | | Attorneys | |
| | | Musicians | |
| | | Unemployed | Employed |
| | Race | Caucasian | Non-Caucasian |
| | Religion | Not religious | Religious |
| | | Jewish | Catholic |
| | | Protestant | Muslim |
| | Economic conditions | Economic recession or depression | Strong economy |
| Lethality of attempt | Plan and means | A plan for suicide (e.g., decision to stockpile pills) | No plan for suicide |
| | | A means of committing suicide (e.g., access to a gun) | No means of suicide |
| | | Sudden appearance of peacefulness in an agitated, depressed patient (he has reached an internal decision to kill himself and is now calm) | |
| | Method | Shooting oneself | Taking pills or poison |
| | | Crashing one's vehicle | Slashing one's wrists |
| | | Hanging oneself | |
| | | Jumping from a high place | |

| table **12.3** The Genetics of Bipolar Disorder | |
|---|---|
| **Group** | **Approximate Occurrence (%)** |
| General population | 1 |
| Person who has one parent or sibling (or dizygotic twin) with bipolar disorder | 20 |
| Person who has two parents with bipolar disorder | 60 |
| Monozygotic twin of a person with bipolar disorder | 75 |

B. The **psychosocial** etiology of depression and dysthymia can include
   1. **Loss of a parent** in childhood.
   2. **Loss of a spouse or child** in adulthood.
   3. **Loss of health.**
   4. **Low self-esteem** and negative interpretation of life events.
   5. "**Learned helplessness**" (i.e., because attempts to escape bad situations in the past have proven futile, the person now feels helpless) (see Chapter 7).

C. Psychosocial factors are **not directly involved** in **the etiology of mania** or hypomania.

# IV. MANAGEMENT

A. **Overview**
   1. Depression is **successfully managed in most patients**.
   2. Only about **25% of patients with depression seek and receive treatment**.
      a. Patients do not seek treatment in part because Americans often believe that mental illness indicates **personal failure or weakness**.
      b. As in other illnesses, **women are more likely than men to seek treatment**.
   3. Untreated episodes of depression and mania are **usually self-limiting** and last approximately 6–12 months and 3 months, respectively.
   4. The **most effective management** of the mood disorders is **pharmacologic**.

B. **Pharmacologic management** (see Chapter 16)
   1. Treatment for depression and dysthymia includes **antidepressant agents** (e.g., heterocyclics, selective serotonin and selective serotonin and norepinephrine reuptake inhibitors [SSRIs and SNRIs], monoamine oxidase inhibitors [MAOIs], and stimulants).

| table **12.4** Differential Diagnosis of Depression | |
|---|---|
| **Medical Conditions** | **Psychiatric and Related Conditions** |
| Cancer, particularly pancreatic and other gastrointestinal tumors | Schizophrenia (particularly after an acute psychotic episode) |
| Viral illness (e.g., pneumonia, influenza, acquired immune deficiency syndrome [AIDS]) | Adjustment disorder |
| Endocrinologic abnormality (e.g., hypothyroidism, diabetes, Cushing's syndrome) | Anxiety disorder |
| | Normal reaction to a life loss, e.g., bereavement |
| Neurologic illness (e.g., Parkinson disease, multiple sclerosis, Huntington disease, dementia, stroke [particularly left frontal]) | Somatoform disorder |
| | Eating disorder |
| Nutritional deficiency (e.g., folic acid, $B_{12}$) | Drug and alcohol abuse (particularly use of sedatives and withdrawal from stimulants) |
| Renal or cardiopulmonary disease | Prescription drug use (e.g., reserpine, steroids, antihypertensives, antineoplastics) |

 2. **Mood stabilizers**
   a. **Lithium** and **anticonvulsants** such as carbamazepine (Tegretol) and divalproex (Depakote) are used to manage bipolar disorder.
   b. Mood stabilizers in doses similar to those used to manage bipolar disorder are the primary treatment for **cyclothymic disorder**.
   c. **Atypical antipsychotics** such as olanzapine (Zyprexa) and risperidone (Risperdal).
   d. **Sedative agents** such as lorazepam (Ativan) are used to manage acute manic episodes because they resolve symptoms quickly.

C. **Psychological management**
   1. Psychological management for depression and dysthymia includes psychoanalytic, interpersonal, family, behavioral, and cognitive therapies (see Chapter 17).
   2. **Psychological management in conjunction with medication is more effective** than either type of management alone.

D. **Electroconvulsive therapy (ECT)** (see Chapter 16). The primary indication for ECT **is major depressive disorder**. It is used when
   1. The symptoms **do not respond to antidepressant medications**.
   2. Antidepressants are too **dangerous or have intolerable side effects**. Thus, ECT may be particularly useful for **elderly patients**.
   3. **Rapid resolution** of symptoms is necessary (e.g., the patient is acutely **suicidal** or **psychotic**).

# Review Test

**Directions:** Each of the numbered items or incomplete statements in this section is followed by answers or by completions of the statement. Select the **one** lettered answer or completion that is **best** in each case.

**1.** A 65-year-old woman, who was diagnosed with advanced lung cancer 3 months ago, has lost 18 pounds, wakes frequently during the night, and has very little energy. Over the past month she has been preoccupied with feelings of guilt about "people I have hurt in my life" and expresses concern that she will die in pain. The sign or symptom most likely to indicate that this patient is experiencing a major depressive episode rather than a normal reaction to life-limiting illness is

(A) weight loss
(B) decreased energy
(C) difficulty sleeping
(D) preoccupation with feelings of guilt
(E) concern about dying in pain

## Questions 2–4

A 20-year-old male college student is taken to the emergency department by police because he tried to enter a state office building to "have a conference with the governor" about conducting a fund drive to "finance my cure for cancer." When police prevent him from entering the building, he becomes irritable and hostile and resists attempts to restrain him.

**2.** The most appropriate diagnosis for this patient is

(A) dysthymic disorder
(B) major depressive disorder
(C) bipolar disorder
(D) hypochondriasis
(E) cyclothymic disorder

**3.** The most effective long-term management for this patient is

(A) a heterocyclic antidepressant
(B) lithium
(C) electroconvulsive therapy
(D) psychotherapy
(E) a monoamine oxidase inhibitor

**4.** This college student has two brothers. The first is his monozygotic twin; the second is 2 years younger. The risks that his first and second brothers will develop bipolar disorder are respectively about

(A) 75% and 60%
(B) 75% and 20%
(C) 60% and 10%
(D) 50% and 10%
(E) 10% and 1%

## Questions 5 and 6

For the past few months, a 28-year-old woman has seemed full of energy and optimism for no obvious reason. Although she gets only about 6 hours of sleep a night, she has been very productive at work. She is talkative and gregarious and relates that she belongs to four clubs and two different sports teams. A few years previously, friends say she was often pessimistic and seemed tired and "washed out." During that period, she continued to work but did not seek out social activities and had little interest in sex. There is no evidence of a thought disorder and the patient denies suicidality or hopelessness. Physical examination including body weight is normal.

**5.** This patient shows evidence of

(A) dysthymic disorder
(B) major depressive disorder
(C) bipolar disorder
(D) hypochondriasis
(E) cyclothymic disorder

**6.** The most effective long-term management for this patient is

(A) a heterocyclic antidepressant
(B) lithium
(C) electroconvulsive therapy
(D) psychotherapy
(E) a monoamine oxidase inhibitor

11. **The answer is I.** The Wisconsin Card Sorting Test is the most appropriate test for evaluating abstract reasoning and problem solving in a patient. In this test a patient is asked to sort 128 response cards that vary in color, form, and number.

12. **The answer is E.** A false belief, in this case that the CIA is listening to one's telephone conversations through the television set, is an example of a delusion. A hallucination is a false perception, and an illusion is a misperception of reality (see also Table 11.1). Clouding of consciousness is the inability to respond to external events, while blunted affect is a decreased display of emotional responses.

**Questions 7 and 8**

A 62-year-old woman whose husband died 6 months ago tells her physician that she believes killing herself would end her suffering. Physical examination is unremarkable.

**7.** Of the following signs and symptoms, which is most likely to be seen in this patient?

(A) Weight gain
(B) Flight of ideas
(C) Auditory hallucinations
(D) Feeling better in the morning than in the evening
(E) Poor grooming

**8.** Analysis of neurotransmitter availability in the brain of this patient is most likely to reveal

(A) increased dopamine
(B) decreased histamine
(C) increased acetylcholine
(D) decreased acetylcholine
(E) decreased serotonin

**9.** A 25-year-old male patient who is slow moving and has a flat affect is put on fluoxetine (Prozac). Within 2 weeks, the patient is showing greatly increased activity level, flight of ideas, and pressured speech. In this patient, the medication has

(A) precipitated a manic episode
(B) had a toxic effect
(C) had a delayed effect
(D) increased anxiety
(E) increased depression

**10.** A 35-year-old physician tells his internist that he has lost interest in playing in the hospital string quartet, an activity he formerly enjoyed. He reports that over the past 3 months he commonly wakes up a few hours before his alarm goes off and cannot fall back to sleep, and has lost 12 pounds without dieting. He states "maybe my family would be better off without me." He says that although he has lots of aches and pains and often feels tired, he feels somewhat better as the day progresses. Physical examination and laboratory studies are unremarkable. The most appropriate diagnosis for this patient is

(A) dysthymic disorder
(B) major depressive disorder
(C) masked depression
(D) hypochondriasis
(E) cyclothymic disorder
(F) malingering
(G) bipolar disorder

**11.** A 28-year-old man comes in complaining of headaches and a variety of other aches and pains that have been present for the past 6 months. He denies that he is sad or hopeless. After a 4-week trial of antidepressant medication, the patient's physical complaints have disappeared. The most appropriate diagnosis for this patient is

(A) dysthymic disorder
(B) major depressive disorder
(C) masked depression
(D) hypochondriasis
(E) cyclothymic disorder
(F) malingering
(G) bipolar disorder

**Questions 12–14**

A 65-year-old Catholic male patient has been abusing alcohol for the past 15 years. His history reveals that his wife recently asked him for a separation.

**12.** Which of the following characteristics is this patient's greatest risk factor for suicide?

(A) Alcoholism
(B) Male sex
(C) Marital separation
(D) Religion
(E) Age

**13.** This man is at the lowest risk for suicide if he works as a

(A) messenger
(B) policeman
(C) physician
(D) lawyer
(E) dentist

**14.** If this patient tries to commit suicide, the method most likely to fail is

(A) shooting himself with a gun
(B) crashing his car
(C) slashing his wrists
(D) jumping from a high place
(E) hanging himself

**15.** The percentage of depressed patients who seek treatment for their symptoms is about

(A) 1%
(B) 5%
(C) 25%
(D) 50%
(E) 75%

**16.** A 15-year-old girl is brought to the emergency room after ingesting 20 acetaminophen tablets. She tells the physician that she tried to commit suicide because she was not admitted to an honors English class. The girl is the president of her grade in school and always tries to be perfect. The most important factor in whether this girl tries to kill herself again is

**(A)** that she is female
**(B)** the method of the suicide attempt
**(C)** that she has major depressive disorder
**(D)** that she tried to commit suicide once
**(E)** her need to be perfect

**17.** When compared with a man, the chances that a woman will develop major depressive disorder, dysthymic disorder, or bipolar disorder over the course of her lifetime are, respectively

**(A)** higher, higher, equal
**(B)** higher, higher, lower
**(C)** higher, equal, higher
**(D)** higher, higher, higher
**(E)** equal, higher, equal
**(F)** equal, higher, lower
**(G)** equal, equal, equal

**18.** A 30-year-old financial consultant tells her doctor that over the past 5 years she has felt "down" most of the time. She relates that when colleagues ask her to dinner or to a get-together she usually says "yes" but then rarely feels like going when the time comes and does not have a good time when she does go. There are no significant physical findings. While the patient denies suicidality, she notes that she never feels really excited or happy about anything. The best diagnosis for this patient at this time is

**(A)** major depressive disorder
**(B)** bipolar I disorder
**(C)** bipolar II disorder
**(D)** dysthymic disorder
**(E)** cyclothymic disorder
**(F)** substance-induced mood disorder
**(G)** mood disorder due to a general medical condition

**19.** A 45-year-old man with bipolar disorder tells his doctor that he has remarried and would like to have a child with his new wife. He is concerned because the 19-year-old daughter that he had with his first wife has just been diagnosed with bipolar disorder. Neither of the patient's wives has bipolar disorder. What is the probability that this patient will have another child with bipolar disorder?

**(A)** 1%
**(B)** 10%
**(C)** 20%
**(D)** 50%
**(E)** 70%

# Answers and Explanations

**The answer is G.** The most likely diagnosis at this time is mood disorder due to a general medical condition. This patient is showing symptoms of hypothyroidism, for example, slowing of cognition, gravelly voice, constipation, dry skin, hair loss, and lag in the relaxation phase of the ankle jerk reflex, in addition to symptoms of major depression (e.g., suicidality). Other mood disorders are diagnosed when there are no medical findings to explain the mood symptoms. For example, major depressive disorder involves at least one SWAG symptom most of the time for a period of at least 2 weeks. Dysthymic disorder involves mild or moderate depression most of the time, occurring over a 2-year period with no discrete episodes of symptoms. Bipolar disorder involves episodes of both mania and depression (bipolar I) or hypomania and depression (bipolar II). Cyclothymic disorder involves episodes of hypomania and dysthymia occurring over a 2-year period with no discrete episodes of symptoms

1. **The answer is D.** The sign or symptom most likely to indicate that this patient is experiencing a major depressive episode rather than a normal reaction to serious illness is her preoccupation with feelings of guilt. Such feelings are more characteristic of depression than sadness about being very ill. The other symptoms that the patient shows (e.g., weight loss, decreased energy, and sleep problems) are characteristic of patients with advanced cancer. Fear of dying in pain is realistic and commonly seen in patients with life-limiting illnesses.

2. **The answer is C. 3. The answer is B. 4. The answer is B.** This patient is most likely to have bipolar I disorder. While this disorder involves episodes of both mania and depression, a single episode of mania defines the illness. The beliefs that one is important enough to demand a conference with the governor and cure cancer are grandiose delusions. Schizophrenic delusions are commonly paranoid in nature. Irritability and hostility are also common in a manic episode. Of the listed treatments, the one most effective for bipolar disorder is lithium. Heterocyclic antidepressants, electroconvulsive therapy, monoamine oxidase inhibitors, and psychotherapy are used primarily to manage depression. Antidepressants and psychotherapy are used to manage dysthymia. The chances of the monozygotic twin and first-degree relative (e.g., brother) of this bipolar patient developing the disorder are about 75% and 20%, respectively.

5. **The answer is E. 6. The answer is B.** This patient shows evidence of cyclothymic disorder. This disorder involves periods of both hypomania (energy and optimism) and dysthymia (pessimism and feeling "washed out") occurring over a 2-year period with no discrete episodes of illness. Of the listed treatments, the one most effective for cyclothymic disorder, as for bipolar disorder, is lithium. Heterocyclic antidepressants, electroconvulsive therapy, monoamine oxidase inhibitors, and psychotherapy are primarily used to manage depression. Antidepressants and psychotherapy are used to manage dysthymia.

7. **The answer is E. 8. The answer is E.** This woman is showing evidence of major depression (note: Suicidality is *not* characteristic of a normal grief reaction). Depressed people typically show poor grooming. She is also more likely to show weight loss, and to feel better in the evening than in the morning. Auditory hallucinations are common in schizophrenia but uncommon in depression. Flight of ideas is characteristic of mania. Analysis of neurotransmitter availability in this patient is most likely to reveal decreased serotonin, commonly reflected in decreased plasma levels of its major metabolite 5-HIAA. Increased dopamine is seen in schizophrenia, and decreased acetylcholine is seen in Alzheimer disease.

9. **The answer is A.** In this depressed patient, the antidepressant fluoxetine has precipitated a manic episode (i.e., greatly increased activity level, flight of ideas, and pressured speech). This indicates that the patient has bipolar disorder rather than major depressive disorder. There is no evidence of increased depression, increased anxiety, or a delayed or toxic effect in this patient.

10. **The answer is B.** This patient is most likely to have major depressive disorder. Evidence for this is that, while there are no physical findings, he has lost interest in his usual activities, wakes up too early in the morning, has vague physical symptoms, shows diurnal variation in symptoms (worse in the morning), has lost a significant amount of weight, and is showing suicidal ideation (e.g., "maybe my family would be better off without me"). Also, his symptoms have been present for a discrete, identified amount of time. Dysthymic disorder involves mild or moderate depression most of the time, occurring over a 2-year period with no discrete episodes of illness. Bipolar disorder involves episodes of both mania and depression. Cyclothymic disorder involves episodes of hypomania and dysthymia occurring over a 2-year period with no discrete episodes of illness. In hypochondriasis, patients believe that normal body functions or minor illnesses are serious or life threatening. People who are malingering fabricate symptoms for obvious gain (e.g., to win a lawsuit) (see Chapter 13).

11. **The answer is C.** This patient's physical complaints (i.e., headaches and other aches and pains) were relieved by antidepressant medication. This indicates that these symptoms were manifestations of masked (hidden) depression rather than hypochondriasis. There is no evidence in this patient of bipolar disorder, dysthymic disorder, cyclothymic disorder, or malingering (see also answer to Question 10).

12. **The answer is E. 13. The answer is A. 14. The answer is C.** Although male sex, alcohol abuse, and marital separation all are risk factors for suicide, the highest risk factor of those mentioned is his advanced age. Catholic religion is associated with a reduced risk of suicide. Nonprofessionals are at a lower suicide risk than professionals. Among professionals, those at the highest risk for suicide are police officers, physicians, lawyers, and dentists. The method of suicide most likely to fail is slashing the wrists or taking pills. Shooting, crashing a car, jumping from a high place, and hanging are more lethal methods of committing suicide.

15. **The answer is C.** Only about 25% of depressed patients seek treatment, although management (antidepressants, psychotherapy, electroconvulsive therapy) is effective in most depressed patients.

16. **The answer is D.** This girl shows a number of risk factors for depression and attempted suicide, including female sex and her excessive need to be perfect. However, the most important factor in whether she tries to kill herself again is that she tried to commit suicide once. Taking pills such as aspirin or acetaminophen is less lethal than other methods, but young people such as this teenager may not know this. Thus, this girl has made a serious suicide attempt. (See also answers to Questions 12–14.)

17. **The answer is A.** When compared with a man, a woman is twice as likely to develop major depressive disorder, and three times as likely to develop dysthymic disorder. Bipolar disorder and cyclothymic disorder occur equally in men and women.

18. **The answer is D.** This best diagnosis for this patient is dysthymic disorder. The patient has had a low mood for years, but although she is never really happy or excited about what should be pleasant experiences, because she is functional. For example, she is working and is not suicidal, it is less likely that she has major depressive disorder (and see also answer to Question 10).

19. **The answer is C.** The likelihood that this man with bipolar disorder will have a child with bipolar disorder is about 20%. The fact that his older child has bipolar disorder is not relevant to the chances that his next child will have the disorder (and see also answer to Question 2).

# chapter 13

# Anxiety Disorders, Somatoform Disorders, and Related Conditions

**Typical Board Question**

A 15-year-old boy is brought to the doctor by his mother for "strange behavior." She reports that her son is often late for school because he spends more than an hour in the shower every morning. When asked about this, he says that he takes a long time because he feels compelled to wash himself in a certain manner, and has to repeat the whole process if he makes a mistake. He knows that this behavior sounds ridiculous, and that it makes him late for school and other activities, but he cannot seem to stop himself from doing it. There are no significant medical findings. Which of the following disorders best fits this clinical picture?

(A) Post-traumatic stress disorder
(B) Hypochondriasis
(C) Obsessive–compulsive disorder
(D) Panic disorder
(E) Somatization disorder
(F) Generalized anxiety disorder
(G) Body dysmorphic disorder
(H) Conversion disorder
(I) Specific phobia
(J) Social phobia
(K) Adjustment disorder
(L) Masked depression

*(See "Answers and Explanations" at end of chapter.)*

# I. ANXIETY DISORDERS

A. **Fear and anxiety**
1. **Fear** is a normal reaction to a known, external source of danger.
2. In **anxiety**, the individual is frightened but the source of the danger is not known, not recognized, or **inadequate to account for the symptoms**.
3. The **physiologic manifestations** of anxiety are similar to those of fear. They include
   a. Shakiness and sweating
   b. Palpitations (subjective experience of tachycardia)
   c. Tingling in the extremities and numbness around the mouth
   d. Dizziness and syncope (fainting)
   e. Gastrointestinal and urinary disturbances (e.g., diarrhea and urinary frequency)
   f. Mydriasis (pupil dilation)

130

B. **Classification and occurrence of the anxiety disorders**
1. The *Diagnostic and Statistical Manual of Mental Disorders, Fourth Edition, Text Revision (DSM-IV-TR)* classification of anxiety disorders includes
   a. Panic disorder (with or without agoraphobia)
   b. Phobias (specific and social)
   c. Obsessive–compulsive disorder (OCD)
   d. Generalized anxiety disorder (GAD)
   e. Post-traumatic stress disorder (PTSD)
   f. Acute stress disorder (ASD)
2. Descriptions of these disorders can be found in **Table 13.1. Adjustment disorder** is not an anxiety disorder but it is included in this table because it is very common and also because it often must be distinguished from PTSD.
3. The anxiety disorders are the **most commonly treated** mental health problems.

C. **The organic basis of anxiety**
1. Neurotransmitters involved in the development of anxiety include norepinephrine (increased activity), serotonin (decreased activity), and g-aminobutyric acid (GABA) (decreased activity) (see Chapter 4).
2. The **locus ceruleus** (site of noradrenergic neurons), **raphe nucleus** (site of serotonergic neurons), caudate nucleus (particularly in OCD), temporal cortex, and frontal cortex are the brain areas likely to be involved in anxiety disorders.
3. Organic causes of symptoms of anxiety include **excessive caffeine intake**, substance abuse, hyperthyroidism, vitamin $B_{12}$ deficiency, hypoglycemia or hyperglycemia, cardiac arrhythmia, anemia, pulmonary disease, and **pheochromocytoma** (adrenal medullary tumor).
4. If the etiology is primarily organic, the diagnoses **substance-induced anxiety disorder** or **anxiety disorder caused by a general medical condition** may be appropriate.

D. **Management of the anxiety disorders**
1. **Antianxiety agents** (see Chapter 16), including benzodiazepines, buspirone, and β-blockers, are used to treat the symptoms of anxiety.
   a. **Benzodiazepines** are fast-acting antianxiety agents.
      (1) Because they carry a high risk of dependence and addiction, they are usually **used for only a limited amount of time** to treat acute anxiety symptoms.
      (2) Because they work quickly, benzodiazepines, particularly **alprazolam (Xanax)**, are used for emergency department management of **panic attacks**.
   b. **Buspirone (BuSpar)** is a non-benzodiazepine antianxiety agent.
      (1) Because of its **low abuse potential**, buspirone is useful as **long-term maintenance** therapy for patients with **GAD**.
      (2) Because it **takes up to 2 weeks to work**, buspirone has little immediate effect on anxiety symptoms.
   c. The **β-blockers**, such as **propranolol (Inderal)**, are used to control **autonomic symptoms** (e.g., tachycardia) in anxiety disorders, particularly for anxiety about performing in public or taking an examination.
2. **Antidepressants** (see Chapter 16)
   a. Antidepressants, including monoamine oxidase inhibitors (MAOIs), tricyclics, and especially **selective serotonin reuptake inhibitors (SSRIs)**, such as paroxetine (Paxil), fluoxetine (Prozac), and sertraline (Zoloft), are the most effective long-term (maintenance) therapy for panic disorder and OCD and have shown efficacy also in PTSD.
   b. Recently, SSRIs (e.g., escitalopram [Lexapro]) and the **selective serotonin and norepinephrine reuptake inhibitors (SNRIs)** venlafaxine (Effexor) and duloxetine (Cymbalta) were approved to treat GAD.
   c. Paroxetine, sertraline, and venlafaxine now also are indicated in the management of **social phobia**.
3. **Psychological management** (see also Chapter 17)
   a. **Systematic desensitization** and **cognitive therapy** (see Chapter 17) are the most effective management for phobias and are useful adjuncts to pharmacotherapy in other anxiety disorders.

| t a b l e    **13.1**    *DSM-IV-TR* Classification of the Anxiety Disorders and Adjustment Disorder |
|---|

**Panic Disorder (with or without Agoraphobia)**

Episodic (about twice weekly) periods of intense anxiety (panic attacks)

Cardiac and respiratory symptoms and the conviction that one is about to die or lose one's mind

Sudden onset of symptoms, increasing in intensity over a period of approximately 10 min, and lasting about 30 min (attacks rarely follow a fixed pattern)

Attacks can be induced by administration of sodium lactate or $CO_2$ (see Chapter 5)

Strong genetic component

More common in young women in their 20s

In panic disorder with agoraphobia, characteristics and symptoms of panic disorder (see above) are associated with fear of open places or situations in which the patient cannot escape or obtain help (agoraphobia)

Panic disorder with agoraphobia is associated with separation anxiety disorder in childhood (see Chapter 15)

**Phobias (Specific and Social)**

In specific phobia, there is an irrational fear of certain things (e.g., elevators, snakes, or closed-in areas)

In social phobia (aka social anxiety disorder), there is an exaggerated fear of embarrassment in social situations (e.g., public speaking, eating in public, using public restrooms)

Because of the fear, the patient avoids the object or situation

Avoidance leads to social and occupational impairment

**Obsessive–Compulsive Disorder (OCD)**

Recurring, intrusive feelings, thoughts, and images (obsessions) that cause anxiety

Anxiety is relieved in part by performing repetitive actions (compulsions)

A common obsession is avoidance of hand contamination and a compulsive need to wash the hands after touching things

Obsessive doubts lead to compulsive checking (e.g., of gas jets on the stove) and counting of objects, obsessive need for symmetry leads to compulsive ordering and arranging, and obsessive concern about discarding valuables leads to compulsive hoarding

Patients usually have insight (i.e., they realize that these thoughts and behaviors are irrational and want to eliminate them)

Usually starts in early adulthood, but may begin in childhood

Genetic factors are involved

Increased in first-degree relatives of Tourette disorder patients

**Generalized Anxiety Disorder**

Persistent anxiety symptoms including hyperarousal and worrying lasting 6 mos or more

Gastrointestinal symptoms are common

Symptoms are not related to a specific person or situation (i.e., free-floating anxiety)

Commonly starts during the 20s

**Post-Traumatic Stress Disorder (PTSD) and Acute Stress Disorder (ASD)**

Symptoms occurring after a catastrophic (life-threatening or potentially fatal event, e.g., war, house fire, serious accident, rape, robbery) affecting the patient or the patient's close friend or relative

Symptoms can be divided into four types:
(1) Reexperiencing (e.g., intrusive memories of the event [flashbacks] and nightmares)
(2) Hyperarousal (e.g., anxiety, increased startle response, impaired sleep, hypervigilance)
(3) Emotional numbing (e.g., difficulty connecting with others)
(4) Avoidance (e.g., survivor's guilt, dissociation, and social withdrawal)

In PTSD, symptoms last for more than 1 mo (sometimes years) and may have a delayed onset

In ASD, symptoms last only between 2 days and 4 wks

**Adjustment Disorder**

Emotional symptoms (e.g., anxiety, depression, or conduct problems) causing social, school, or work impairment occurring within 3 mos and lasting less than 6 mos after a serious life event (e.g., divorce, bankruptcy, changing residence) but do not meet full criteria for a mood or anxiety disorder

Symptoms can persist for more than 6 mos in the presence of a chronic stressor

Not diagnosed if the symptoms represent typical bereavement

**b.** Behavioral therapies, such as flooding and implosion, also are useful.
**c.** Support groups (e.g., victim survivor groups) are particularly useful for ASD and PTSD.

# II. SOMATOFORM DISORDERS

**A. Characteristics and classification**
1. Somatoform disorders are characterized by **physical symptoms without explainable organic cause**.
2. The patient thinks that the symptoms have an organic cause but the symptoms are believed to be **psychological**, and thus are unconscious expressions of unacceptable feelings (see Chapter 6).
3. Most somatoform disorders are **more common in women**, although **hypochondriasis occurs equally** in men and women.
4. The *DSM-IV-TR* **categories** of somatoform disorders and their characteristics are listed in Table 13.2.

**B. Differential diagnosis**
1. The most important differential diagnosis of the somatoform disorders is **unidentified organic disease**.
2. Factitious disorder (see below), malingering (faking or feigning illness), and masked depression (see Chapter 12) also must be excluded.

**C. Management**
1. Effective strategies for managing patients with somatoform disorders include
   a. Forming a **good physician–patient relationship** (e.g., scheduling regular monthly appointments, providing reassurance)
   b. Providing a **multidisciplinary approach** including other medical professionals (e.g., pain management, mental health services)
   c. Identifying and **decreasing the social difficulties** in the patient's life that may intensify the symptoms
2. **Antianxiety** and **antidepressant agents, hypnosis**, and **behavioral relaxation therapy** also may be useful.

**table  13.2** *DSM-IV-TR* Classification of the Somatoform Disorders

| Classification | Characteristics |
| --- | --- |
| Somatization disorder | History over years of at least two gastrointestinal symptoms (e.g., nausea), four pain symptoms, one sexual symptom (e.g., menstrual problems), and one pseudoneurological symptom (e.g., paralysis)<br>Onset before 30 yrs of age |
| Hypochondriasis | Exaggerated concern with health and illness lasting at least 6 mos<br>Concern persists despite medical evaluation and reassurance<br>More common in middle and old age<br>Goes to many different doctors seeking help ("doctor shopping") |
| Conversion disorder | Sudden, dramatic loss of sensory or motor function (e.g., blindness, paralysis), often associated with a stressful life event<br>More common in unsophisticated adolescents and young adults<br>Patients appear relatively unworried ("la belle indifférence") |
| Body dysmorphic disorder | Excessive focus on a minor or imagined physical defect<br>Symptoms are not accounted for by anorexia nervosa (see Chapter 14)<br>Onset usually in the late teens |
| Pain disorder | Intense acute or chronic pain not explained completely by physical disease and closely associated with psychological stress<br>Onset usually in the 30s and 40s |

| table | 13.3 | Factitious Disorder, Factitious Disorder by Proxy, and Malingering |

| Disorder | Characteristics |
|---|---|
| Factitious disorder (formerly Munchausen syndrome) | Conscious simulation of physical or psychiatric illness to gain attention from medical personnel<br>Undergoes unnecessary medical and surgical procedures<br>Has a "grid abdomen" (multiple crossed scars from repeated surgeries) |
| Factitious disorder by proxy | Conscious simulation of illness in another person, typically in a child by a parent, to obtain attention from medical personnel<br>Is a form of child abuse (see Chapter 18) because the child undergoes unnecessary medical and surgical procedures<br>Must be reported to child welfare authorities (state social service agency) |
| Malingering | Conscious simulation or exaggeration of physical or psychiatric illness for financial (e.g., insurance settlement) or other obvious gain (e.g., avoiding incarceration)<br>Avoids treatment by medical personnel<br>Health complaints cease as soon as the desired gain is obtained |

## III. FACTITIOUS DISORDER (FORMERLY MUNCHAUSEN SYNDROME), FACTITIOUS DISORDER BY PROXY, AND MALINGERING

A. **Characteristics**
  1. While individuals with somatoform disorders truly believe that they are ill, patients with factitious disorders and malingering **feign mental** or **physical illness**, or actually **induce physical illness** in themselves or others for psychological gain (factitious disorder) or tangible gain (malingering) (Table 13.3).
  2. Patients with factitious disorder often have worked in the medical field (e.g., nurses, technicians) and know how to persuasively simulate an illness.
  3. Malingering is not a psychiatric disorder.

B. **Feigned symptoms** most commonly include abdominal pain, fever (by heating the thermometer), blood in the urine (by adding blood from a needle stick), induction of tachycardia (by drug administration), skin lesions (by injuring easily reached areas), and seizures.

C. When confronted by the physician with the fact that no organic cause can be found, patients with factitious disorder or patients who are malingering typically become **angry and abruptly leave the situation**.

# Review Test

**Directions:** Each of the numbered items or incomplete statements in this section is followed by answers or by completions of the statement. Select the **one** lettered answer or completion that is **best** in each case.

## Questions 1–3

A 23-year-old medical student comes to the emergency room with elevated heart rate, sweating, and shortness of breath. The student is convinced that she is having an asthma attack and that she will suffocate. The symptoms started suddenly during a car ride to school. The student has had episodes such as this on at least three previous occasions over the past 2 weeks and now is afraid to leave the house even to go to school. She has no history of asthma and, other than an increased pulse rate, physical findings are unremarkable.

**1.** Of the following, the most effective immediate treatment for this patient is

(A) an antidepressant
(B) a support group
(C) a benzodiazepine
(D) buspirone
(E) a β-blocker

**2.** Of the following, the most effective long-term management for this patient is

(A) an antidepressant
(B) a support group
(C) a benzodiazepine
(D) buspirone
(E) a β-blocker

**3.** The neural mechanism most closely involved in the etiology of this patient's symptoms is

(A) nucleus accumbens hyposensitivity
(B) ventral tegmental hypersensitivity
(C) ventral tegmental hyposensitivity
(D) locus ceruleus hypersensitivity
(E) peripheral autonomic hypersensitivity

**4.** A 35-year-old woman who was raped 5 years ago has recurrent vivid memories of the incident accompanied by intense anxiety. These memories frequently intrude during her daily activities, and nightmares about the event often wake her. Her symptoms intensified when a coworker was raped 2 months ago. Of the following, the most effective long-term management for this patient is

(A) an antidepressant
(B) a support group
(C) a benzodiazepine
(D) buspirone
(E) a β-blocker

## Questions 5 and 6

A 45-year-old woman says that she frequently feels "nervous" and often has an "upset stomach," which includes heartburn, indigestion, and diarrhea. She has had this problem since she was 25 years of age and notes that other family members also are "tense and nervous."

**5.** Which of the following additional signs or symptoms is this patient most likely to show?

(A) Flight of ideas
(B) Hallucinations
(C) Tingling in the extremities
(D) Ideas of reference
(E) Neologisms

**6.** Of the following, the most effective long-term management for this patient is

(A) alprazolam (Xanax)
(B) psychotherapy
(C) propranolol (Inderal)
(D) buspirone (BuSpar)
(E) diazepam (Valium)

**7.** A 39-year-old woman claims that she injured her hand at work. She asserts that the pain caused by her injury prevents her from working. She has no further hand problems after she receives a $30,000 workers' compensation settlement. This clinical presentation is an example of

(A) factitious disorder
(B) conversion disorder
(C) factitious disorder by proxy
(D) somatization disorder
(E) somatoform pain disorder
(F) malingering

**8.** Which of the following events is most likely to result in post-traumatic stress disorder (PTSD)?

(A) Divorce
(B) Bankruptcy
(C) Diagnosis of diabetes mellitus
(D) Changing residence
(E) Robbery at knifepoint

**Questions 9 and 10**

A 39-year-old woman takes her 6-year-old son to a physician's office. She says that the child often experiences episodes of breathing problems and abdominal pain. The child's medical record shows many office visits and four abdominal surgical procedures, although no abnormalities were ever found. Physical examination and laboratory studies are unremarkable. When the doctor confronts the mother with the suspicion that she is fabricating the illness in the child, the mother angrily grabs the child and leaves the office immediately.

**9.** This clinical presentation is an example of

(A) factitious disorder
(B) conversion disorder
(C) factitious disorder by proxy
(D) somatization disorder
(E) somatoform pain disorder
(F) malingering

**10.** In this situation, what is the first thing the physician should do?

(A) Take the child aside and ask him how he feels.
(B) Call a pediatric pulmonologist to determine the cause of the dyspnea.
(C) Call a pediatric gastroenterologist to determine the cause of the abdominal pain.
(D) Notify the appropriate state social service agency to report the physician's suspicions.
(E) Wait until the child's next visit before taking any action.

**Questions 11–18**

For each of the following cases, select the disorder which best fits the clinical picture.

(A) Post-traumatic stress disorder
(B) Hypochondriasis
(C) Obsessive–compulsive disorder
(D) Panic disorder
(E) Somatization disorder
(F) Generalized anxiety disorder
(G) Body dysmorphic disorder
(H) Conversion disorder
(I) Specific phobia
(J) Social phobia
(K) Adjustment disorder
(L) Masked depression

**11.** A 45-year-old woman has a 20-year history of vague physical complaints including nausea, painful menses, and loss of feeling in her legs. Physical examination and laboratory workup are unremarkable. She says that she has always had physical problems but her doctors never seem to identify their cause.

**12.** Three months after moving, a teenager who was formerly outgoing and a good student seems sad, loses interest in making friends, and begins to do poor work in school. His appetite is normal and there is no evidence of suicidal ideation.

**13.** A 29-year-old man experiences sudden right-sided hemiparesis, but appears unconcerned. He reports that just before the onset of weakness, he saw his girlfriend with another man. Physical examination fails to reveal evidence of a medical problem.

**14.** A 41-year-old man says that he has been "sickly" for most of his life. He has seen many doctors but is angry with most of them because they ultimately referred him for psychological help. He now fears that he has stomach cancer because his stomach makes noises after he eats. Physical examination is unremarkable and body weight is normal.

**15.** A 41-year-old man says that he has been "sickly" for the past 3 months. He fears that he has stomach cancer. The patient is unshaven and appears thin and slowed down. Physical examination, including a gastrointestinal workup, is unremarkable except that there is an unexplained loss of 15 pounds since his last visit 1 year ago.

**16.** A 28-year-old woman seeks facial reconstructive surgery for her "sagging" eyelids. She rarely goes out in the daytime because she believes that this characteristic makes her look "like a grandmother." On physical examination, her eyelids appear completely normal.

**17.** A 29-year-old man is upset because he must take a client to dinner in a restaurant. Although he knows the client well, he is so afraid of making a mess while eating that he says he is not hungry and sips from a glass of water instead of ordering a meal.

**18.** A 29-year-old man tells the doctor that he has been so "nervous" and upset since his girlfriend broke up with him 1 month ago that he had to quit his job and stay at home. The man has no history of medical or psychiatric disorders, although his father has a history of bipolar disorder, his mother has a history of alcoholism, and his younger brother was in rehab for drug abuse the previous year.

**19.** A 35-year-old nurse is brought to the emergency room after fainting outside of a patient's room. The nurse notes that she has had fainting episodes before and that she often feels weak and shaky. Laboratory studies reveal hypoglycemia, very high insulin level, and suppressed plasma C peptide. Which of the following best fits this clinical picture?

(A) A sleep disorder
(B) An anxiety
(C) A somatoform disorder
(D) Malingering
(E) An endocrine disorder
(F) A factitious disorder

**20.** A 22-year-old man is brought into the emergency room by the police. The policeman tells the physician that the man was caught while attempting to rob a bank. When the police told him to freeze and drop his gun, the man dropped to the floor and could not speak, but remained conscious. When the doctor attempts to interview him, the patient repeatedly falls asleep. The history reveals that the patient's brother has narcolepsy. Which of the following best fits this clinical picture?

(A) A sleep disorder
(B) A seizure disorder
(C) A somatoform disorder
(D) Malingering
(E) An endocrine disorder
(F) A factitious disorder

**21.** A 12-year-old boy is admitted to the hospital with a diagnosis of "pain of unknown origin." His parents tell the physician that the child has complained about pain in his legs for about 1 month. Neurologic and orthopedic examinations fail to identify any pathology. The history reveals that the child was hospitalized on two previous occasions for other pain symptoms for which no cause was found. After 4 days in the hospital, the nurse reports that the child shows little evidence of pain and seems "remarkably content." She also reports that she found a medical textbook in the boy's bedside table with a bookmark in the section entitled "skeletal pain of unknown origin." Which of the following best describes symptom production and motivation in this case?

(A) Symptom production conscious, motivation primarily conscious
(B) Symptom production unconscious, motivation primarily conscious
(C) Symptom production conscious, motivation primarily unconscious
(D) Symptom production unconscious, motivation primarily unconscious

**22.** A 40-year-old man tells his physician that he is often late for work because he has difficulty waking up on time. He attributes this problem to the fact that he gets out of bed repeatedly during the night to recheck the locks on the doors and to be sure the gas jets on the stove are turned off. His lateness is exacerbated by his need to count all of the traffic lights along the route. If he suspects that he missed a light, he becomes quite anxious and must then go back and recount them all. Physical examination and laboratory studies are unremarkable. Of the following, the most effective long-term management for this patient is most likely to be

**(A)** an antidepressant
**(B)** an antipsychotic
**(C)** a benzodiazepine
**(D)** buspirone
**(E)** a $\beta$-blocker

**23.** The mother of a 4-year-old child with diabetes takes the child to the pediatrician to "be checked" at least 3 times per week. She watches the child at all times and does not let him play outside. She also measures and remeasures his food portions three times at every meal. The mother understands that this behavior is excessive but states that she is unable to stop doing it. The most appropriate pharmacological treatment for this mother is

**(A)** diazepam
**(B)** buspirone
**(C)** clomipramine
**(D)** haloperidol
**(E)** propranolol

# Answers and Explanations

## Typical Board Question

**The answer is C.** This 15-year-old who must wash himself in a certain manner each day, is showing evidence of OCD. OCD is a disorder in which one is compelled to engage in repetitive non-productive behavior which, as in this patient, impairs function (e.g., the patient is late for school and activities). The fact that this teenager has insight, that is, he knows that what he is doing is "ridiculous," also is characteristic of OCD.

1. **The answer is C. 2. The answer is A. 3. The answer is D.** This patient is showing evidence of panic disorder with agoraphobia. Panic disorder is characterized by panic attacks, which include increased heart rate, dizziness, sweating, shortness of breath, and fainting, and the conviction that one is about to die. Attacks commonly occur twice weekly, last about 30 minutes, and are most common in young women, such as this patient. This young woman has also developed a fear of leaving the house (agoraphobia) which occurs in some patients with panic disorder. While the most effective immediate treatment for this patient is a benzodiazepine because it works quickly, the most effective long-term (maintenance) management is an antidepressant, particularly a selective serotonin reuptake inhibitor (SSRI) such as paroxetine (Paxil). The neural etiology most closely involved in panic disorder with agoraphobia is hypersensitivity of the locus ceruleus.

4. **The answer is B.** This patient is most likely to have post-traumatic stress disorder (PTSD). This disorder, which is characterized by symptoms of anxiety and intrusive memories and nightmares of a life-threatening event such as rape, can last for many years in chronic form and may have been intensified in this patient by re-experiencing her own rape through the rape of her coworker. The most effective long-term management for this patient is a support group, in this case a rape survivor's group. Pharmacologic treatment is useful as an adjunct to psychological management in PTSD.

5. **The answer is C. 6. The answer is D.** This patient is most likely to have generalized anxiety disorder (GAD). This disorder, which includes chronic anxiety and, often, gastrointestinal symptoms is more common in women and often starts in the 20s. Genetic factors are seen in the observation that other family members have similar problems with anxiety. Additional signs or symptoms of anxiety that this patient is likely to show include tingling in the extremities and numbness around the mouth, often resulting from hyperventilation. Flight of ideas, hallucinations, ideas of reference, and neologisms are psychotic symptoms, which are not seen in the anxiety disorders or the somatoform disorders. Of the choices, the most effective long-term management for this patient is buspirone because, unlike the benzodiazepines alprazolam and diazepam, it does not cause dependence or withdrawal symptoms with long-term use. The antidepressants venlafaxine and duloxetine and SSRIs also are effective for long-term management of GAD. Psychotherapy and β-blockers can be used as adjuncts to treat GAD, but are not the most effective long-term treatments.

7. **The answer is F.** This presentation is an example of malingering, feigning illness for obvious gain (the $30,000 workers' compensation settlement). Evidence for this is that the woman has no further hand problems after she receives the money. In conversion disorder, somatization disorder, factitious disorder, and factitious disorder by proxy there is no obvious or material gain related to the symptoms.

8. **The answer is E.** Robbery at knifepoint, a life-threatening event, is most likely to result in post-traumatic stress disorder (PTSD). While life events such as divorce, bankruptcy, illness, and changing residence are stressful, they are rarely life-threatening. Psychological symptoms occurring after such less severe events may result in adjustment disorder, not PTSD.

9. **The answer is C. 10. The answer is D.** This presentation is an example of factitious disorder by proxy. The mother has feigned the child's illness (episodes of breathing problems and abdominal pain) for attention from medical personnel. This faking has resulted in four abdominal surgical procedures in which no abnormalities were found. Since she knows she is lying, the mother will become angry and flee when confronted with the truth. The first thing the physician must do is to notify the state social service agency since factitious disorder by proxy is a form of child abuse. Waiting until the child's next visit before acting could result in the child's further injury or even death. Calling in specialists may be appropriate after the physician reports his suspicions to the state. It is not appropriate to take the child aside and ask him how he really feels. He probably is not aware of his mother's behavior.

11. **The answer is E.** This woman with a 20-year history of unexplained vague and chronic physical complaints probably has somatization disorder. This can be distinguished from hypochondriasis, which is an exaggerated worry about normal physical sensations and minor ailments (see also answers to Questions 12–18).

12. **The answer is K.** This teenager, who was formerly outgoing and a good student and now seems sad, loses interest in making friends, and begins to do poor work in school, probably has adjustment disorder (with depressed mood). It is likely that he is having problems adjusting to his new school. In contrast to adjustment disorder, in masked depression the symptoms are more severe and often include significant weight loss or suicidality (see also TBQ and answer to Question 18).

13. **The answer is H.** This man, who experiences a sudden neurological symptom triggered by seeing his girlfriend with another man, is showing evidence of conversion disorder. This disorder is characterized by an apparent lack of concern about the symptoms (i.e., la belle indifférence).

14. **The answer is B.** This man, who says that he has been "sickly" for most of his life and fears that he has stomach cancer, is showing evidence of hypochondriasis, exaggerated concern over normal physical sensations (e.g., stomach noises) and minor ailments. There are no physical findings nor obvious evidence of depression in this patient.

15. **The answer is L.** This man probably has masked depression. In contrast to the hypochondriacal man in the previous question, evidence for depression in this patient includes the fact that, in addition to the somatic complaints, he shows symptoms of depression (e.g., he is not groomed, appears slowed down [psychomotor retardation], and has lost a significant amount of weight).

16. **The answer is G.** This woman probably has body dysmorphic disorder, which is characterized by over-concern about a physical feature (e.g., "sagging" eyelids in this case), despite normal appearance.

17. **The answer is J.** This man probably has social phobia. He is afraid of embarrassing himself in a public situation (e.g., getting food on his face while eating dinner in front of others in a restaurant).

18. **The answer is K.** The most likely explanation for this clinical picture that includes symptoms of anxiety which begin after a life stressor (e.g., a romantic break-up) is adjustment disorder (with anxiety). The absence of a previous history and the brief duration indicates that this is not an anxiety disorder and the fact that the stressor was not life-threatening rules out PTSD and ASD. The family history is not likely to be related to this patient's symptoms in this case.

19. **The answer is F.** The triad of hypoglycemia, very high insulin level, and suppressed plasma C peptide indicates that this nurse has self-administered insulin, a situation known as factitious hyperinsulinism. In hyperinsulinism due to medical causes, for example, insulinoma (pancreatic B-cell tumor), plasma C peptide is typically increased, not decreased. Factitious disorder is more common in people associated with the health professions. There is no evidence in this woman of a sleep disorder, anxiety disorder, somatoform disorder, or endocrine disorder such as diabetes. Because there is no obvious or practical gain for this woman in being ill, malingering is unlikely.

20. **The answer is D.** When there is financial or other obvious gain to be obtained from an illness, the possibility that the person is malingering must be considered. In this case, a man who has committed a crime is feigning symptoms of narcolepsy to avoid prosecution. Knowledge of the details of his brother's illness has taught him how to feign the cataplexy (sudden loss of motor control) and daytime sleepiness associated with narcolepsy (see Chapter 7).

21. **The answer is C.** This clinical presentation is an example of factitious disorder (note: Most psychiatric diagnoses disorders can also be made in children). In contrast to patients with somatoform disorders who really believe that they are ill, patients with factitious disorder are conscious of the fact that they are feigning their illness. Pain is one of the most commonly feigned symptoms and this patient's nighttime reading is providing him with specific knowledge of how to feign the symptoms realistically. Although he is consciously producing his symptoms, this boy is not receiving tangible benefit for his behavior. Thus, in contrast to individuals who are consciously feigning illness for obvious gain, that is, malingering (see also answer to Question 20), the motivation for this patient's pain-faking behavior is primarily unconscious.

22. **The answer is A.** This man's repeated checking and counting behavior indicates that he has OCD (and see the TBQ). The most effective long-term management for OCD is an antidepressant, particularly a selective serotonin reuptake inhibitor (SSRI) such as fluvoxamine (Luvox) or a heterocyclic agent such as clomipramine. Antianxiety agents such as benzodiazepines (e.g., diazepam) and buspirone, and $\beta$-blockers such as propranolol are more commonly used for the management of acute or chronic anxiety. Antipsychotic agents such as haloperidol may be useful as adjuncts but do not substitute for SSRIs or clomipramine in OCD.

23. **The answer is C.** The need to check and recheck the child's portions and repeatedly take him to the doctor indicates that, as in Question 22 and the TBQ, this patient is showing symptoms of OCD. The fact that she knows that her behavior is excessive ("insight") is typical of patients with OCD. As noted in Answer 22, the most effective long-term management for OCD is an antidepressant such as clomipramine.

# chapter 14

# Cognitive, Personality, Dissociative, and Eating Disorders

**Typical Board Question**

The mother of a 25-year-old man who was diagnosed with AIDS 1 year ago, reports that her son had been doing well until this morning when she observed him sitting up in bed, punching the air and grabbing at insects, although none were present. The patient's $CD_4$ count is <100 cells/mm$^3$ and his temperature is 103°F. The mother is concerned about these symptoms because the patient's elder brother has schizophrenia. This clinical picture is most consistent with

- **(A)** AIDS dementia
- **(B)** delirium caused by cryptococcal meningitis
- **(C)** schizophrenia
- **(D)** brief psychotic disorder
- **(E)** amnestic disorder

*(See "Answers and Explanations" at end of chapter.)*

# I. COGNITIVE DISORDERS

**A. General characteristics**

1. Cognitive disorders (formerly called organic mental syndromes) involve problems in **memory**, orientation, level of **consciousness**, and other intellectual functions.
   a. These difficulties are due to abnormalities in neural chemistry, structure, or physiology **originating in the brain** or **secondary to systemic illness**.
   b. Patients with cognitive disorders may also show **psychiatric symptoms** (e.g., depression, anxiety, hallucinations, delusions, and illusions; see Table 8.2) which are secondary to the cognitive problems.
   c. The major cognitive disorders are **delirium, dementia**, and **amnestic disorder**. Characteristics and etiologies of these disorders can be found in Table 14.1 and below.

**B. Delirium**

1. Delirium is a syndrome which includes **confusion** and **clouding of consciousness** that result from central nervous system impairment.
2. It usually occurs in the course of an **acute medical illness** such as encephalitis or meningitis but is also seen in drug abuse and withdrawal, particularly withdrawal from alcohol ("delirium tremens").
3. It is common in **surgical and coronary intensive care** units and in **elderly debilitated patients**.

table **14.1** Characteristics and Etiologies of Cognitive Disorders

| Characteristic | Delirium | Dementia | Amnestic Disorder |
|---|---|---|---|
| Hallmark | Impaired consciousness | Loss of memory and intellectual abilities | Loss of memory with few other cognitive problems |
| Etiology | CNS disease (e.g., Huntington or Parkinson disease) CNS trauma CNS infection (e.g., meningitis) Systemic disease (e.g., hepatic, cardiovascular) High fever Substance abuse Substance withdrawal HIV infection Prescription drug overdose (e.g., atropine) | Alzheimer disease Vascular disease (15%–30% of all dementias) CNS disease (e.g., Huntington or Parkinson disease) CNS trauma CNS infection (e.g., HIV or Creutzfeldt–Jakob disease) Lewy body dementia Pick disease (frontotemporal dementia) | Thiamine deficiency due to long-term alcohol abuse, leading to destruction of mediotemporal lobe structures (e.g., mammillary bodies) Temporal lobe trauma, vascular disease, or infection (e.g., herpes simplex encephalitis) |
| Occurrence | More common in children and the elderly Most common etiology of psychiatric symptoms in medical and surgical hospital units | More common in the elderly Seen in about 20% of individuals over the age of 85 | More common in patients with a history of alcohol abuse |
| Associated physical findings | Acute medical illness Autonomic dysfunction Abnormal EEG (fast wave activity or generalized slowing) | No medical illness Little autonomic dysfunction Normal EEG | No medical illness Little autonomic dysfunction Normal EEG |
| Associated psychological findings | Impaired consciousness Illusions, delusions (often paranoid) or hallucinations (often visual and disorganized) "Sundowning" (symptoms much worse at night) Anxiety with psychomotor agitation | Normal consciousness Psychotic symptoms uncommon in early stages Depressed mood "Sundowning" Personality changes in early stages (in Pick disease) | Normal consciousness Psychotic symptoms uncommon in early stages Depressed mood Little diurnal variability Confabulation (untruths told to hide memory loss) |
| Course | Develops quickly Fluctuating course with lucid intervals | Develops slowly Progressive downhill course | Develops slowly Progressive downhill course if drinking continues |
| Management and prognosis | Removal of the underlying medical problem will allow the symptoms to resolve Increase orienting stimuli Delirium must be ruled out before dementia can be diagnosed | No effective treatment, rarely reversible Pharmacotherapy and supportive therapy to treat associated psychiatric symptoms Acetylcholinesterase inhibitors and NMDA receptor antagonists (for Alzheimer disease) Antihypertensive or anticlotting agent (for vascular dementia) Provide a structured environment | No effective treatment, rarely reversible Pharmacotherapy and supportive therapy to manage associated psychiatric symptoms Vitamin B$_1$ for acute symptoms |

CNS, central nervous system; HIV, human immunodeficiency virus; EEG, electroencephalogram  NMDA, N-methyl-D-aspartate.

## C. Dementia

1. Dementia involves the **gradual loss of intellectual abilities** without impairment of consciousness.

2. Dementia of Alzheimer type (hereinafter **Alzheimer disease**) is the **most common type** of dementia (50%–65% of all dementias). Other types of dementia include vascular dementia (10%–15% of dementias), Lewy body dementia, and dementia caused by HIV infection (see I.E below).

## D. Alzheimer disease

1. **Diagnosis**

   a. Patients with Alzheimer disease show a **gradual loss of memory and intellectual abilities**. Their psychiatric symptoms include inability to control impulses and lack of judgment as well as depression and anxiety.

| table 14.2 | Memory Problems in the Elderly: A Comparison of Alzheimer Disease, Pseudodementia, and Normal Aging | | | |
|---|---|---|---|---|
| **Condition** | **Etiology** | **Clinical Example** | **Major Manifestations** | **Medical Interventions** |
| Alzheimer disease | Brain dysfunction | A 65-year-old former banker cannot remember to turn off the gas jets on the stove nor can he name the object in his hand (a comb) | Severe memory loss Other cognitive problems Decrease in IQ Disruption of normal life | Structured environment Acetylcholinesterase inhibitors Ultimately, nursing home placement |
| Pseudodementia (depression that mimics dementia) | Depression of mood | A 65-year-old dentist cannot remember to pay her bills. She also appears to be physically "slowed down" (psychomotor retardation) and very sad | Moderate memory loss Other cognitive problems No decrease in IQ Disruption of normal life | Antidepressants Electroconvulsive therapy (ECT) Psychotherapy |
| Normal aging | Minor changes in the normal aging brain | A 65-year-old woman forgets new phone numbers and names but functions well living on her own | Minor forgetfulness Reduction in the ability to learn new things quickly No decrease in IQ No disruption of normal life | No medical intervention Practical and emotional support from the physician |

   **b.** Later in the illness, symptoms include confusion and psychosis that progress to coma and **death (usually within 8–10 years of diagnosis)**.
   **c.** For patient management and prognosis, it is important to make the distinction between **Alzheimer disease** and both **pseudodementia** (depression that mimics dementia) and behavioral changes associated with **normal aging** (Table 14.2).
2. **Genetic associations** in Alzheimer disease include:
   **a.** Abnormalities of **chromosome 21** (Down syndrome patients ultimately develop Alzheimer disease).
   **b.** Abnormalities of **chromosomes 1 and 14** (sites of the presenilin 2 and presenilin 1 genes, respectively) implicated particularly in **early onset** Alzheimer disease (i.e., occurring before the age of 65).
   **c.** Possession of at least one copy of the apolipoprotein $E_4$ **(apoE₄)** gene on chromosome 19.
   **d.** Gender—there is a higher occurrence of Alzheimer disease in **women**.
3. **Neurophysiological factors** include:
   **a.** Decreased activity of acetylcholine (Ach) and reduced brain levels of choline acetyl-transferase (i.e., the enzyme needed to synthesize Ach; see Chapter 4).
   **b.** Abnormal processing of amyloid precursor protein.
   **c.** Overstimulation of the N-methyl-D-aspartate (NMDA) receptor by **glutamate** leading to an influx of calcium, nerve cell degeneration and cell death (see Chapter 4, Question 25).
4. **Gross anatomical brain changes** include:
   **a.** **Enlargement of brain ventricles.**
   **b.** Diffuse atrophy and flattening of brain sulci.
5. **Microscopic anatomical brain changes** include:
   **a.** **Amyloid plaques** and **neurofibrillary tangles** (also seen in other neurodegenerative diseases, Down syndrome and, to a lesser extent, in normal aging).
   **b.** Loss of cholinergic neurons in the basal forebrain.
   **c.** Neuronal loss and degeneration in the hippocampus and cortex.
6. Alzheimer disease has a **progressive, irreversible, downhill** course. The most effective initial interventions involve **providing a structured environment**, including visual-orienting cues. Such cues include labels over the doors of rooms identifying their function; daily posting of the day of the week, date, and year; daily written activity schedules; and practical safety measures (e.g., disconnecting the stove).
7. **Pharmacologic** interventions include:
   **a.** **Acetylcholinesterase inhibitors** (e.g., tacrine [Cognex], donepezil [Aricept], rivastigmine [Exelon], and galantamine [Razadyne]) to temporarily **slow the progression** of the disease. However, these agents cannot restore function that has already been lost.

    **b.** Memantine (Namenda), an **NMDA antagonist**, decreases the influx of glutamate and thus slows deterioration in patients with moderate to severe Alzheimer disease.

    **c. Psychotropic agents** are used to treat associated symptoms of anxiety, depression, or psychosis. Since **antipsychotics** are associated with **increased mortality** in elderly demented patients (particularly those with Lewy body dementia, see later), they should be used with extreme caution.

**E. Other dementias**

  **1. Vascular dementia**

    **a.** It is caused by multiple, small cerebral infarctions usually resulting from cardiovascular disorders such as hypertension or atherosclerosis.

    **b.** In contrast to Alzheimer disease, vascular dementia has a higher risk for men and is more likely to cause motor symptoms.

    **c.** The primary intervention is the management of the cardiovascular disorder (e.g., antihypertensives, anticoagulants) to prevent further infarcts leading to deterioration in cognitive functioning.

  **2. Lewy body dementia**

    **a.** Gradual, progressive loss of cognitive abilities as well as hallucinations (often visual) and the motor characteristics of Parkinson disease. Also associated with REM sleep behavior disorder (see Chapter 10).

    **b.** Pathology includes amyloid plaques but, in contrast to Alzheimer disease, few neurofibrillary tangles.

    **c.** Patients typically have **adverse responses to antipsychotic medications**.

  **3. HIV dementia**

    **a.** Dementia due to cortical atrophy, inflammation, and demyelination resulting from direct infection of the brain with HIV. Supportive measures are the primary management.

    **b.** Must be differentiated, in HIV patients, from delirium caused by cerebral lymphoma or opportunistic brain infection. Such delirium is often reversible with chemotherapeutic or antibiotic agents.

## II. PERSONALITY DISORDERS

**A. Characteristics**

  **1.** Individuals with personality disorders (PDs) show **chronic, lifelong, rigid, unsuitable patterns of relating to others** that cause social and occupational difficulties (e.g., few friends, job loss).

  **2.** Persons with PDs generally are not aware that they are the cause of their own problems (**do not have "insight"**), do not have frank psychotic symptoms, and **do not seek psychiatric help**.

**B. Classification**

  **1.** Personality disorders are categorized by the *Diagnostic and Statistical Manual of Mental Disorders, Fourth Edition, Text Revision (DSM-IV-TR)* into *clusters:* **A** (paranoid, schizoid, schizotypal); **B** (histrionic, narcissistic, borderline, and antisocial); and **C** (avoidant, obsessive-compulsive, and dependent); and not otherwise specified (**NOS**) (passive-aggressive).

  **2.** Each cluster has its own hallmark characteristics and genetic or familial associations (e.g., relatives of people with PDs have a higher likelihood of having certain disorders) (Table 14.3).

  **3.** For the *DSM-IV-TR* diagnosis, a PD must be present by early adulthood. Antisocial PD cannot be diagnosed until the age of 18; prior to this age, the diagnosis is conduct disorder (see Chapter 15).

| t a b l e    **14.3** | *DSM-IV-TR* Classification and Characteristics of Personality Disorders |
|---|---|
| **Personality Disorder** | **Characteristics** |
| ***Cluster A*** | |
| *Hallmark* | Avoids social relationships, is "peculiar" but not psychotic |
| *Genetic or familial association* | Psychotic illnesses |
| Paranoid | Distrustful, suspicious, litigious |
| | Attributes responsibility for own problems to others |
| | Interprets motives of others as malevolent |
| | Collects guns |
| Schizoid | Long-standing pattern of voluntary social withdrawal |
| | Detached, restricted emotions, lacks empathy, has no thought disorder |
| Schizotypal | Peculiar appearance |
| | Magical thinking (i.e., believing that one's thoughts can affect the course of events) |
| | Odd thought patterns and behavior without frank psychosis |
| ***Cluster B*** | |
| *Hallmark* | Dramatic, emotional, inconsistent |
| *Genetic or familial association* | Mood disorders, substance abuse, and somatoform disorders |
| Histrionic | Theatrical, extroverted, emotional, sexually provocative, "life of the party" |
| | Shallow, vain |
| | In men, "Don Juan" dress and behavior |
| | Cannot maintain intimate relationships |
| Narcissistic | Pompous, with a sense of special entitlement |
| | Lacks empathy for others |
| Antisocial | Refuses to conform to social norms and shows no concern for others |
| | Associated with conduct disorder in childhood and criminal behavior in adulthood ("psychopaths" or "sociopaths") |
| Borderline | Erratic, impulsive, unstable behavior and mood |
| | Feeling bored, alone, and "empty" |
| | Suicide attempts for relatively trivial reasons |
| | Self-mutilation (cutting or burning oneself) |
| | Often comorbid with mood and eating disorders |
| | Mini-psychotic episodes (i.e., brief periods of loss of contact with reality) |
| ***Cluster C*** | |
| *Hallmark* | Fearful, anxious |
| *Genetic or familial association* | Anxiety disorders |
| Avoidant | Overly sensitive to criticism or rejection |
| | Feelings of inferiority, socially withdrawn |
| Obsessive-compulsive | Perfectionistic, orderly, inflexible |
| | Stubborn and indecisive |
| | Ultimately inefficient |
| Dependent | Allows other people to make decisions and assume responsibility for them |
| | Poor self-confidence, fear of being deserted and alone |
| | May tolerate abuse by domestic partner |
| ***Not Otherwise Specified*** | |
| Passive-aggressive | Procrastinates and is inefficient |
| | Outwardly agreeable and compliant but inwardly angry and defiant |

C. **Management**
   1. For those who seek help, individual and group psychotherapy may be useful.
   2. Pharmacotherapy also can be used to manage symptoms such as depression and anxiety, that may be associated with the PDs.

# III. DISSOCIATIVE DISORDERS

A. **Characteristics**
   1. The dissociative disorders are characterized by abrupt but temporary **loss of memory (amnesia) or identity**, or by feelings of detachment owing to psychological factors.

| t a b l e   **14.4** | *DSM-IV-TR* Classification and Characteristics of Dissociative Disorders |
|---|---|

| Classification | Characteristics |
|---|---|
| Dissociative amnesia | Failure to remember important information about oneself after a stressful life event<br>Amnesia usually resolves in minutes or days but may last years |
| Dissociative fugue | Amnesia combined with sudden wandering from home after a stressful life event<br>Adoption of a different identity |
| Dissociative identity disorder (formerly multiple personality disorder) | At least two distinct personalities ("alters") in an individual<br>More common in women (particularly those sexually abused in childhood)<br>In a forensic (e.g., jail) setting, malingering and alcohol abuse must be considered and excluded |
| Depersonalization disorder | Recurrent, persistent feelings of detachment from one's own body, the social situation, or the environment (derealization) when stressed<br>Understanding that these perceptions are only feelings, i.e., normal reality testing |
| Dissociative disorder not otherwise specified | Dissociative symptom (e.g., trance-like state, memory loss) (1) in persons exposed to intense coercive persuasion (e.g., brainwashing) or (2) indigenous to particular locations or cultures (e.g., "Amok" in Indonesia) |

2. In contrast to the cognitive disorders in which memory loss is caused by biological brain dysfunction (see Section I), dissociative disorders are related to **disturbing emotional experiences** in the patient's **recent or remote past**.

B. **Classification and management**
1. The **DSM-IV-TR** categories of dissociative disorders are listed in Table 14.4.
2. Management of the dissociative disorders includes **hypnosis and drug-assisted interviews** (see Chapter 5) as well as long-term **psychoanalytically oriented psychotherapy** (see Chapter 17) to recover "lost" (repressed) memories of disturbing emotional experiences.

# IV. OBESITY AND EATING DISORDERS

A. **Obesity**
1. Overview
   a. Obesity is defined as being **more than 20% over ideal weight** on the basis of common height and weight charts or having a **body mass index (BMI)** (body weight in kg/height in m$^2$) **of 30** or higher (Figure 14.1).
   b. At least **25% of adults** are obese and an increasing number of children are overweight (at or above the 95th percentile of BMI for age) in the United States.
   c. Obesity is **not an eating disorder**. **Genetic factors** are most important in obesity; adult weight is closer to that of biologic rather than adoptive parents.
   d. Obesity is more common in lower socioeconomic groups and is associated with **increased risk** for cardiorespiratory, sleep, and orthopedic problems; hypertension; and diabetes mellitus.
2. Management
   a. Most weight loss achieved using commercial dieting and weight loss programs is **regained within a 5-year period**.
   b. **Bariatric surgery** (e.g., gastric bypass, gastric banding) is initially effective but of limited value for maintaining long-term weight loss.
   c. Pharmacologic agents for weight loss include **orlistat (Xenical, Alli)**, a pancreatic lipase inhibitor that limits the breakdown of dietary fats, and **phentermine (Ionamin)**, a sympathomimetic amine that decreases appetite.
   d. A combination of **sensible dieting and exercise** is the most effective to way to maintain long-term weight loss.

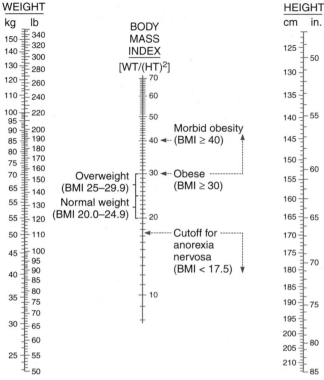

FIGURE 14.1. BMI. BMI is calculated by placing a straight edge between the body-weight column (left) and the height column (right) and reading the BMI from the point at which the straight edge crosses the BMI column.

**B. Eating disorders: Anorexia nervosa and bulimia nervosa**

   **1.** In anorexia nervosa and bulimia nervosa, the patient shows abnormal behavior associated with food despite **normal appetite**.

   **2.** The **subtypes of anorexia nervosa** are the **restricting type** (e.g., excessive dieting) and, in 50% of the patients, the **binge eating purging type** (e.g., excessive dieting plus binge eating [consuming large quantities of high-calorie food at one time] and purging [e.g., vomiting, or misuse of laxatives, diuretics, and enemas]).

   **3.** The **subtypes of bulimia nervosa** are the **purging type** (e.g., binge eating and purging) and **non-purging type** (e.g., binge eating and excessive dieting or exercising but no purging).

   **4.** The purging type of either anorexia nervosa or bulimia nervosa is associated with **electrolyte abnormalities**. Specific electrolyte abnormalities are related to the type of purging seen.

   **a.** Low potassium (hypokalemia), low sodium, and high bicarbonate (metabolic alkalosis) levels are seen with **vomiting or diuretic abuse**.

   **b.** Low potassium, high chloride, and low bicarbonate levels (together known as hyperchloremic metabolic acidosis) are seen with **laxative abuse**.

   **5.** Eating disorders are **more common in women**, in **higher socioeconomic groups**, and in the **United States** (compared with other developed countries).

   **6.** Physical and psychological characteristics and management of anorexia nervosa and bulimia nervosa can be found in Table 14.5.

| table **14.5** | Physical and Psychological Characteristics and Management of Anorexia Nervosa and Bulimia Nervosa | | |

| Disorder | Physical Characteristics | Psychological Characteristics | Management (in Order of Highest to Lowest Utility) |
|---|---|---|---|
| Anorexia nervosa | Extreme weight loss (15% or more of normal body weight)<br>Amenorrhea (three or more consecutive missed menstrual periods)<br>Electrolyte disturbances<br>Hypercholesterolemia<br>Mild anemia and leukopenia<br>Lanugo (downy body hair on the trunk)<br>Melanosis coli (blackened area of the colon if there is laxative abuse)<br>Osteoporosis<br>Cold intolerance<br>Syncope | Refusal to eat despite normal appetite because of an overwhelming fear of being obese<br>Belief that one is fat when very thin<br>High interest in food-related activities (e.g., cooking)<br>Simulates eating<br>Lack of interest in sex<br>Was a "perfect child" (e.g., good student)<br>Interfamily conflicts (e.g., patient's problem draws attention away from parental marital problem or an attempt to gain control to separate from the mother)<br>Excessive exercising ("hypergymnasia") | Hospitalization directed at reinstating nutritional condition (starvation and compensatory behavior such as purging can result in metabolic abnormalities [e.g., hypokalemia] leading to death)<br>Family therapy (aimed particularly at normalizing the mother–child relationship)<br>Group psychotherapy in an inpatient eating disorders program |
| Bulimia nervosa | Relatively normal body weight<br>Esophageal varices caused by repeated vomiting<br>Tooth enamel erosion due to gastric acid in the mouth<br>Swelling or infection of the parotid glands<br>Metacarpal–phalangeal calluses (Russell sign) from the teeth because the hand is used to induce gagging<br>Electrolyte disturbances<br>Menstrual irregularities | Binge eating (in secret) of high-calorie foods, followed by vomiting or other purging behavior to avoid weight gain<br>Depression<br>"Hypergymnasia" | Cognitive and behavioral therapies<br>Average to high doses of antidepressants, particularly SSRIs; fluoxetine is the only FDA-approved agent; bupropion is contraindicated<br>Group psychotherapy in an inpatient or outpatient eating disorders program |

# Review Test

**Directions:** Each of the numbered items or incomplete statements in this section is followed by answers or by completions of the statement. Select the **one** lettered answer or completion that is **best** in each case.

**1.** A 20-year-old man states that he is uncomfortable around women. He says that he gets anxious when he is with a woman and "just does not know what to say to her." The patient, a high school graduate, reports that he has a few male friends with whom he "hangs out" and is doing well in his job in construction. This clinical picture is most consistent with which of the following?

**(A)** Schizoid personality disorder
**(B)** Schizotypal personality disorder
**(C)** Avoidant personality disorder
**(D)** Asperger disorder
**(E)** Normal shyness

**2.** A 75-year-old man with a 3-year history of Alzheimer disease has recently become disoriented when the lights are turned off at night. He wanders about the apartment at night and his wife is concerned that he will injure himself while she is sleeping. The Folstein Mini-Mental State Exam shows that the patient is disoriented regarding time and place and has poor short-term memory. Physical examination is unremarkable and the patient is not currently taking any medication. What is the most appropriate first recommendation for the management of this patient?

**(A)** Ask the wife to increase home nighttime lighting
**(B)** Prescribe donepezil for the patient
**(C)** Prescribe haloperidol for the patient
**(D)** Prescribe methylphenidate for the wife so that she can stay alert during the night
**(E)** Recommend that the patient be put in mechanical restraints at bedtime

**3.** The mother of an obese 12-year-old boy tells the physician that the "child is not eating well." What is the physician's best response to the mother's statement?

**(A)** What do you mean by "not eating well"?
**(B)** The child looks like he is eating well enough.
**(C)** There are a number of diets available that are excellent for children.
**(D)** Increased exercising may be the answer to your son's weight problem.
**(E)** Diet plus exercise is the most effective management for obesity.

**4.** In Alzheimer disease patients, the major effect on neurotransmitter systems of tacrine, donepezil, rivastigmine, and galantamine is to

**(A)** increase dopamine availability
**(B)** decrease dopamine availability
**(C)** increase Ach availability
**(D)** decrease Ach availability
**(E)** decrease serotonin availability

### Questions 5 and 6

A 78-year-old retired female physician reports that she has been confused and forgetful over the past 10 months. She also has difficulty sleeping, her appetite is poor, and she has lost 20 pounds. Questioning reveals that her 18-year-old dog died 10 months ago.

**5.** At this time, the most appropriate diagnosis for this patient is

**(A)** delirium
**(B)** pseudodementia
**(C)** Alzheimer disease
**(D)** dissociative fugue
**(E)** amnestic disorder

**6.** Of the following, the most appropriate initial intervention for this patient is

**(A)** antipsychotic medication
**(B)** provision of a structured environment
**(C)** antidepressant medication
**(D)** donepezil
**(E)** reassurance

**Questions 7 and 8**

A 75-year-old man is brought to the emergency department after being burned in a house fire. This is the patient's third emergency visit in 2 months. His other visits occurred after he inhaled natural gas when he left the stove on without a flame, and because he fell down the stairs after wandering out of the house in the middle of the night. There is no evidence of physical illness and no history of substance abuse. His wife is distressed and begs the doctor to let her husband come home.

**7.** This patient is showing evidence of

**(A)** delirium
**(B)** pseudodementia
**(C)** Alzheimer disease
**(D)** dissociative fugue
**(E)** amnestic disorder

**8.** Of the following, the most appropriate initial intervention for this patient is

**(A)** antipsychotic medication
**(B)** provision of a structured environment
**(C)** antidepressant medication
**(D)** donepezil
**(E)** reassurance

**9.** A 43-year-old woman says that when she is under stress, she often feels as if she is "outside of herself" and is watching her life as though it were a play. She knows that this perception is only a feeling and that she is really living her life. This woman is showing evidence of

**(A)** dissociative amnesia
**(B)** dissociative fugue
**(C)** dissociative identity disorder
**(D)** depersonalization disorder
**(E)** schizophrenia

**10.** A 28-year-old stockbroker who is married and has two children usually dresses conservatively. She receives a letter containing a recent photograph of herself in a skimpy black leather outfit. She does not remember the man who signed the letter, or posing for the photograph. This woman is showing evidence of

**(A)** dissociative amnesia
**(B)** dissociative fugue
**(C)** dissociative identity disorder
**(D)** depersonalization disorder
**(E)** schizophrenia

**11.** A 30-year-old single woman who has been smoking three packs of cigarettes a day for the last 10 years asks the physician to help her stop smoking. The doctor asks the patient why she smokes so much. The patient responds, "I always feel very alone and empty inside; I smoke to fill myself up." The patient reveals that she sometimes cuts the skin on her arms with a knife in order to "feel something." She also notes that when she is upset, she often uses cocaine and has sex with men whom she does not know well. After these episodes she typically feels even more alone and empty. Which of the following is the most characteristic defense mechanism used by people with this woman's personality characteristics?

**(A)** Displacement
**(B)** Intellectualization
**(C)** Denial
**(D)** Reaction formation
**(E)** Splitting

**12.** The elderly parents of a 45-year-old mildly mentally retarded patient tell the physician that their son began to have difficulty identifying familiar objects and people about 6 months ago. Physical examination reveals that the patient is short in stature, has a protruding tongue, flat facies, hypotonia, and a thick neck. The chromosomal abnormality most likely to be responsible for this clinical picture is most likely to be associated with chromosome

**(A)** 1
**(B)** 4
**(C)** 14
**(D)** 19
**(E)** 21

**13.** An 18-year-old student who is about 10 pounds overweight tells her physician that she has decided to go on a low carbohydrate diet that she read about in a book. She says that the book guarantees that people who follow the diet will lose at least 25 pounds in 3 weeks. The doctor's best statement to the patient at this time is

**(A)** That is nonsense, you can't lose that much weight in only 3 weeks.

**(B)** You may lose the weight but you will end up gaining back even more weight.

**(C)** Please tell me more about the book that you read.

**(D)** You may be showing signs of an eating disorder.

**(E)** Many people your age have eating disorders.

**14.** Two days after a 23-year-old man is rescued from a burning building he has no memory of the fire or of the few hours before or after it. Physical examination is unremarkable. The most likely explanation for this clinical picture is

**(A)** posttraumatic stress disorder

**(B)** dissociative amnesia

**(C)** adjustment disorder

**(D)** early onset Alzheimer disease

**(E)** subarachnoid hemorrhage

**15.** A physician conducts a yearly physical examination on a typical 85-year-old patient. Which of the following mental characteristics is the doctor most likely to see in this patient?

**(A)** Impaired consciousness

**(B)** Abnormal level of arousal

**(C)** Minor forgetfulness

**(D)** Psychosis

**(E)** Depression

## Questions 16 and 17

A 21-year-old ballet dancer, who is 5 feet 7 inches tall and has weighted 95 pounds (BMI = 14.5) for the past year, tells the doctor that she needs to lose another 15 pounds to pursue a career in dance. Her mood appears good. Findings on physical examination are normal except for excessive growth of downy body hair. She reports that she has not menstruated in more than 3 years.

**16.** Which of the following is most likely to characterize this female?

**(A)** Lack of interest in preparing food

**(B)** Embarrassment about her appearance

**(C)** Lack of appetite

**(D)** Conflict with her mother

**(E)** Poor school performance

**17.** Which of the following disorders is this patient at the highest risk for in the future?

**(A)** Dermatitis

**(B)** Osteoarthritis

**(C)** Osteoporosis

**(D)** Pancreatic cancer

**(E)** Biliary atresia

**18.** A physician would like to prescribe an antidepressant to treat her 24-year-old male patient who has bulimia. Which of the following agents should be avoided in this patient?

**(A)** Desipramine

**(B)** Fluoxetine

**(C)** Bupropion

**(D)** Tranylcypromine

**(E)** Paroxetine

## Questions 19–26

For each patient below choose the most appropriate personality disorder

**(A)** Borderline personality disorder

**(B)** Histrionic personality disorder

**(C)** Obsessive-compulsive personality disorder

**(D)** Avoidant personality disorder

**(E)** Antisocial personality disorder

**(F)** Dependent personality disorder ·

**(G)** Dissociative identity disorder

**(H)** Paranoid personality disorder

**(I)** Passive-aggressive personality disorder

**(J)** Narcissistic personality disorder

**(K)** Schizotypal personality disorder

**(L)** Schizoid personality disorder

**19.** A 38-year-old man asks his doctor to refer him to a physician who attended a top-rated medical school. He says that he knows the doctor will not be offended because she will understand that he is "better" than her other patients.

**20.** A 20-year-old female college student tells the doctor that because she was afraid to be alone, she tried to commit suicide after a man with whom she had had two dates did not call her again. After the interview, she tells him that all of the other doctors she has seen were terrible and that he is the only doctor who has ever understood her problems.

**21.** Whenever a 28-year-old woman comes to the doctor's office, she brings gifts for the receptionist and the nurses. When she hears that one of the nurses has taken another job, she begins to sob loudly. When the doctor sees her, she reports that she is so warm that she must have "a fever of at least 106°F."

**22.** Two weeks after a 50-year-old, overweight, hypertensive woman agreed to start an exercise program, she gained 4 pounds. She reports that she has not exercised yet because "the gym was too crowded."

**23.** The parents of a 26-year-old woman say that they are concerned about her because she has no friends and spends most of her time hiking in the woods and working on her computer. The doctor examines her and finds that she is content with her solitary life and has no evidence of a thought disorder.

**24.** A 22-year-old medical student is unable to stop studying until she has memorized the entire set of notes for each of her courses. Making comprehensive lists of all the subjects she must study also takes up her study time. Because of this, she is constantly behind in her work and in danger of failing her courses.

**25.** A 40-year-old patient with bruises on his arms, neck, and back tells the doctor that his lover often berates him and physically abuses him. He begs the doctor not to interfere because he is afraid that the man will desert him and that he will be alone.

**26.** A 20-year-old female college student who was unable to answer a teacher's question in class drops out of school the next day.

# Answers and Explanations

## Typical Board Question

**The answer is B.** This clinical picture that includes the sudden onset of a psychiatric symptom (i.e., visual hallucinations) coinciding with the onset of a high fever in a relatively recently diagnosed (1 year) AIDS patient is most consistent with delirium caused by an opportunistic infection of the brain such as cryptococcal meningitis. Psychotic illnesses such as schizophrenia, brief psychotic disorder, or AIDS dementia cannot be diagnosed if the symptoms (as in this patient) can be explained by an acute medical illness. Also, AIDS dementia occurs in the late stages of the disease and would be characterized primarily by gradually worsening cognitive functioning (e.g., memory loss) as well as motor symptoms. Amnestic disorder is often associated with a history of alcoholism and has a gradual, progressive course.

1. **The answer is E.** This clinical picture is most consistent with normal shyness. Although this 20-year-old patient is somewhat anxious around women, the fact that he has friends and is doing well in his job makes it unlikely that he has a personality disorder or Asperger disorder (see Chapter 15).

2. **The answer is A.** The most appropriate first recommendation for the management of this patient is to ask the wife to increase home nighttime lighting. Lighting will improve the patient's ability to negotiate the apartment at night and so reduce his nocturnal disorientation. Keeping the wife awake is not practical or positive for her and mechanical restraints should be avoided if possible (see also answers to Questions 7 and 8).

3. **The answer is A.** The physician's best response to the mother's statement is to get more information, for example, "What do you mean by not eating well?" Recommending changes in diet or exercise or commenting on the child's appearance are not appropriate until you find out more about the mother's perception of the problem.

4. **The answer is C.** Low levels of Ach are associated with the symptoms of Alzheimer disease. Tacrine, donepezil, rivastigmine, and galantamine are acetylcholinesterase inhibitors (i.e., they block the breakdown of Ach, increasing its availability). These agents can thus be effective in slowing down the progression of the illness. They do not restore the function the patient has already lost.

5. **The answer is B. 6. The answer is C.** The best explanation for this patient's symptoms is pseudodementia—depression that mimics dementia. In the elderly, depression is often associated with cognitive problems as well as sleep and eating problems. Evidence for depression is provided by the fact that this patient's symptoms began with the loss of an important relationship (i.e., the death of her dog). Delirium and dementia are caused by physiological abnormalities. Dissociative fugue involves wandering away from home, and amnestic disorder is associated with a history of alcoholism. The most effective intervention for this depressed patient is antidepressant medication. When the medication relieves the depressive symptoms, her memory will improve. Antipsychotic medication, provision of a structured environment, acetylcholinesterase inhibitors such as donepezil, and simple reassurance are not appropriate for this patient.

7. **The answer is C. 8. The answer is B.** This patient is showing evidence of Alzheimer disease. He is having accidents because he is forgetful (e.g., forgetting to turn off the gas jet), and wanders out of the house because he does not know which is the closet or bathroom door and which is the outside door. There is no evidence of a medical cause for his symptoms, as there would be in delirium. There is no evidence of depression, as

in pseudodementia, or of a history of alcohol abuse, as in amnestic disorder. The most effective initial intervention for this patient is provision of a structured environment (e.g., giving the patient visual cues for orientation [labeling doors for function]) and taking practical measures (e.g., removing the gas stove). Donepezil can then be used to slow the progression of his illness. Other medications and reassurance may be useful for symptoms such as psychosis, depression, and anxiety, but will have little effect on the patient's forgetful and potentially dangerous behavior.

9. **The answer is D.** This woman, who feels as if she is "outside of herself," watching her life as though it were a play, is showing evidence of depersonalization disorder, a persistent feeling of detachment from one's own body or the social situation. In contrast to psychotic disorders such as schizophrenia (see Chapter 11), this woman is aware that this perception is only a feeling and that she is really living her life.

10. **The answer is C.** This stockbroker is showing evidence of dissociative identity disorder (formerly multiple personality disorder). She does not remember the man who signed the letter or posing for the photograph because these events occurred when she was showing another personality. Dissociative amnesia involves a failure to remember important information about oneself, and dissociative fugue is amnesia combined with sudden wandering from home and taking on a different identity. Depersonalization disorder is a persistent feeling of detachment from one's own body, the social situation, or the environment (derealization) (and see also answer to Question 9).

11. **The answer is E.** This woman, who has always felt empty and alone (not merely lonely), shows evidence of borderline personality disorder. Borderline patients typically use splitting (see Chapter 6) as a defense mechanism. Self-injurious behavior and impulsive behavior (e.g., drug abuse, sex with multiple partners) also are characteristic of people with this personality disorder.

12. **The answer is E.** This patient with mild mental retardation and associated physical findings probably has Down syndrome, which is associated with chromosome 21. Down syndrome patients often develop Alzheimer disease in middle age, which explains the memory loss that this patient displays.

13. **The answer is C.** The doctor's best statement to the patient at this time is, "Please tell me more about the book that you read." It is important to get as much information as possible from the patient before deciding on a course of action (see also Chapter 21).

14. **The answer is B.** The most likely explanation for this clinical picture, for example, having no memory of a traumatic event with no physical findings, is dissociative amnesia. In PTSD and in adjustment disorder there is no frank memory loss. Subarachnoid hemorrhage, a hemorrhage in the space between the arachnoid space and the pia mater, typically presents with a "thunderclap" headache, vomiting, or other neurologic symptoms.

15. **The answer is C.** This typical 85-year-old patient is likely to show minor forgetfulness, such as forgetting new names and phone numbers. Impaired consciousness, psychosis, and abnormal level of arousal are seen in delirium, which is associated with a variety of physical illnesses. As in younger people, in the elderly depression is an illness (see Chapter 12), not a natural consequence of typical aging.

16. **The answer is D. 17. The answer is C.** This woman is already underweight yet wants to lose more weight, and she has developed lanugo (growth of downy body hair) and amenorrhea (absence of menses). These findings indicate that she has anorexia nervosa. Since dancers and gymnasts often must be small and slim, these activities are closely associated with the development of anorexia nervosa. Anorexia is also characterized by family conflicts, particularly with the mother; normal appetite; high interest in food and cooking; low sexual interest; good school performance; and excessive exercising. Patients who have anorexia nervosa for an extended period (5 years in this young woman) are at high risk for osteoporosis.

18. **The answer is C.** Bupropion is contraindicated in eating disorder patients who also purge because it can lower the seizure threshold. The only antidepressant which is FDA approved for patients with bulimia nervosa is fluoxetine.

19. **The answer is J.** This 38-year-old man, who asks to be referred to a physician who attended a top-rated medical school because he is "better" than other patients, is showing evidence of narcissistic personality disorder (see also answers to Questions 20–26).

20. **The answer is A.** This 20-year-old college student, who made a suicide attempt after a relatively trivial relationship broke up and who uses splitting as a defense mechanism (e.g., all of the other doctors she has seen were terrible and this doctor is perfect), is showing evidence of borderline personality disorder.

21. **The answer is B.** This 28-year-old woman who brings gifts for the receptionist and the nurses because she needs to have everyone pay attention to her is showing evidence of histrionic personality disorder. Patients with this personality disorder tend to exaggerate their physical symptoms for dramatic effect (e.g., "a fever of at least 106°F").

22. **The answer is I.** This 50-year-old woman, who agreed to start an exercise program and then makes weak excuses for her failure to follow the program, is showing evidence of passive-aggressive personality disorder. She did not really want to follow the doctor's exercise program (was inwardly defiant) but agreed to do it (was outwardly compliant).

23. **The answer is L.** This 26-year-old woman, who shows no evidence of a thought disorder, has no friends, and spends most of her time at solitary pursuits, is showing evidence of schizoid personality disorder. Patients with schizoid personality disorder are typically content with their solitary lifestyle.

24. **The answer is C.** This medical student, who must constantly make lists and review and memorize her notes, is showing evidence of obsessive-compulsive personality disorder. This behavior is ultimately inefficient and has resulted in her academic problems.

25. **The answer is F.** This abused man is showing evidence of dependent personality disorder. He tolerates his partner's abuse because of his overriding fear of being deserted by his lover, being alone, and having to make his own decisions.

26. **The answer is D.** This 20-year-old female college student shows evidence of avoidant personality disorder. She is so overwhelmed by what she perceives as criticism and rejection that she drops out of school rather than face her teacher and classmates again.

# chapter 15

# Psychiatric Disorders in Children

## Typical Board Question

The parents of an 8-year-old boy report that his behavior at home is problematic. He refuses do his chores and often fights with his 6-year-old brother and 11-year-old sister. His teachers report that he is well-behaved at school, is working at the expected level, and gets along well with the other children. Medical examination is unremarkable. The most likely explanation for this picture is

**(A)** oppositional defiant disorder
**(B)** attention deficit/hyperactivity disorder
**(C)** social difficulties in the family
**(D)** conduct disorder
**(E)** typical, age-appropriate behavior

*(See "Answers and Explanations" at end of chapter.)*

## I. PERVASIVE DEVELOPMENTAL DISORDERS OF CHILDHOOD

### A. Overview

1. Pervasive developmental disorders (e.g. autistic disorder, Asperger disorder, Rett disorder, childhood disintegrative disorder) are characterized by the **failure to acquire** or the **early loss** of **social skills** and **difficulties with language**, resulting in lifelong **problems** in **social and occupational functioning**.

2. These disorders are **not reversible**. Management involves **behavioral therapy** to increase social and communicative skills, decrease behavior problems (e.g., self-injury), and improve self-care skills, as well as supportive therapy and counseling to parents (see Chapter 17).

### B. Autism spectrum disorders (ASD)

1. Characteristics of **autistic disorder**, a severe form of ASD, include
   a. Significant **problems with communication** (despite normal hearing).
   b. Significant **problems forming social relationships** (including those with caregivers).
   c. Restricted range of interests; **do not play imaginative games**.
   d. **Repetitive, purposeless behavior** (e.g., spinning, self-injury).
   e. Below-normal intelligence in 25%–75% of children with autistic disorder.
   f. **Unusual abilities** in some children (e.g., exceptional memory or calculation skills). These are referred to as **savant skills**.

2. **Asperger disorder** (a mild form of ASD) involves
   a. Significant problems forming social relationships.

**157**

   **b.** Repetitive behavior and **intense interest in obscure subjects** (e.g., models of 1940s farm tractors).

   **c.** In contrast to autistic disorder, in Asperger disorder there is **no developmental language delay**. However, conversational language skills are often impaired.

3. **Occurrence of ASD**

   **a.** They occur in about 13 children per 10,000.

   **b.** They begin **before age 3 years**.

   **c.** The disorders are four to five times **more common in boys**.

4. Abnormalities that give clues for the **neurobiological etiology** (no psychological causes have been identified) of ASD include

   **a.** **Cerebral dysfunction;** 25% develop **seizures**.

   **b.** A history of **perinatal complications**.

   **c.** A **genetic component** (e.g., higher concordance rate in monozygotic than in dizygotic twins).

   **d.** Evidence of total **brain** as well as **amygdale overgrowth** during the first few years of life.

   **e.** Abnormalities in the hippocampus, fewer Purkinje cells in the cerebellum.

   **f.** Less circulating **oxytocin** and dysregulation of **serotonin** synthesis.

C. **Other pervasive developmental disorders**

1. **Rett disorder** involves

   **a.** **Diminished social, verbal**, and **cognitive development** after up to 4 years of normal functioning.

   **b.** Occurrence **only in girls** (Rett disorder is X-linked, specifically Xq28, and affected males die before birth).

   **c.** Stereotyped, **hand-wringing** movements; ataxia.

   **d.** Breathing problems.

   **e.** Mental retardation.

   **f.** Motor problems later in the illness.

2. **Childhood disintegrative disorder** involves

   **a.** **Diminished social, verbal, cognitive**, and **motor development** after at least 2 years of normal functioning.

   **b.** Mental retardation.

## II. ATTENTION DEFICIT/HYPERACTIVITY DISORDER AND DISRUPTIVE BEHAVIOR DISORDERS OF CHILDHOOD

A. **Overview**

1. **Attention deficit/hyperactivity disorder (ADHD)** and the **disruptive behavior disorders (e.g., conduct disorder and oppositional defiant disorder)** are characterized by **inappropriate behavior** that causes difficulties in social relationships and school performance.

2. There is **no frank mental retardation**.

3. These disorders are not uncommon and are seen more often **in boys**.

4. **Differential diagnosis** includes **mood disorders and anxiety disorders**.

5. If the behavioral abnormalities **occur only in one setting** (e.g., only at home or only at school), these disorders are not diagnosed, rather, relationship problems (e.g., with either parents or teachers) must be explored.

6. Characteristics and prognoses of these disorders can be found in Table 15.1.

B. **Etiology**

1. **Genetic factors** are involved. Relatives of children with conduct disorder and ADHD have an increased incidence of these disorders and of **antisocial personality disorder** and **substance abuse**.

2. Although evidence of serious structural problems in the brain is not present, children with conduct disorder and ADHD may have **minor brain dysfunction**.

| table **15.1** | Characteristics and Prognosis of Attention Deficit Hyperactivity Disorder, Conduct Disorder, and Oppositional Defiant Disorder | |
|---|---|---|
| **Attention Deficit Hyperactivity Disorder (ADHD)** | **Conduct Disorder** | **Oppositional Defiant Disorder** |
| **Characteristics (must be present in at least 2 settings, e.g., at home and at school)** | | |
| Hyperactivity Inattention Impulsivity Carelessness Propensity for accidents History of excessive crying, high sensitivity to stimuli, and irregular sleep patterns in infancy | Behavior that grossly violates social norms (e.g., torturing animals, stealing, truancy, fire setting) | Behavior that, while defiant, negative, and noncompliant, does not grossly violate social norms (e.g., anger, argumentativeness, resentment toward authority figures) |
| Symptoms present before age 7 | Can begin in childhood (ages 6–10) or adolescence (no symptoms prior to age 10) | Gradual onset, usually before age 8 |
| **Prognosis** | | |
| Hyperactivity is the first symptom to disappear as the child reaches adolescence Risk for conduct disorder and oppositional defiant disorder | Risk for criminal behavior, antisocial personality disorder, substance abuse, and mood disorders in adulthood | A significant number of cases progress to conduct disorder |
| Most children show remission by adulthood | Most children show remission by adulthood | Most children show remission by adulthood |

3. Substance abuse, serious parental discord, and mood disorders, are seen in some parents of children with these disorders; these children are also **more likely to be abused** by parents or caretakers.
4. There is **no scientific basis** for claims of an association between ADHD and either improper diet (e.g., excessive sugar intake) or food allergy (e.g., artificial colors or flavors).

C. **Management**
 1. Pharmacologic treatment for **ADHD** consists of use of central nervous system (CNS) **stimulants** including methylphenidate (Ritalin, Concerta), dextroamphetamine sulfate (Dexedrine), a combination of amphetamine/dextroamphetamine (Adderall), and dexmethylphenidate (Focalin). Atomoxetine (Strattera) is a **norepinephrine reuptake inhibitor** also indicated for ADHD.
  a. For ADHD, CNS stimulants apparently help **reduce activity level and increase attention span** and the ability to concentrate; antidepressants also may be useful.
  b. Since stimulant drugs **decrease appetite** (see Chapter 9), they may inhibit growth and lead to **failure to gain weight**; both growth and weight usually return to normal once the child stops taking the medication.
 2. **Family therapy** is the most effective management for conduct disorder and oppositional defiant disorder (see Chapter 17).

## III. OTHER DISORDERS OF CHILDHOOD

A. **Tourette disorder**
 1. Tourette disorder is characterized by **involuntary movements and vocalizations (tics)** that may include the involuntary use of profanity (coprolalia). While these behaviors can be controlled briefly, they must ultimately be expressed.
 2. The disorder, which is **lifelong and chronic**, begins before age 18. It usually starts with a motor tic (e.g., facial grimacing) that appears between ages 7 and 8.
 3. The disorder is three times **more common in males** and has a **strong genetic component**.
 4. There is a genetic relationship **between** Tourette disorder and both **ADHD** and **obsessive–compulsive disorder** (see Chapter 13).

**5.** While the manifestations are behavioral, the **etiology** of Tourette disorder is neurologic. It is believed to involve dysfunctional regulation of dopamine in the **caudate nucleus** and is commonly managed with typical **antipsychotic agents** (e.g., haloperidol, pimozide) as well as atypical agents, (e.g., risperidone). In milder cases, alpha-2 adrenergic agonists agents such as clonidine also are helpful.

**B. Separation anxiety disorder**
  **1.** Often incorrectly called school phobia, because the child refuses to go to school, this disorder is characterized by an **overwhelming fear of loss of a major attachment figure**, particularly the mother.
  **2.** The child often complains of **physical symptoms** (e.g., stomach pain or headache) to avoid going to school and leaving the mother.
  **3.** The most effective management of a child with this disorder is to have the mother accompany the child to school and then, when the child is more comfortable, gradually decrease her time spent at school.
  **4.** Individuals with a history of separation anxiety disorder in childhood are at greater risk for anxiety disorders in adulthood, particularly **agoraphobia**.

**C. Selective mutism**
  **1.** Children (more commonly girls) with this rare disorder **speak in some social situations** (e.g., at home) **but not in others** (e.g., at school); the child also may whisper or communicate with hand gestures.
  **2.** Selective mutism must be distinguished from typical shyness.

**D. Elimination disorders: Enuresis and encopresis**
  **1.** Typically, most children are bowel and bladder trained by age 3 years.
  **2.** The elimination disorders **encopresis** (soiling) and **enuresis** (wetting) are not diagnosed until after age 4 years and 5 years, respectively.
  **3.** After medical factors (e.g., urinary tract infection) are ruled out, the most common cause of enuresis is **physiological immaturity** (see Chapter 1).
  **4.** **Management** of nighttime enuresis (in order of utility) includes
    **a.** **Restricting fluids** after dinner.
    **b.** Use of **a bell and pad** apparatus. A pad that can sense moisture is placed under the child at night. If the pad becomes wet, a buzzer goes off which wakens the child. By negative reinforcement (see Chapter 7) the child eventually wakes before wetting at night.
    **c.** Use of a pharmacologic agent such as **desmopressin** acetate (a synthetic analog of antidiuretic hormone) or a cyclic antidepressant such as **imipramine** at bedtime. Both agents reduce nocturnal urine output; desmopressin is preferred because it has fewer adverse effects.

# Review Test

**Directions:** Each of the numbered items or incomplete statements in this section is followed by answers or by completions of the statement. Select the **one** lettered answer or completion that is **best** in each case.

## Questions 1 and 2

Since the age of 8, a 15-year-old girl with normal intelligence and interactive skills has shown a number of repetitive motor movements. She recently has begun to have outbursts in which she curses and shrieks. When asked if she can control the vocalizations and movements she says, "For a short time only; it is like holding your breath—eventually you have to let it out." Medical evaluation is unremarkable.

**1.** This child is showing evidence of

**(A)** autism spectrum disorders (ASD)
**(B)** Rett disorder
**(C)** attention deficit hyperactivity disorder (ADHD)
**(D)** Tourette disorder
**(E)** selective mutism

**2.** The most effective management of the unwanted vocalizations and movements is

**(A)** an antipsychotic
**(B)** an antidepressant
**(C)** family therapy
**(D)** a stimulant
**(E)** individual psychotherapy

**3.** A 4-year-old child who has never spoken voluntarily shows no interest in or connection to his parents, other adults, or other children. Medical examination and otological testing are unremarkable. The child's mother tells the doctor that he persistently turns on the taps to watch the water running and that he screams and struggles fiercely when she tries to dress him. Which of the following disorders best fits this clinical picture?

**(A)** ASD
**(B)** Rett disorder
**(C)** ADHD
**(D)** Tourette disorder
**(E)** Selective mutism

## Questions 4–7

A 9-year-old boy with normal intelligence frequently gets into trouble at school because he blurts out answers, interrupts the teacher, disturbs the other students, and cannot seem to sit still in class. He also frequently injures himself during play and rarely sits through an entire meal at home. His siblings say that he is "a real pest." However, the child does his schoolwork well and behaves well when he is alone with his tutor.

**4.** The best explanation for this child's behavior is

**(A)** oppositional defiant disorder
**(B)** ADHD
**(C)** social difficulties in the family
**(D)** conduct disorder
**(E)** typical, age-appropriate behavior

**5.** Which of the following is most closely involved in the etiology of this child's problem?

**(A)** Food allergy
**(B)** Improper diet
**(C)** Neurologic dysfunction
**(D)** Excessive punishment
**(E)** Excessive leniency

**6.** Of the following, the most effective management for this child is

**(A)** lithium
**(B)** a stimulant
**(C)** an antidepressant
**(D)** a sedative
**(E)** psychotherapy

**7.** This boy is at a higher risk than other children to develop which of the following disorders?

**(A)** Tourette disorder
**(B)** Separation anxiety disorder
**(C)** Bipolar disorder
**(D)** Conduct disorder
**(E)** Schizophrenia

**8.** After starting first grade, a 7-year-old boy often complains of feeling ill and refuses to go to school. There are no medical findings. At home, the child is appropriately interactive with his parents and, when friends visit, he plays well with them. At first his parents let him stay at home, but they are becoming increasingly concerned that he is falling behind in his schoolwork. The parents want to hire a home tutor for the child. What is the pediatrician's next step in management?

**(A)** Advise the parents to go to school with the child and, over days, gradually decrease the time they spend there.
**(B)** Advise the parents to allow the child to stay at home until he indicates that he is comfortable separating from the parents.
**(C)** Advise the parents to ignore the school refusal, bring the child to school, and tell him what time they will pick him up.
**(D)** Reassure the parents that hiring a home tutor for the current school year is best for the child.
**(E)** Prescribe an antianxiety agent for the child to be given only on school days.

**9.** A 9-year-old boy with normal intelligence has a history of fighting with other children and catching and torturing birds, squirrels, and rabbits. When asked why he engages in this behavior, he says, "It's just fun." Developmental history and medical examination are unremarkable. The best explanation of this child's behavior is

**(A)** oppositional defiant disorder
**(B)** ADHD
**(C)** social difficulties in the family
**(D)** conduct disorder
**(E)** normal age-appropriate behavior

**Questions 10 and 11**

Concerned parents of a 7-year-old boy bring their child to the pediatrician for evaluation. They note that ever since he was an infant, their son has never wanted to be held, cries whenever he is bathed, and becomes very upset when his daily routine is changed in any way. Although the child cannot yet read, his parents remark that he can identify the state of origin of any car license plate and almost exclusively plays with replicas of car license plates. The child's speaks in complete sentences and has a good vocabulary, but his behavior seems odd and he does not make eye contact when spoken to. Medical evaluation is unremarkable.

**10.** As an adolescent, this boy is likely to have the most difficulty in which of the following areas?

**(A)** Paying attention in school
**(B)** Concentrating on relevant stimuli
**(C)** Caring for pets
**(D)** Making friends
**(E)** Controlling his activity level

**11.** The major characteristic that suggests that this child has Asperger disorder rather than autistic disorder is that this child does **not** show

**(A)** restricted interests
**(B)** special abilities
**(C)** focus on keeping up routines
**(D)** problems in peer relationships
**(E)** language delay

**12.** The parents and teacher of a 7-year-old boy note that he frequently shrugs his shoulders. Often he blinks his eyes excessively and, at other times, shouts out words for no reason. In adulthood this child is at risk to develop which of the following conditions?

**(A)** A seizure disorder
**(B)** Obsessive–compulsive disorder
**(C)** Conduct disorder
**(D)** Schizophrenia
**(E)** ASD

**13.** The parents of a 10-year-old child report that the child is still wetting the bed. The child is very upset about this because he would like to go away to summer camp but is afraid that he will wet the bed there as well. Physical examination is unremarkable and the child is otherwise developing typically for his age. Behavioral interventions such as limiting fluids before bed and the bell and pad apparatus have not been effective. At this time, which of the following is the best choice for pharmacologic management of enuresis in this child

**(A)** Imipramine
**(B)** Diazepam
**(C)** Desmopressin acetate
**(D)** Acetaminophen
**(E)** Aspirin

# Answers and Explanations

**The answer is C.** The most likely explanation for why this child misbehaves at home but not at school is that there are social difficulties in the family, for example, problems in the relationship between the mother and father. In contrast, children with conduct disorder show behavior that violates social norms (e.g., stealing), children with ADHD have trouble controlling their behavior, and children with oppositional defiant disorder have problems dealing with authority figures. In these disorders behavioral difficulties are present both at home and at school.

1. **The answer is D. 2. The answer is A.** This girl is most likely to have Tourette disorder, a chronic neurologic condition with behavioral manifestations such as unwanted motor activity and vocalizations. The vocalizations and motor tics can be controlled only briefly and then they must be expressed. ASD and Rett disorder are pervasive developmental disorders of childhood, that are characterized by abnormal social interaction and speech. ADHD involves normal development of speech and social interaction but difficulty paying attention or sitting still. Selective mutism involves voluntary absence or decrease in speaking in social situations. The most effective management for Tourette disorder is antipsychotic medication, such as haloperidol. There is no evidence that antidepressants or stimulants are helpful for control of motor or vocal tics. Psychotherapy can help patients with Tourette disorder deal with the social problems their disorder may cause, but is not the most effective management for the symptoms of the disorder.

3. **The answer is A.** This child, who has never spoken voluntarily and who shows no interest in or connection to his parents, other adults, or other children despite normal hearing, probably has ASD. He turns on the tap to watch the water running because, as with many children with ASD, repetitive motion calms him. Any change in his environment, such as being dressed, leads to intense discomfort, struggling, and screaming (see also answer to Question 1).

4. **The answer is B. 5. The answer is C. 6. The answer is B. 7. The answer is D.** This 9-year-old boy who gets into trouble at school because he disturbs the teacher and the other students, has behavioral difficulties at home and with siblings, and cannot seem to sit still is showing evidence of ADHD (see also answer to Question 1). Children with ADHD can often learn well when there are few distractions (e.g., alone with a tutor). Children with conduct disorder show behavior that violates social norms (e.g., stealing). In contrast, children with ADHD have trouble controlling their behavior but do not intentionally cause harm. Children with oppositional defiant disorder have problems dealing with authority figures but not with other children or animals. ADHD is believed to result from neurologic dysfunction. Although anecdotal evidence has been put forward, scientific studies have not revealed an association between ADHD and either improper diet (e.g., excessive sugar intake) or food allergy (e.g., to artificial colors or flavors). The disorder also is not a result of parenting style (e.g., excessive punishment or leniency). However, in part because of their difficult behavior, children with ADHD are more likely to be physically abused by parents. The most effective management for children with ADHD is use of central nervous system stimulants including methylphenidate (Ritalin), and dextroamphetamine sulfate (Dexedrine). Lithium is used to treat bipolar disorder, antidepressants are used primarily to treat depression, and sedatives are used primarily to treat anxiety. While psychotherapy may help the parents and child deal with the behavioral symptoms, it is not the most effective management since the disorder is caused by neurologic dysfunction. Children with ADHD are at higher risk than other children for oppositional defiant disorder and conduct disorder.

8. **The answer is A.** This child is showing evidence of separation anxiety disorder. By the age of 3 to 4 years children should be able to spend some time away from parents in a school setting. The pediatrician's best recommendation is for the parents to go to school with the child and, over days, gradually decrease the time they spend there. Allowing the child to stay at home or hiring a home tutor will just increase the child's difficulty separating from his parents. Pharmacologic therapy is not the first choice in the management of this child.

9. **The answer is D.** This child is showing evidence of conduct disorder. Children with this disorder have little or no concern for others or for animals (e.g., this child finds torturing animals "fun") (see also answer to Question 4).

10. **The answer is D. 11. The answer is E.** This child who does not want to be held, cries when his environment is changed (e.g., when bathed), and does not make eye contact is likely to have ASD. Children with ASD have great difficulty with interpersonal relations. Problems with attention and concentration are more characteristic of ADHD. Children with conduct disorder tend to have poor self-control and to break societal rules. Hyperactivity may be present but is not specifically associated with ASD. The major characteristic that differentiates autistic disorder from Asperger disorder is that in the former but not in the latter, there is developmental language delay. This child shows relatively normal language development, so Asperger disorder is more likely than autistic disorder in this case. Restricted or unusual interests (here, intense focus on state license plates), special abilities, focus on keeping up routines and problems in peer relationships are characteristic of both disorders.

12. **The answer is B.** This child who shows evidence of Tourette disorder is at risk to develop obsessive–compulsive disorder (OCD) in adulthood. Both disorders involve dysfunction of the caudate nucleus. Seizure disorders, conduct disorder, schizophrenia, and ASD are not particularly associated with Tourette disorder (see also answer to Question 1).

13. **The answer is C.** The best choice for the pharmacologic management of bedwetting in an older child such as this is desmopressin acetate. Imipramine is also useful in managing enuresis but has more side effects. Diazepam (a benzodiazepine), used to treat anxiety, and acetaminophen and aspirin, used in the management of minor pain, are not useful in managing enuresis.

# chapter 16

# Biologic Therapies: Psychopharmacology

**Typical Board Question**

A 40-year-old man comes to the emergency department with a 4-day history of vomiting and diarrhea. The patient has elevated blood pressure, and body temperature as well as myclonus, and muscular rigidity. Except for a slightly elevated white blood count, blood and urine tests are within normal limits and there is no evidence of infection. The patient, who has been on 40 mg/daily of fluoxetine for years, has recently started to take a new medication for back pain. Which of the following pain medications is most likely to have been prescribed for this patient?

**(A)** Oxycodone
**(B)** Hydrocodone
**(C)** Gabapentin
**(D)** Tramadol
**(E)** Ibuprofen

*(See "Answers and Explanations" at end of chapter.)*

## I. OVERVIEW

A. **Neurotransmitter abnormalities** are involved in the etiology of many psychiatric illnesses (e.g., psychotic disorders, mood disorders, anxiety disorders) (see Chapter 4).

B. Although normalization of neurotransmitter levels by **pharmacologic agents** can ameliorate many of the symptoms, these agents **do not cure** psychiatric disorders.

C. Psychopharmacologic agents may also be useful in the **treatment of symptoms of certain medical conditions** (e.g., gastrointestinal problems, pain, seizures).

## II. ANTIPSYCHOTIC AGENTS

A. **Overview**
   1. Antipsychotic agents (formerly called neuroleptics or major tranquilizers) are used in the treatment of **schizophrenia** as well as in the treatment of psychotic symptoms associated with other psychiatric and physical disorders.
   2. Antipsychotics are also used medically to treat nausea, hiccups, intense anxiety and agitation, and Tourette disorder.

3. Although antipsychotics commonly are taken daily by mouth, nonadherent patients can be treated with long-acting **"depot"** forms, such as **haloperidol decanoate or fluphenazine decanoate** administered intramuscularly every 2–4 weeks.
4. Antipsychotic agents can be classified as **traditional (i.e., typical) or atypical** depending on their mode of action and side effect profile.

B. **Traditional** antipsychotic agents
1. Traditional antipsychotic agents act primarily by **blocking central dopamine-2 ($D_2$)** receptors.
2. Although negative symptoms of schizophrenia, such as withdrawal, may improve with continued treatment, traditional antipsychotic agents are **most effective against positive symptoms**, such as hallucinations and delusions (see Chapter 11).
3. **Adverse effects** of antipsychotics
   a. **Low-potency** agents (e.g., chlorpromazine (Thorazine), thioridazine [Mellaril]) are associated primarily with **non-neurologic** adverse effects (Table 16.1). Because there are better choices (e.g., atypical agents), low-potency agents are now rarely used.
   b. **High-potency** agents (e.g., haloperidol [Haldol], trifluoperazine [Stelazine], fluphenazine [Prolixin], perphenazine [Trilafon], thiothixene [Navane], and molindone [Moban]) are associated primarily with **neurologic** adverse effects (Table 16.1).
   c. Agents related to antipsychotics such as the dopamine receptor antagonist **metoclopromide** (Reglan) which is used to reduce nausea and vomiting in medical patients, can have similar adverse effects, for example, akathisia and extrapyramidal symptoms (EPS) (Table 16.1).

C. **Atypical** antipsychotic agents (e.g., clozapine [Clozaril], risperidone [Risperdal], olanzapine [Zyprexa], quetiapine [Seroquel], ziprasidone [Geodon], aripiprazole [Abilify], paliperidone [Invega]), iloperidone (Fanapt), asenapine (Saphris), and lurasidone (Latuda)
1. In contrast to traditional antipsychotic agents, a major mechanism of action of atypical antipsychotics appears to be on **serotonergic systems**. They also affect dopaminergic receptors in addition to $D_2$ (e.g., $D_1$, $D_3$, and $D_4$).
2. Many of the atypical antipsychotics are also indicated to treat **bipolar disorder**.

table **16.1**  Adverse Effects of Typical Antipsychotic Agents

| System | Adverse Effects |
| --- | --- |
| *Non-neurologic Adverse Effects—More Common with Traditional, Low-Potency Agents* | |
| Circulatory | Orthostatic (postural) hypotension |
| | Electrocardiogram abnormalities (prolongation of QT and PR intervals) |
| Endocrine | Increase in prolactin level resulting in gynecomastia (breast enlargement), galactorrhea, erectile dysfunction, amenorrhea, and decreased libido |
| Hematologic | Leukopenia, agranulocytosis |
| Hepatic | Jaundice, elevated liver enzyme levels |
| Dermatologic | Skin eruptions, photosensitivity, and blue-gray skin discoloration |
| Ophthalmologic | Irreversible retinal pigmentation (particularly thioridizine) |
| Anticholinergic | Peripheral effects: dry mouth, constipation, urinary retention, and blurred vision |
| | Central effects: agitation and disorientation |
| Antihistaminergic | Weight gain and sedation |
| *Neurologic Adverse Effects—More Common with Traditional, High-Potency Agents* | |
| Extrapyramidal | Pseudoparkinsonism (muscle rigidity, shuffling gait, resting tremor, mask-like facial expression) |
| | Akathisia (subjective feeling of motor restlessness) |
| | Acute dystonia (prolonged muscular spasms; more common in men under age 40) |
| | Treat with anticholinergic (e.g., benztropine) or antihistaminergic (e.g., diphenhydramine) agent |
| Other | Tardive dyskinesia (abnormal writhing movements of the tongue, face, and body; more common in women and after at least 6 months of treatment); to treat, substitute low-potency or atypical antipsychotic agent. Is rarely reversible |
| | Neuroleptic malignant syndrome (high fever, sweating, increased pulse and blood pressure, dystonia, apathy; more common in men and early in treatment; mortality rate about 20%); to treat, stop agent, give a skeletal muscle relaxant (e.g., dantrolene), and provide medical support |
| | Decreased seizure threshold |

| table 16.2 | Adverse Effects of Atypical Antipsychotic Agents | | | | | | | | |
|---|---|---|---|---|---|---|---|---|---|
| Adverse Effect | Aripiprazole | Clozapine | Olanzapine | Risperidone | Quetiapine | Ziprasidone | Asenapine | Iloperidone | Lurasidone | Paliperidone |
| Weight gain and diabetes | ± | ++++ | +++ | ++ | ++ | + | ± | + | ± | ± |
| EPS and prolactin elevation | ± | ± | ± | ++ | ± | ± | ++ | ± | +++ | + |
| Sedation | ± | ++++ | +++ | ++ | +++ | —+ | ++ | ++ | +++ | ± |
| Increased QT interval | ± | ± | ++ | + | ++ | +–++ | ++ | ++++ | ± | ++ |

EPS, extrapyramidal symptoms ; ± = few if any, + = mild, ++ = moderate, +++ = severe, ++++ = very severe.

3. **Advantages** of atypical agents over traditional agents
   a. Atypical agents, particularly clozapine, may be **more effective** when used to treat the **negative**, chronic, and refractory **symptoms** of schizophrenia (see Chapter 11).
   b. They are **less likely to cause adverse neurological symptoms** and dystonias (Table 16.1) and so are now the **first-line** agents for treating chronic psychiatric disorders such as schizophrenia.
4. **Disadvantages** of atypical agents
   a. Atypical agents may increase the likelihood of blood dyscrasias such as **agranulocytosis** (very low granulocyte count leading to severe infections), with **clozapine** as the most problematic agent.
   b. They may also increase the likelihood of **seizures**, anticholinergic side effects, and pancreatitis.
   c. Some atypical agents have more adverse effects than others. Table 16.2 provides the adverse effects for different atypical agents with respect to **weight gain and type 2 diabetes, EPS and prolactin elevation, sedation**, and cardiovascular effects such as **prolongation of the QT interval**.

## III. ANTIDEPRESSANT AGENTS

### A. Overview

1. **Heterocyclic antidepressants (HCAs), selective serotonin reuptake inhibitors (SSRIs), selective serotonin** and **norepinephrine reuptake inhibitors (SNRIs), monoamine oxidase inhibitors (MAOIs),** and **atypical antidepressants** are used to treat depression. These agents also have other clinical uses (Table 16.3).
2. All antidepressants are believed to increase the availability of serotonin and/or norepinephrine in the synapse via inhibition of reuptake mechanisms (HCAs, SSRIs, SNRIs) or blockade of MAO (MAOIs), which ultimately leads to **downregulation of postsynaptic receptors** and improvement in mood (see Chapter 4).
3. All antidepressants take about **3–6 weeks to work** and all have **equal efficacy**.
4. While heterocyclics were once the mainstay of management, because of their more positive side effect profile, **SSRIs** (e.g., fluoxetine [Prozac]) are now used as **first-line agents**.
5. Antidepressant agents **do not elevate mood in nondepressed people** and **have no abuse potential**. They can, however, **precipitate manic episodes** in potentially bipolar patients.
6. **Stimulants**, such as methylphenidate or dextroamphetamine, also may be useful in treating depression. They work quickly, and thus may help to improve mood in terminally ill or elderly patients. They are also useful in patients with depression refractory to other

| t a b l e   **16.3** | Antidepressant Agents (Grouped Alphabetically by Category) | |
|---|---|---|
| **Agent (Current or Former Brand Name)** | **Effects** | **Clinical Uses in Addition to Depression (FDA Indications)** |
| ***Heterocyclic Agents (HCAs)*** | | |
| Amitriptyline (Elavil) | Sedating<br>Anticholinergic<br>Prolonged QT interval | Depression with insomnia<br>Chronic pain |
| Clomipramine (Anafranil) | Most serotonin-specific of the HCAs | Obsessive–compulsive disorder (OCD) |
| Doxepin (Adapin, Sinequan) | Sedating, antihistaminergic<br>Anticholinergic | Peptic ulcer disease<br>Pruritis, i.e., itching |
| Imipramine (Tofranil) | Orthostatic hypotension<br>Prolonged QT interval | Panic disorder with agoraphobia<br>Enuresis<br>Eating disorders |
| Maprotiline (Ludiomil) | May cause seizures | Anxiety with depressive features |
| Nortriptyline (Aventyl, Pamelor) | Least likely of the HCAs to cause orthostatic hypotension | Depression in the elderly<br>Pruritus<br>Patients with cardiac diseases |
| Protriptyline (Vivactil) | Stimulating | ADHD<br>Narcolepsy |
| ***Selective Serotonin Reuptake Inhibitors (SSRIs)*** | | |
| Citalopram (Celexa) | More cardiotoxic than other SSRIs<br>Low cytochrome P450 effects | OCD (paroxetine, sertraline, fluoxetine)<br>Panic disorder (paroxetine, sertraline, fluoxetine) |
| Escitalopram (Lexapro) | Most serotonin-specific of the SSRIs<br>Low cytochrome P450 effects<br>Fewer side effects than citalopram<br>Rapid symptom relief | Chronic pain<br>Paraphilias<br>Generalized anxiety disorder (paroxetine and escitalopram) |
| Fluoxetine (Prozac, Sarafem) | May cause agitation and insomnia initially<br>Sexual dysfunction<br>May uniquely cause some weight loss | Social phobia (paroxetine, sertraline)<br>Premenstrual dysphoria (Sarafem, sertraline)<br>PTSD (paroxetine, sertraline) |
| Fluvoxamine (Luvox) | Currently indicated only for OCD | Bulimia nervosa (fluoxetine) |
| Paroxetine (Paxil) | Most sedating SSRI<br>Most anticholinergic SSRIs<br>Sexual dysfunction | Premature ejaculation<br>Body dysmorphic disorder |
| Sertraline (Zoloft) | Most likely of the SSRIs to cause gastrointestinal disturbances (e.g., diarrhea)<br>Sexual dysfunction | |
| ***Selective Serotonin and Norepinephrine Reuptake Inhibitors (SNRIs)*** | | |
| Duloxetine (Cymbalta) | Rapid symptom relief<br>Few sexual side effects | Generalized anxiety disorder<br>Social phobia |
| Venlafaxine (Effexor) | Rapid symptom relief<br>Few sexual side effects<br>Low cytochrome P450 effects<br>Increased diastolic blood pressure at higher doses | Panic disorder<br>Chronic pain (SNRIs) |
| ***Monoamine Oxidase Inhibitors (MAOIs)*** | | |
| Isocarboxazid (Marplan)<br>Tranylcypromine (Parnate)<br>Phenelzine (Nardil) | Hyperadrenergic crisis precipitated by ingestion of pressor amines in tyramine-containing foods or sympathomimetic drugs | Geriatric depression<br>Atypical depression<br>Pain disorders<br>Eating disorders<br>Panic disorder |
| Selegiline (Emsam: transdermal patch) | Orthostatic hypotension | Social phobia |
| ***Other Antidepressants*** | | |
| Amoxapine (Asendin) | Antidopaminergic effects (e.g., parkinsonian symptoms, galactorrhea, sexual dysfunction)<br>Most dangerous in overdose | Depression with psychotic features |
| Bupropion (Wellbutrin, Zyban, Contrave) | Insomnia<br>Seizures: Avoid in eating disorder patients who purge<br>Sweating<br>Few adverse sexual effects | Smoking cessation (Zyban)<br>Seasonal affective disorder<br>SSRI induced sexual dysfunction<br>Adult ADHD<br>Obesity (Contrave) |
| Mirtazapine (Remeron) | Increased appetite<br>Few adverse sexual effects | Insomnia |
| Trazodone (Desyrel, Oleptro) | Sedation<br>Priapism<br>Hypotension | Insomnia |
| Vilazodone (Viibryd) | Fewer adverse sexual effects | Only indicated for major depressive disorder |

treatment and in those at risk for the development of adverse effects of other agents for depression. Disadvantages include their addiction potential.

7. **Thyroid hormones** can be used also in the management of mood disorders.
   a. Levothyroxine (Synthroid) is a synthetic form of thyroxine ($T_4$) which has mood stabilizing effects in patients with bipolar disorder.
   b. Liothyronine (Cytomel) is a synthetic form of $T_4$'s metabolically active form triiodothyronine ($T_3$) which can augment the effects of antidepressants.

B. **Heterocyclic Agents**

   1. **HCAs block reuptake of norepinephrine** and **serotonin** at the synapse. Some also block reuptake of dopamine.
      a. These agents also block muscarinic acetylcholine receptors, resulting in **anticholinergic effects** (e.g., dry mouth, blurred vision, urine retention, constipation); they are contraindicated in patients with **glaucoma**.
      b. Histamine receptors also are blocked by heterocyclic agents, resulting in antihistaminergic effects (e.g., **weight gain** and **sedation**).
   2. Other adverse effects include cardiovascular effects, such as orthostatic hypotension, and QT prolongation, and neurologic effects, such as tremor, weight gain, and sexual dysfunction.
   3. Heterocyclics are **dangerous in overdose.**

C. **SSRIs and SNRIs**

   1. **SSRIs selectively block the reuptake of serotonin only; SNRIs block the reuptake of both serotonin and norepinephrine.**
   2. SSRIs and SNRIs have little effect on acetylcholine, or histamine systems.
   3. Because of this selectivity, **SSRIs** and **SNRIs cause fewer side effects** and are **safer** in **overdose**, in the **elderly**, and in **pregnancy** than heterocyclics or MAOIs.
   4. SNRIs may work more quickly (e.g., in 2–3 weeks) and cause fewer sexual side effects than SSRIs.

D. **MAOIs**

   1. MAOIs inhibit the breakdown of neurotransmitters by monoamine oxidase A ($MAO_A$) in the brain in an irreversible reaction.
   2. These agents may be particularly useful in the management of **atypical depression** (see Chapter 12) and treatment resistance to other agents.
   3. A major drawback of using MAOIs is **a potentially fatal reaction** when they are taken in conjunction with certain foods or medications. This reaction occurs because
      a. **MAO metabolizes tyramine, a pressor**, in the gastrointestinal tract.
      b. If MAO is inhibited, ingestion of **tyramine-rich foods** (e.g., aged cheese, beer, wine, broad beans, beef or chicken liver, and smoked or pickled meats or fish) or **sympathomimetic drugs** (e.g., ephedrine, methylphenidate [Ritalin], phenylephrine [Neo-Synephrine], pseudoephedrine [Sudafed]) can increase tyramine levels.
      c. Increase in tyramine can cause elevated blood pressure, sweating, headache, and vomiting (i.e., the **noradrenergic** or **hypertensive crisis**), which in turn can lead to **stroke** and **death**.
   4. Other adverse effects of MAOIs are similar to those of the heterocyclics, including danger in overdose.
   5. **The serotonin syndrome**
      a. MAOIs and SSRIs or HCAs used together as well as MAOIs used along with serotonergic analgesics such as **meperidine** (Demerol) or **tramadol** (Ultram) can cause a potentially fatal drug–drug interaction, the serotonin syndrome.
      b. This syndrome is characterized by **high fever**, autonomic instability, headache, seizures, delirium, nausea, diarrhea, vomiting, and muscular rigidity.
      c. To avoid this reaction, the recommended **washout period** for an SSRI or an HCA before starting an MAOI is 5 weeks and 2 weeks, respectively.

## IV. MOOD STABILIZERS

A. **Lithium** (carbonate and citrate)
1. Lithium is a mood stabilizer used to **prevent both** the manic and depressive phases of bipolar disorder.
2. It may be used also to **increase the effectiveness of antidepressant agents** in depressive illness and to **control aggressive behavior** (see Chapter 20).
3. **Adverse effects** of chronic use of lithium include:
   a. congenital abnormalities (particularly of the cardiovascular system e.g., **Ebstein's anomaly**)
   b. hypothyroidism
   c. tremor
   d. renal dysfunction leading to diabetes insipidus
   e. cardiac conduction problems
   f. gastric distress
   g. mild cognitive impairment
4. Lithium **takes 2–3 weeks to work**. Antipsychotics or benzodiazepines rather than lithium are therefore the initial treatment for psychotic symptoms in an acute manic episode.
5. Because of potential **toxicity**, blood levels of lithium must be maintained at **0.8–1.2 mEqL**.

B. **Anticonvulsants: carbamazepine (Tegretol), oxcarbamazepine (Trileptal), valproic acid (Depakene, Depakote), and others**
1. Anticonvulsants are also used to manage bipolar disorder, particularly **rapid cycling bipolar disorder** (i.e., more than four episodes annually), and **mixed episodes** (mania and depression occurring concurrently).
2. **Carbamazepine** may be associated with severe adverse effects, such as **aplastic anemia** and **agranulocytosis**.
3. **Valproic acid** may be particularly useful for treating bipolar symptoms resulting from cognitive disorders (see Chapter 14) and for prophylaxis of migraine headaches.
4. Adverse effects of valproic acid include gastrointestinal and liver problems, congenital neural tube defects (e.g., **spina bifida**), and alopecia (hair loss).
5. **Other anticonvulsant agents** that appear to have mood-stabilizing effects include lamotrigine (Lamictal), gabapentin (Neurontin), topiramate (Topamax), and tiagabine (Gabitril).

C. **Atypical antipsychotics** are also indicated in the management of bipolar disorder.

## V. ANTIANXIETY AGENTS

A. **Benzodiazepines (BZs)**
1. BZs activate binding sites on the **γ-aminobutyric acid A (GABA$_A$) receptor**, thereby decreasing neuronal and muscle cell firing.
2. These agents have a short, intermediate, or long onset and duration of action and may be used to treat disorders other than anxiety disorders (Table 16.4).
3. Their characteristics of action are related to their clinical indications and their potential for abuse; for example, short-acting agents are good hypnotics (sleep inducers) but have a higher potential for abuse than longer acting agents.
4. BZs commonly cause **sedation** but have few other adverse effects in adults.
5. **Tolerance** and **dependence** may occur with chronic use of these agents.
6. **Flumazenil** (Mazicon, Romazicon) is a BZ receptor antagonist that can reverse the effects of BZs in cases of overdose or when BZs (e.g., midazolam [Versed]) are used for sedation during medical or surgical procedures.

| table 16.4 | Antianxiety Agents (Listed Alphabetically by Duration of Action within Category) | |
|---|---|---|
| **Agent (Brand Name)** | **Duration of Action** | **Clinical Uses in Addition to Anxiety** |
| *Benzodiazepines* | | |
| Clorazepate (Tranxene) | Short | Adjunct in management of partial seizures |
| Triazolam (Halcion) | Short | Insomnia |
| Alprazolam (Xanax) | Intermediate | Depression, panic disorder, social phobia |
| Lorazepam (Ativan) | Intermediate | Psychotic agitation, alcohol withdrawal, acute control of seizures |
| Temazepam (Restoril) | Intermediate | Insomnia |
| Chlordiazepoxide (Librium) | Long | Alcohol withdrawal (particularly for agitation) |
| Clonazepam (Klonopin) | Long | Seizures, mania, social phobia, panic disorder, obsessive-compulsive disorder |
| Diazepam (Valium) | Long | Muscle relaxation, analgesia, seizures, alcohol withdrawal (particularly for seizures) |
| Flurazepam (Dalmane) | Long | Insomnia |
| *Non-benzodiazepines* | | |
| Ramelteon (Rozerem) | Short | Indicated only for insomnia |
| Zaleplon (Sonata) | Short | Indicated only for insomnia |
| Zolpidem (Ambien) | Short (longer acting "CR" version available) | Indicated only for insomnia |
| Eszopiclone (Lunesta) | Intermediate | Indicated only for insomnia |
| Buspirone (BuSpar) | Very long | Anxiety in the elderly, generalized anxiety disorder |

B. **Non-benzodiazepines**

1. **Buspirone** (BuSpar), an azaspirodecanedione, is not related to the BZs.
   a. In contrast to BZs, buspirone is nonsedating and is **not associated with dependence, abuse**, or **withdrawal** problems.
   b. It is used primarily to treat conditions causing chronic anxiety, in which BZ-dependence can become a problem (e.g., **generalized anxiety disorder**) (see Chapter 13).
   c. Buspirone **takes up to 2 weeks to work** and may not be acceptable to patients who are accustomed to taking the fast-acting BZs for their symptoms.
2. **Zolpidem** (Ambien), **zaleplon** (Sonata), **eszopiclone** (Lunesta), and **ramelteon** (Rozerem) are short-acting agents used primarily to treat insomnia (see Chapter 10). Like the BZs, the first three of these agents act on the $GABA_A$ receptor. In contrast, ramelteon is a **selective melatonin agonist**.
3. **Antihypertensives** such as $\beta$-blockers (block both $\alpha_1$- and $\beta_2$-adrenergic receptors) such as propranolol (Inderal) and $\alpha_2$-adrenergic receptor antagonists such as clonidine (Catapres) decrease autonomic hyperarousal and are used to treat symptoms of anxiety (e.g., tachycardia), particularly in patients with social phobias such as fear of public speaking.

# VI. PSYCHOACTIVE MEDICATIONS IN PREGNANCY

A. When women of childbearing age have psychiatric symptoms, there are often questions as to whether to administer psychoactive medications during pregnancy.

B. The potential benefits of many psychoactive agents may warrant their use during pregnancy. Table 16.5 lists the Food and Drug Administration (**FDA**) pregnancy categories for psychoactive agents. For example, most antidepressants and antipsychotics are in FDA pregnancy category C. In contrast, because BZs may cause breathing difficulties, "floppy" muscles and other adverse effects in newborns of mothers who use them during pregnancy, these agents are in FDA pregnancy **categories D and X**.

| table 16.5 | Psychoactive Agents by FDA Pregnancy Category (listed alphabetically within type of agent) | | | |
|---|---|---|---|---|
| Pregnancy Category | Antipsychotics | Antidepressants | Mood stabilizers | Antianxiety agents |
| A | None | None | None | None |
| B | Clozapine<br>Lurasidone | Bupropion<br>Maprotiline | None | Buspirone<br>Zolpidem |
| C | Aripiprazole<br>Asenapine<br>Chlorpromazine<br>Fluphenazine<br>Haloperidol<br>Iloperidone<br>Loxapine<br>Olanzapine<br>Paliperidone<br>Perphenazine<br>Pimozide<br>Quetiapine<br>Risperidone<br>Thioridazine<br>Thiothixene<br>Trifluoperazine<br>Ziprasidone | Amitriptyline<br>Amoxapine<br>Citalopram<br>Clomipriamine<br>Desipramine<br>Doxepin<br>Duloxetine<br>Escitalopram<br>Fluoxetine<br>Fluvoxamine<br>Imipramine<br>Mirtazapine<br>Nortriptyline<br>Protriptyline<br>Sertraline<br>Trazadone<br>Venlafaxine | Lamotrigine | Eszopiclone<br>Zaleplon |
| D | None | Paroxetine | Carbamazepine<br>Lithium<br>Valproic acid | Alprazolam<br>Chlordiazepoxide<br>Clonazepam<br>Clorazepate<br>Diazepam<br>Lorazepam<br>Oxazepam |
| X | None | None | None | Flurazepam<br>Temazepam<br>Triazolam |

Category **A.** No risk to the fetus in animal or human studies
Category **B.** No or slight risk to the fetus in animal studies, no risk seen in human studies
Category **C.** Risk to the fetus in animals; no adequate studies in humans. Potential benefit may warrant use in pregnancy.
Category **D.** Risk to the fetus in humans. Potential benefit may warrant use in pregnancy.
Category **X.** Human fetal risk outweighs potential benefits.

# VII. ELECTROCONVULSIVE THERAPY AND RELATED THERAPIES

A. Uses of electroconvulsive therapy (ECT)
   1. ECT provides **rapid, effective, safe** treatment for some psychiatric disorders.
      a. It is most commonly used to treat **major depressive disorder** that is **refractory to antidepressants**.
      b. ECT may be indicated also for serious depression when rapid symptom resolution is imperative because of **psychotic symptoms** or **suicide risk** (see Chapter 12).
      c. ECT is particularly useful for treating **depression in the elderly** because it may be safer than long-term use of antidepressant agents. It also may be used to treat depression during pregnancy.
   2. The mechanism of action of ECT is not known but may be related to alteration of neurotransmitter function in a manner similar to that of treatment with psychoactive agents.

B. Administration
   1. ECT involves the induction of a **generalized seizure**, lasting 25–60 seconds, by **passing an electric current across the brain**.

    **2.** Prior to seizure induction, the patient is **premedicated** (e.g., with atropine), then administered a short-acting general anesthesia (e.g., methohexital) and a muscle relaxant (e.g., succinylcholine) to prevent injury during the seizure.

    **3.** Improvement in mood typically **begins after a few ECT treatments**. A maximum response to ECT is usually seen after 5–10 treatments given over a 2–3-week period.

**C. Problems associated with ECT**

    **1.** The major adverse effects of ECT are **memory problems**.

    **2.** **Increased intracranial pressure** or recent (within 2 weeks) **myocardial infarction** is relative **contraindication** for ECT.

    **3.** The mortality rate associated with ECT is very low and is comparable to that associated with the induction of general anesthesia.

**D. Other somatic therapies**

**Transcranial magnetic stimulation (TMS)** is a therapy in which an electric current is applied to the scalp to generate a magnetic field about 2 cm deep that stimulates cortical interneurons lying parallel to the brain surface. TMS has been approved by the FDA and appears to be useful in patients with major depressive disorder and obsessive–compulsive disorder.

# Review Test

**Directions:** Each of the numbered items or incomplete statements in this section is followed by answers or by completions of the statement. Select the **one** lettered answer or completion that is **best** in each case.

**Questions 1 and 2**

**1.** A 22-year-old man with schizophrenia who has been taking an antipsychotic for the past 3 months reports that recently he has experienced an uncomfortable sensation in his arms and legs during the day and must constantly move them. Because of this, he can sit still for only a few minutes at a time. This medication side effect is best described as

**(A)** restless legs syndrome
**(B)** neuroleptic malignant syndrome
**(C)** akathisia
**(D)** tardive dyskinesia
**(E)** acute dystonia
**(F)** pseudoparkinsonism

**2.** The antipsychotic agent that this patient is most likely to be taking is

**(A)** risperidone
**(B)** thioridazine
**(C)** olanzapine
**(D)** haloperidol
**(E)** clozapine

**Questions 3 and 4**

A 54-year-old woman with schizophrenia who has been taking a high-potency antipsychotic agent for the past 5 years has begun to show involuntary chewing and lip-smacking movements.

**3.** This sign indicates that the patient is experiencing a side effect of antipsychotic medication known as

**(A)** restless legs syndrome
**(B)** neuroleptic malignant syndrome
**(C)** akathisia
**(D)** tardive dyskinesia
**(E)** acute dystonia
**(F)** pseudoparkinsonism

**4.** The side effect described in question 3 is best treated initially

**(A)** by changing to a low-potency or atypical antipsychotic agent
**(B)** with an antianxiety agent
**(C)** with an antidepressant agent
**(D)** with an anticonvulsant
**(E)** by stopping the antipsychotic agent

**Questions 5 and 6**

A 25-year-old patient who has taken haloperidol for the past 2 months is brought to the hospital with a temperature of 104°F, blood pressure of 190/110, and muscular rigidity.

**5.** These signs indicate that the patient has an antipsychotic medication side effect known as

**(A)** restless legs syndrome
**(B)** neuroleptic malignant syndrome
**(C)** akathisia
**(D)** tardive dyskinesia
**(E)** acute dystonia
**(F)** pseudoparkinsonism

**6.** The side effect described in question 5 is best treated initially

**(A)** by changing to a low-potency antipsychotic agent
**(B)** with an antianxiety agent
**(C)** with an antidepressant agent
**(D)** with an anticonvulsant
**(E)** by stopping the antipsychotic agent

**7.** A 26-year-old man comes to the emergency department with elevated blood pressure, sweating, headache, and vomiting. His companion tells the physician that the patient became ill at a party where he ate pizza and drank alcoholic punch. The drug that this patient is most likely to be taking is

**(A)** fluoxetine
**(B)** lithium
**(C)** nortriptyline
**(D)** tranylcypromine
**(E)** haloperidol

**8.** A 30-year-old woman tells the physician that she must drive the route she takes home from work each day at least three times to be sure that she did not hit an animal in the road. Of the following, the most appropriate long-term pharmacological management for this patient is

**(A)** a high-potency antipsychotic agent
**(B)** an anticholinergic agent
**(C)** an antianxiety agent
**(D)** an antidepressant agent
**(E)** lithium

**9.** A 45-year-old woman presents with the symptoms of a major depressive episode. The patient has never previously taken an antidepressant. Her physician decides to prescribe fluoxetine (Prozac). The most likely reason for this choice is that, when compared to a heterocyclic antidepressant, fluoxetine

**(A)** is more effective
**(B)** works faster
**(C)** has fewer side effects
**(D)** is less likely to be abused
**(E)** is long lasting

**10.** The best choice of antianxiety agent for a 40-year-old woman with generalized anxiety disorder and a history of benzodiazepine abuse is

**(A)** zolpidem
**(B)** flurazepam
**(C)** clonazepam
**(D)** buspirone
**(E)** chlordiazepoxide
**(F)** bupropion

**11.** A 40-year-old businessman who has been a physician's patient for the past 5 years asks her for a medication to help him sleep on an overnight flight to Australia. Of the following, the best agent for this use is

**(A)** zaleplon
**(B)** flurazepam
**(C)** clonazepam
**(D)** buspirone
**(E)** chlordiazepoxide
**(F)** bupropion

**12.** A 57-year-old male patient with a history of alcoholism has decided to stop drinking. Of the following, the agent most commonly used to treat anxiety and agitation associated with the initial stages of alcohol withdrawal is

**(A)** zaleplon
**(B)** flurazepam
**(C)** clonazepam
**(D)** buspirone
**(E)** chlordiazepoxide
**(F)** bupropion

**13.** Which of the following psychotropic agents is most likely to be abused?

**(A)** Diazepam
**(B)** Haloperidol
**(C)** Fluoxetine
**(D)** Buspirone
**(E)** Lithium

**14.** An 80-year-old man is brought to the emergency room by his wife. The man, who has a history of depression and suicidal behavior, refuses to eat and states that life is not worth living anymore. Consultations with his primary care physician and a consulting psychiatrist reveal that the patient has not responded to at least three different antidepressant medications that he has taken in adequate doses and for adequate time periods in the past 2 years. The most appropriate next step in the management of this patient is to recommend

**(A)** diazepam
**(B)** electroconvulsive therapy (ECT)
**(C)** psychotherapy
**(D)** buspirone
**(E)** lithium

**15.** A 30-year-old man with schizophrenia has been very withdrawn and apathetic for more than 10 years. He now is taking an antipsychotic agent that is helping him to be more outgoing and sociable. However, the patient is experiencing seizures, and agranulocytosis. The antipsychotic agent that this patient is most likely to be taking is

(A) risperidone
(B) thioridizine
(C) olanzapine
(D) haloperidol
(E) clozapine

**Questions 16 and 17**

A 30-year-old patient is brought to the emergency department after being found running down the street naked. He is speaking very quickly and tells the physician that he has just given his clothing and all of his money to a homeless man. He states that God spoke to him and told him to do this. His history reveals that he is a practicing attorney who is married with three children.

**16.** The most effective immediate management for this patient is

(A) lithium
(B) fluoxetine
(C) amitriptyline
(D) diazepam
(E) haloperidol

**17.** The most effective long-term management for this patient is

(A) lithium
(B) fluoxetine
(C) amitriptyline
(D) diazepam
(E) haloperidol

**18.** What is the most appropriate agent for a doctor to recommend for a 34-year-old, overweight, depressed patient who needs to take an antidepressant but is afraid of gaining weight?

(A) Venlafaxine
(B) Tranylcypromine
(C) Trazodone
(D) Doxepin
(E) Amoxapine
(F) Fluoxetine
(G) Nortriptyline
(H) Imipramine

**19.** What is the antidepressant agent most likely to cause persistent erections (priapism) in a 40-year-old male patient?

(A) Venlafaxine
(B) Tranylcypromine
(C) Trazodone
(D) Doxepin
(E) Amoxapine
(F) Fluoxetine
(G) Nortriptyline
(H) Imipramine

**20.** Which of the following antidepressant agents is most likely to cause gynecomastia and parkinsonian symptoms in a 45-year-old male patient?

(A) Venlafaxine
(B) Tranylcypromine
(C) Trazodone
(D) Doxepin
(E) Amoxapine
(F) Fluoxetine
(G) Nortriptyline
(H) Imipramine

**21.** What is the most appropriate antidepressant agent for rapid relief of the symptoms of depression in a 25-year-old woman?

(A) Venlafaxine
(B) Tranylcypromine
(C) Trazodone
(D) Doxepin
(E) Amoxapine
(F) Fluoxetine
(G) Nortriptyline
(H) Imipramine

**22.** Which of the following antidepressant agents is most likely to cause extreme sedation?

(A) Venlafaxine
(B) Tranylcypromine
(C) Trazodone
(D) Doxepin
(E) Amoxapine
(F) Fluoxetine
(G) Nortriptyline
(H) Imipramine

**23.** A 30-year-old woman who is taking an antipsychotic medication reports that she has been experiencing fluid discharge from the nipples. Which of the following hormones is most likely to be responsible for this problem?

(A) Progesterone
(B) Testosterone
(C) Prolactin
(D) Estrogen
(E) Cortisol

**24.** A 35-year-old man who has been taking haloperidol for the last year develops a resting tremor, mask-like facial expression, and difficulty initiating body movements. After reducing the haloperidol dose, the next step the physician should take to relieve these symptoms is to give the patient

(A) a high-potency antipsychotic agent
(B) an anticholinergic agent
(C) an antianxiety agent
(D) an antidepressant agent
(E) lithium

**25.** A 45-year-old man presents in the emergency room with sinus tachycardia (112/bpm), flattening of T waves and prolonged QT interval. The patient tells the physician that he is taking "nerve pills." Which of the following medications is this patient most likely to be taking?

(A) Bupropion
(B) Fluoxetine
(C) Lorazepam
(D) Valproic acid
(E) Imipramine

**26.** A 45-year-old woman with schizophrenia has been taking an atypical antipsychotic for the past year. Since starting the medication she has gained 35 pounds, has developed diabetes mellitus, and shows a prolonged QT interval. Because of these medication side effects her physician would like to switch her to a different atypical agent. Of the following atypical agents, which is likely to be the best choice for this patient?

(A) Quetiapine
(B) Ziprasidone
(C) Aripiprazole
(D) Clozapine
(E) Olanzapine

**27.** A resident is called to assess an oncology patient on a general medical floor who has developed a muscle spasm causing her neck to twist uncontrollably to the left. The intern evaluates the patient's list of medications and concludes that her new symptoms are probably due to which of the following?

(A) Aspirin
(B) Digoxin
(C) Erythromycin
(D) Fluoxetine
(E) Metoclopramide

**28.** A 23-year-old man with a diagnosis of schizophrenia, paranoid type, has been maintained on a low dose of haloperidol for the past 3 years. For the past month, his symptoms of paranoia and auditory hallucinations have been more prominent, and his psychiatrist decides to increase his dose of haloperidol. The patient's mother calls the psychiatrist, concerned that he seems slower than usual and has a fine resting tremor of his upper extremities. Furthermore, the patient complains that he feels "stiff." This clinical picture suggests that the patient is experiencing which of the following?

(A) Benign essential tremor
(B) Antipsychotic-induced parkinsonism
(C) Neuroleptic malignant syndrome
(D) Parkinson disease
(E) Tardive dyskinesia

**29.** A 32-year-old woman and her husband tell the physician that they want to have a baby but they are concerned about the impact this will have on the wife's emotional state. She has had three major depressive episodes within the past 10 years which have been treated successfully with antidepressant medication. The woman is concerned that she may become depressed while pregnant and will be unable to take any medication because of the pregnancy. Which of the following is the most appropriate response by the physician?

(A) "Depression associated with pregnancy is unrelated to major depression; therefore, you are not at greater risk for being depressed while pregnant."

(B) "The risk for depression is greatest after delivery and depression during pregnancy can often be safely treated."

(C) "The risk for depression is greatest during pregnancy, but ECT is quite safe."

(D) "Since you have been symptom-free for the past year, you should not be at greatest risk for depression than the normal population."

(E) "We will need to follow you closely since the suicide rate is higher for women who are pregnant than for women who are not pregnant."

# Answers and Explanations

**The answer is D.** Combinations of tramadol (Ultram) a serotonergic analgesic with SSRIs such as fluoxetine can lead to the symptoms this patient shows, that is, the serotonin syndrome. Opioids such as oxycodone and hydrocodone, mood stabilizers such as gabapentin or ibuprofen are unlikely to produce this syndrome when combined with an SSRI.

1. **The answer is C. 2. The answer is D.** The symptom that this patient describes is akathisia, a subjective, uncomfortable feeling of motor restlessness related to use of some antipsychotics. Restless legs syndrome also involves uncomfortable sensations in the legs, but it is a sleep disorder (see Chapter 10), which causes difficulty falling and staying asleep. Other antipsychotic side effects include neuroleptic malignant syndrome (high fever, sweating, increased pulse and blood pressure, and muscular rigidity), pseudoparkinsonism (muscle rigidity, shuffling gait, resting tremor, and mask-like facial expression), and tardive dyskinesia (involuntary movements including chewing and lip-smacking). High-potency antipsychotics, such as haloperidol, are more likely to cause these neurologic side effects than low-potency agents such as thioridizine, or atypical agents, such as risperidone, olanzapine, and clozapine.

3. **The answer is D. 4. The answer is A.** These involuntary chewing and lip-smacking movements indicate that the patient has developed tardive dyskinesia, a serious side effect of treatment with antipsychotic medication (see also answer to Question 1). Tardive dyskinesia usually occurs after at least 6 months of starting a high-potency antipsychotic and is best treated by changing to a low-potency or atypical agent; stopping the antipsychotic medication will exacerbate the symptoms.

5. **The answer is B. 6. The answer is E.** High body temperature and blood pressure, and muscular rigidity indicate that the patient has developed an antipsychotic medication side effect known as neuroleptic malignant syndrome (see also answer to Question 1). Neuroleptic malignant syndrome is seen most commonly with high-potency antipsychotic treatment and is best relieved by stopping the antipsychotic medication, providing medical support, and administering dantrolene, a muscle relaxant. After recovering from this life-threatening condition, the patient can be put on an atypical agent since they are less likely than high potency agents such as haloperidol to cause this dangerous side effect.

7. **The answer is D.** This patient who became ill at a pizza party is most likely to be taking tranylcypromine, a monoamine oxidase inhibitor (MAOI). These agents can cause a hypertensive crisis if certain foods (e.g., aged cheese, smoked meats, beer, and wine) are ingested. A patient who eats in an unfamiliar place (e.g., a party) may unwittingly ingest forbidden foods. This patient ate pizza that probably contained aged Parmesan cheese and drank punch that probably contained red wine. This resulted in a hypertensive crisis (e.g., elevated blood pressure, sweating, headache, and vomiting). Fluoxetine, lithium, nortriptyline, and haloperidol do not interact negatively with food.

8. **The answer is D.** The most effective pharmacological treatment for this patient who has obsessive–compulsive disorder is an antidepressant, particularly a selective serotonin reuptake inhibitor (see Chapter 13). Antipsychotics, antianxiety agents, and lithium are less appropriate than an antidepressant for this patient.

9. **The answer is C.** The doctor decides to give this patient fluoxetine because, when compared to a heterocyclic antidepressant, SSRIs such as fluoxetine have fewer side effects. Heterocyclics and SSRIs have equal efficacy, equivalent speed of action, and equivalent length of action. Neither SSRIs nor heterocyclics are likely to be abused.

10. **The answer is D.** The best choice of antianxiety agent for a 40-year-old patient with generalized anxiety disorder and a history of BZ abuse is buspirone, a non-benzodiazepine with very low abuse potential. Benzodiazepines such as flurazepam, clonazepam, and chlordiazepoxide have higher abuse potential than buspirone. Bupropion is an antidepressant, which is also used for smoking cessation. Zolpidem is a non-benzodiazepine sleep agent.

11. **The answer is A.** Zaleplon, a non-benzodiazepine sleep agent, is the best choice to aid sleep on an overnight flight. Benzodiazepines have higher abuse potential than agents such as zaleplon. Buspirone has little abuse potential but does not cause sedation, and, in any case, takes weeks to work. Bupropion is an antidepressant agent and is non-sedating.

12. **The answer is E.** Because it is long acting and has relatively low abuse potential for a BZ, chlordiazepoxide is the antianxiety agent most commonly used to treat the anxiety and agitation associated with the initial stages of alcohol withdrawal.

13. **The answer is A.** Of the listed agents, BZs such as diazepam are most likely to be abused. Antipsychotics such as haloperidol, antidepressants such as fluoxetine, mood stabilizers such as lithium, and non-benzodiazepines such as buspirone (see also answer to Question 10) have little or no abuse potential.

14. **The answer is B.** The most appropriate next step is to recommend a course of electroconvulsive therapy (ECT) for this elderly, severely depressed patient. ECT is a safe, fast, effective treatment for major depression. Diazepam, lithium, buspirone, and psychotherapy will not be effective as ECT in relieving this patient's suicidal depression quickly.

15. **The answer is E.** The antipsychotic agent that this patient is most likely to be taking is clozapine. Like other atypical agents, clozapine is more effective against negative symptoms (e.g., withdrawal) than traditional agents such as haloperidol. However, clozapine is also is more likely to cause seizures and agranulocytosis than traditional agents or other atypicals, such as risperidone and olanzapine.

16. **The answer is E. 17. The answer is A.** This patient's good employment and relationship history suggest that his psychotic symptoms are an acute manifestation of a manic episode. While the most effective immediate treatment for this patient is a fast-acting, high-potency antipsychotic agent, such as haloperidol, to control his hallucinations and delusions, lithium, which takes 2–3 weeks to work, would be more effective for long-term maintenance. Fluoxetine, amitriptyline, and diazepam are less appropriate primary treatments for this bipolar patient.

18. **The answer is F.** In contrast to most antidepressant agents, which are associated with weight gain, fluoxetine (Prozac) is associated with some weight loss. Thus it is the most appropriate antidepressant agent for a patient who is afraid of gaining weight.

19. **The answer is C.** Trazodone is the agent most likely to cause priapism in this patient.

20. **The answer is E.** Amoxapine has antidopaminergic action and, thus, is the agent most likely to cause gynecomastia as well as parkinsonian symptoms in this patient.

21. **The answer is A.** SNRIs may work more quickly than other antidepressants and, as such, venlafaxine is a good choice for rapid relief of depressive symptoms in this young woman.

22. **The answer is C.** Trazadone not only causes priapism (see also answer to Question 19) but also is highly sedating. It is thus often used in patients who have depression with insomnia.

23. **The answer is C.** Prolactin is the hormone responsible for galactorrhea, fluid discharge from the nipples. Galactorrhea is more common with the use of low-potency antipsychotic agents.

24. **The answer is B.** This patient is showing evidence of pseudoparkinsonism, a neurologic side effect caused by excessive blockade of postsynaptic dopamine receptors during treatment with high-potency antipsychotics, such as haloperidol. Because dopamine normally suppresses acetylcholine activity, giving the patient an anticholinergic agent (e.g., benztropine) will serve to increase dopaminergic activity and relieve the patient's symptoms. Antianxiety agents such as benzodiazepines can be used as adjuncts to anticholinergics, but antidepressants and lithium are not effective for reversing parkinsonian symptoms caused by antipsychotics.

25. **The answer is E.** TCAs such as imipramine cause sinus tachycardia, flat T waves, prolonged QT interval and depressed ST segments. Bupropion, fluoxetine, lorazepam, and valproic acid are less likely to cause these cardiovascular effects.

26. **The answer is C.** Because of her weight gain, type 2 diabetes and cardiovascular problem, the best choice of atypical antipsychotic agent for this patient now is aripiprazole. Clozapine and olanzapine carry high risk and ziprasidone and aripiprazole carry low risk for weight gain and diabetes. However, ziprasidone prolongs the QT interval and so should be avoided in this patient.

27. **The answer is E.** Metoclopramide (Reglan), a gastric motility agent and antiemetic, is often used to control nausea and vomiting in cancer patients receiving chemotherapy. It has antidopaminergic properties and can cause acute dystonic reactions such as are occurring in this patient. Management includes stopping the metoclopramide and providing an anticholinergic agent, such as benztropine, or an antihistamine, such as diphenhydramine, both of which are usually given in intramuscular form for immediate effect. Aspirin, digoxin, erythromycin, and fluoxetine are unlikely to cause dystonic reactions.

28. **The answer is B.** This patient who is slowed down and has a fine resting tremor of his upper extremities and stiffness is showing evidence of antipsychotic-induced parkinsonism, often a side effect of high doses of high-potency antipsychotics such as haloperidol. Benign essential tremor and Parkinson disease are not related to antipsychotic medication. Although they can both be side effects of haloperidol treatment, neuroleptic malignant syndrome and tardive dyskinesia are characterized by high fever and abnormal tongue and facial movements respectively.

29. **The answer is B.** The most appropriate response for the physician is to tell the patient that the risk for depression is greater after than before delivery and that depression during pregnancy can often be safely treated. Most antidepressants are in pregnancy Category C but two, bupropion and maprotiline, are in Category B. Discussing differential suicide rates is not a helpful intervention. In any case the suicide rate is lower for women who are pregnant than for those who are not pregnant. While ECT is quite safe in pregnancy, psychopharmacology is less invasive and usually preferred.

# chapter 17

# Psychological Therapies

**Typical Board Question**

A 5-year-old child, who, at age 2 years was playing with a large dog when a ceiling tile fell on her head, is now so afraid of dogs that she refuses to go to the park because dogs are there. Medical examination is unremarkable and the child's motor, social, and cognitive development are typical for her age. To manage the child's fear of dogs, the physician first recommends that her father carry a small toy dog very gradually toward her while she is listening to her favorite CD. Which of the following psychological therapies does this example illustrate?

**(A)** Implosion
**(B)** Biofeedback
**(C)** Aversive conditioning
**(D)** Token economy
**(E)** Flooding
**(F)** Systematic desensitization
**(G)** Cognitive/behavioral therapy

*(See "Answers and Explanations" at end of chapter.)*

## I. PSYCHOANALYSIS AND RELATED THERAPIES

**A. Overview**
   **1.** Psychoanalysis and related therapies (e.g., psychoanalytically oriented psychotherapy, brief dynamic psychotherapy) are psychotherapeutic treatments based on Freud's concepts of the **unconscious mind, defense mechanisms**, and **transference reactions** (see Chapter 6).
   **2.** The central strategy of these therapies is to **uncover experiences** that are **repressed in the unconscious mind** and integrate them into the person's conscious mind and personality.

**B. Techniques used to recover repressed experiences include:**
   **1. Free association**
      **a.** In psychoanalysis, the person **lies on a couch** in a reclined position facing away from the therapist and says whatever comes to mind (free association).
      **b.** In therapies related to psychoanalysis, the person sits in a chair and talks while facing the therapist.
   **2. Interpretation of dreams** is used to examine unconscious conflicts and impulses.
   **3. Analysis of transference reactions** (i.e., the person's unconscious responses to the therapist) is used to examine important past relationships (see Chapter 6).

**C.** People who are appropriate for using psychoanalysis and related therapies should have the following characteristics:
   **1.** Are younger than 40 years of age.

2. Are intelligent and not psychotic.
3. Have good relationships with others (e.g., no evidence of antisocial or borderline personality disorder).
4. Have a stable life situation (e.g., not be in the midst of divorce).
5. Have the time and money to spend on treatment.

D. In **psychoanalysis**, people receive treatment **4–5 times weekly for 3–4 years**; related therapies are briefer and more direct (e.g., brief dynamic psychotherapy is limited to 12–40 weekly sessions).

## II. BEHAVIORAL THERAPIES

A. Behavioral therapies are based on **learning theory** (see Chapter 7), that is, symptoms are relieved by unlearning maladaptive behavior patterns and altering negative thinking patterns.

B. In contrast to psychoanalysis and related therapies, the person's history and **unconscious conflicts are irrelevant**, and thus are not examined in behavioral therapies.

C. Characteristics of specific behavioral therapies (e.g., systematic desensitization, aversive conditioning, flooding and implosion, token economy, biofeedback, and cognitive/behavioral therapy) can be found in Table 17.1.

table **17.1** Behavioral Therapies: Uses and Strategies

| Most Common Use | Strategy |
|---|---|
| **Systematic Desensitization** | |
| Management of phobias (irrational fears; see Chapter 13) | In the past, through the process of classical conditioning (see Chapter 7), the person associated an innocuous object with a fear-provoking stimulus until the innocuous object became frightening<br>In the present, increasing doses of the fear-provoking stimulus are paired with a relaxing stimulus to induce a relaxation response<br>Because one cannot simultaneously be fearful and relaxed (reciprocal inhibition), the person shows less anxiety when exposed to the fear-provoking stimulus in the future |
| **Aversive Conditioning** | |
| Management of paraphilias (e.g., pedophilia) or addictions (e.g., smoking) | Classical conditioning is used to pair a maladaptive but pleasurable stimulus with an aversive or painful stimulus (e.g., a shock) so that the two become associated<br>The person ultimately stops engaging in the maladaptive behavior because it automatically provokes an unpleasant response |
| **Flooding and Implosion** | |
| Management of phobias | The person is exposed to an actual (flooding) or imagined (implosion) overwhelming dose of the feared stimulus<br>Through the process of habituation (see Chapter 7) the person becomes accustomed to the stimulus and is no longer afraid |
| **Token Economy** | |
| To increase positive behavior in a person who is severely disorganized (e.g., psychotic), autistic, or mentally retarded | Through the process of operant conditioning (see Chapter 7), desirable behavior (e.g., shaving, hair combing) is reinforced by a reward or positive reinforcement (e.g., the token)<br>The person increases the desirable behavior to gain the reward |
| **Biofeedback** | |
| To manage hypertension, Raynaud disease, migraine and tension headaches, chronic pain, fecal incontinence, and temporomandibular joint pain | Through the process of operant conditioning, the person is given ongoing physiologic information (e.g., blood pressure measurement), which acts as reinforcement (e.g., when blood pressure drops)<br>The person uses this information along with relaxation techniques to control visceral changes (e.g., heart rate, blood pressure, smooth muscle tone) |
| **Cognitive/Behavioral Therapy** | |
| To manage mild to moderate depression, somatoform disorders, eating disorders | Weekly, for 15–25 wks, the person is helped to identify distorted, negative thoughts about him- or herself<br>The person replaces these negative thoughts with positive, self-assuring thoughts and symptoms improve |

# III. OTHER THERAPIES

Other therapies include group, family, marital/couples, supportive and interpersonal therapy as well as stress management techniques. Specific uses of these therapies can be found in Table 17.2.

A. **Group therapy**
   1. **Groups with therapists**
      a. Groups of about eight people with a common problem or negative life experience usually meet weekly for 1–2 hours; sharing the therapist reduces cost.
      b. Members of the group provide the opportunity to express feelings as well as **feedback, support**, and **friendship** to each other.
      c. **The therapist has little input.** He or she facilitates and observes the members' interpersonal interactions.
   2. **Leaderless groups**
      a. In a leaderless group, **no one person is in authority**.
      b. Members of the group provide each other with **support and practical help** for a shared problem (e.g., alcoholism, loss of a loved one, a specific illness).
      c. Twelve-step groups like **Narcotics Anonymous** (NA) and **Overeaters Anonymous** (OA) are based on the **Alcoholics Anonymous** (AA) leaderless group model (see Chapter 9).

B. **Family therapy**
   1. **Family systems theory**
      a. Family therapy is based on the family systems idea that psychopathology in one family member (i.e., the identified patient) reflects **dysfunction of the entire family system**.
      b. Because all members of the family cause behavioral changes in other members, **the family (not the identified patient) is really the patient**.
      c. **Strategies** of family therapy include identifying **dyads** (i.e., subsystems between two family members), **triangles** (i.e., dysfunctional alliances between two family members against a third member), and **boundaries** (i.e., barriers between subsystems) that may be too rigid or too permeable.
   2. **Specific techniques** are used in family therapy.
      a. **Mutual accommodation** is encouraged. This is a process in which family members work toward meeting each other's needs.
      b. **Normalizing boundaries** between subsystems and reducing the likelihood of triangles is encouraged.

| t a b l e  **17.2** | Uses of Group, Family, Marital/Couples, Supportive, Interpersonal, and Stress Management Therapies |
|---|---|
| **Type of Therapy** | **Targeted Population** |
| Group therapy | People with a common problem (e.g., rape victims)<br>People with personality disorders or other interpersonal problems<br>People who have trouble interacting with therapists as authority figures in individual therapy |
| Family therapy | Children with behavioral problems<br>Families in conflict<br>People with eating disorders or substance abuse |
| Marital/couples therapy | Domestic partners with communication or psychosexual problems<br>Domestic partners with differences in values |
| Supportive therapy | People who are experiencing a life crisis<br>Chronically mentally ill people dealing with ordinary life situations |
| Interpersonal therapy | People with emotional difficulties owing to problems with interpersonal skills |
| Stress management | People with anxiety disorders or stress-related illnesses (e.g., headaches, hypertension) |

    **c. Redefining "blame"** (i.e., encouraging family members to reconsider their own responsibility for problems) is another important technique.

C. **Supportive and interpersonal therapy**
1. Supportive therapy is aimed not at insight into problems, but rather at helping people feel protected and supported during life crises (e.g., serious illness of a loved one). For **people** with chronic mental illnesses, supportive therapy may be used over many years along with medication.
2. Based on the idea that psychiatric problems such as anxiety and depression are based on difficulties in dealing with others, interpersonal therapy aims to develop **interpersonal skills** in 12–16 weekly sessions.

# Review Test

**Directions:** Each of the numbered items or incomplete statements in this section is followed by answers or by completions of the statement. Select the **one** lettered answer or completion that is **best** in each case.

**1.** A 30-year-old man who is afraid to ride in an elevator is put into a relaxed state and then shown a film of people entering elevators in a high-rise building. This method of management is based primarily on

**(A)** reciprocal inhibition
**(B)** classical conditioning
**(C)** aversive conditioning
**(D)** operant conditioning
**(E)** stimulus generalization

**2.** A 28-year-old woman joins 10 other women who have been abused by their husbands. The women meet weekly and are led by a psychotherapist who is trained in domestic violence issues. This type of therapy is best described as

**(A)** group therapy
**(B)** leaderless group therapy
**(C)** brief dynamic psychotherapy
**(D)** family therapy
**(E)** supportive therapy

**3.** A 9-year-old boy who is angry and resentful toward adults (oppositional defiant disorder; see Chapter 15) meets with a therapist for 2 hours each week, along with his parents and his sister. After 6 months, the boy's oppositional behavior toward adults has improved. This type of therapy is best described as

**(A)** group therapy
**(B)** leaderless group therapy
**(C)** brief dynamic psychotherapy
**(D)** family therapy
**(E)** supportive therapy

**4.** Ten arthritis patients meet once per week to talk with each other and to inform each other of new devices and services to help disabled people with everyday tasks. This type of therapy is best described as

**(A)** group therapy
**(B)** leaderless group therapy
**(C)** brief dynamic psychotherapy
**(D)** family therapy
**(E)** supportive therapy

**5.** A 50-year-old male hypertensive patient is given ongoing blood pressure readings as he uses mental relaxation techniques to try to lower his blood pressure. After four sessions using this technique, his blood pressure is lower. This method of blood pressure reduction is based primarily on

**(A)** reciprocal inhibition
**(B)** classical conditioning
**(C)** aversive conditioning
**(D)** operant conditioning
**(E)** stimulus generalization

**6.** A 35-year-old man who is afraid of heights is instructed to stand in the observation tower of the Empire State Building and look down from the window until he is no longer afraid. After three visits to the tower each lasting 1 hour, the man is no longer afraid of heights. Which of the following management techniques does this example illustrate?

**(A)** Implosion
**(B)** Biofeedback
**(C)** Aversive conditioning
**(D)** Token economy
**(E)** Flooding
**(F)** Systematic desensitization
**(G)** Cognitive/behavioral therapy

7. A man who is afraid to drive is told to imagine driving a car from the northernmost border to the southernmost border of the state of New Jersey. Eventually, he is able to drive without fear. Which of the following management techniques does this example illustrate?

(A) Implosion
(B) Biofeedback
(C) Aversive conditioning
(D) Token economy
(E) Flooding
(F) Systematic desensitization
(G) Cognitive/behavioral therapy

8. A 30-year-old depressed man is told to replace each self-deprecating thought with a mental image of victory and praise. Over the next few months, his depression gradually lifts. Which of the following management techniques does this example illustrate?

(A) Implosion
(B) Biofeedback
(C) Aversive conditioning
(D) Token economy
(E) Flooding
(F) Systematic desensitization
(G) Cognitive/behavioral therapy

9. A 42-year-old man with sexual interest in children (pedophilia) is given an electric shock each time he is shown a videotape of children. Later, he feels tense around children and avoids them. Which of the following management techniques does this example illustrate?

(A) Implosion
(B) Biofeedback
(C) Aversive conditioning
(D) Token economy
(E) Flooding
(F) Systematic desensitization
(G) Cognitive/behavioral therapy

10. Each time she combs her hair and brushes her teeth, a 20-year-old woman with a pervasive developmental disorder receives a coupon that can be exchanged for dessert in the cafeteria. Her grooming behavior subsequently improves. Which of the following psychological management techniques does this example illustrate?

(A) Implosion
(B) Biofeedback
(C) Aversive conditioning
(D) Token economy
(E) Flooding
(F) Systematic desensitization
(G) Cognitive/behavioral therapy

11. The major reason that patients who could benefit from psychoanalytically oriented psychotherapy do not receive it is that they often

(A) do not want to reveal their histories to strangers
(B) do not want to reveal their personal problems to strangers
(C) believe that it is expensive and time consuming
(D) have little interest in exploring their childhoods
(E) do not feel comfortable in the therapeutic setting

# Answers and Explanations

## Typical Board Question

**The answer is F.** The management technique described here is systematic desensitization. In this example, the child made an erroneous negative association between dogs and pain when she was injured in the presence of the dog. In systematic desensitization, increasing doses of the frightening stimulus (e.g., dogs) are paired with a relaxing stimulus (e.g., the favorite CD) to provoke a relaxation response in situations involving the frightening stimulus. Later in treatment, this child will be exposed to a live dog. Flooding is a management technique for phobias in which a person is exposed to an overwhelming dose of the feared stimulus or situation until he or she is no longer fearful. In implosion, a person is exposed to an imagined, rather than actual, overwhelming dose of a feared stimulus or situation. In biofeedback, a person is given ongoing physiologic information, which acts as reinforcement. In aversive conditioning, a maladaptive but pleasurable stimulus is paired with a painful stimulus so that the two become associated and the maladaptive behavior disappears. In token economy, the desired behavior is reinforced by a reward or token and the person increases her behavior to gain the reward. In cognitive/behavioral therapy, a person is helped to identify distorted, negative thoughts and to replace them with positive, self-assuring thoughts.

1. **The answer is B.** This method of management, systematic desensitization, is based on classical conditioning. The film of people entering elevators in a high-rise building is paired with relaxation. After continued pairing of elevators and relaxation, elevators will no longer induce fear. Later on in treatment, the person will be encouraged to look into a real elevator and finally to ride in one (and see the TBQ).

2. **The answer is A.** This type of therapy is best described as group therapy, a management technique in which people with a common problem (e.g., victims of abuse) get together with a psychotherapist. In leaderless groups there is no therapist or other person in authority; members of the group provide each other with support and practical help for a shared problem. Brief dynamic psychotherapy is a form of psychoanalytically oriented therapy in which a person works with a therapist to gain insight into the cause of his or her problems. In supportive therapy, a therapist helps a person feel protected and supported during life crises.

3. **The answer is D.** This type of therapy, in which a child with a behavior problem and his family meet with a therapist, is best described as family therapy. Family therapy is based on the idea that psychopathology in one family member (e.g., a child) reflects dysfunction of the entire family system (see also answer to Question 2).

4. **The answer is B.** This type of therapy, in which patients with a particular illness (e.g., arthritis) meet for communication and practical help, is best described as leaderless group therapy (see also answer to Question 2).

5. **The answer is D.** The technique described here (i.e., biofeedback) is based primarily on operant conditioning (see Chapter 7 for a discussion of classical conditioning, stimulus generalization, and operant conditioning). Reciprocal inhibition is the mechanism that prevents one from feeling two opposing emotions at the same time (e.g., relaxation and fear), and is associated with systematic desensitization (see TBQ and answer to Question 1). In aversive conditioning, classical conditioning is used to pair a maladaptive but pleasurable stimulus with an aversive or painful stimulus so that the two become associated and the person stops engaging in the maladaptive behavior.

6. **The answer is E.** The management technique described here is flooding, a treatment technique for phobias. In flooding, a person is exposed to an overwhelming dose of the feared stimulus or situation—in this case, heights—until he or she is no longer afraid.

7. **The answer is A.** The management technique described here is implosion, a management technique related to flooding (see also answer to Question 6) in which the person is instructed to imagine extensive exposure to a feared stimulus (driving a car—or New Jersey, depending on your outlook) until he or she is no longer afraid.

8. **The answer is G.** The management technique described here is cognitive/behavioral therapy, a short-term behavioral management technique in which the person is instructed to replace each negative thought with a positive mental image.

9. **The answer is C.** The management technique described here is aversive conditioning, in which a maladaptive but pleasurable stimulus (for this man, sexual interest in children) is paired with painful stimulus (e.g., a shock) so that the two become associated. The person now associates sexual interest in children with pain and stops this maladaptive behavior.

10. **The answer is D.** The management technique described here is token economy. In token economy, the desired behavior (e.g., grooming) is reinforced by a token (e.g., a coupon that can be exchanged for dessert) and the person increases her behavior to gain the reward (e.g., dessert).

11. **The answer is C.** The major reason that patients who could benefit from psychoanalytically oriented psychotherapy do not receive it is that they often believe it is expensive and time consuming. Less commonly, people do not want to reveal their histories and personal problems to strangers, are not interested in exploring their childhoods, or feel uncomfortable in the therapeutic setting.

# 18 The Family, Culture, and Illness

**Typical Board Question**

A 40-year-old Japanese woman born and living in Tokyo has been experiencing stomach bleeding and, after an endoscopy, is diagnosed with gastric cancer. Upon hearing this news, the woman's identical twin sister, who has been living in the United States for 20 years, and works out at the gym three times per week, has an endoscopy. The results of the sister's test are unremarkable and no evidence of gastric cancer is found. The most likely explanation for this difference in disease between the twins is that

- **(A)** gastric cancer is unrelated to genetic factors
- **(B)** environmental factors are likely to play a role in the development of gastric cancer
- **(C)** testing techniques for gastric cancer are better in Japan than in the United States
- **(D)** exercise can prevent gastric cancer
- **(E)** a high nitrate diet is probably responsible for gastric cancer

*(See "Answers and Explanations" at end of chapter.)*

## I. OVERVIEW OF THE FAMILY

A. **Definition**
  1. A group of people related by **blood, adoption**, or **marriage** is a family.
  2. The interpersonal relationships in families play a significant role in the health of family members.

B. **Types of families**
  1. The **traditional nuclear family** includes a mother, a father, and dependent children (i.e., under age 18) living together in one household.
  2. Other types of families include cohabiting heterosexual and gay-parent families and single-parent families.
  3. The **extended family** includes family members, such as grandparents, aunts, uncles, and cousins, who live outside the household.

## II. DEMOGRAPHICS AND CURRENT TRENDS

A. **Marriage and children**
  1. In the United States, the average **age of first marriage** is about **25** years for **women** and **27** years for **men**.
  2. Most people 30–54 years of age are married.

**table  18.1**  Percentage of White, African American and Latino Children Living in Different Family Types in 2010

| Ethnic Group | Married Parents (%) | Single Mother (%) | Single Father (%) | No Parent (%) |
|---|---|---|---|---|
| White American | 71.5 | 18.3 | 3.5 | 3.4 |
| African American | 34.7 | 49.7 | 3.6 | 7.5 |
| Hispanic American (Latino) | 60.9 | 26.3 | 2.7 | 4.0 |

3. A good marriage is an important predictor of health. Married people are **mentally** and **physically healthier** and have higher self-esteem than unmarried people.
4. Approximately **50% of children** live in families with **two working parents**; only about **25% of children live in the "traditional family,"** in which the father works outside of the home and the mother is a full-time homemaker.
5. Raising children is expensive. The total cost of raising a child to age 17 in the United States is currently more than $200,000. Post-secondary education can effectively double this figure.

B. Divorce and single-parent families
  1. **Close to half of all marriages in the United States end in divorce.**
    a. Factors associated with divorce include short courtship, lack of family support, pre-marital pregnancy, marriage during teenage years, divorce in the family, differences in religion or socioeconomic background, and serious illness or death of a child.
    b. **Physicians have a higher divorce rate** than people in other occupations. Much of this difference may be a result of the lifestyle and stresses associated with a career in medicine.
  2. **Single-parent families**
    a. Single-parent families often have **lower incomes** and **less social support** and, therefore, face increased chances of physical and mental illness.
    b. While many unmarried mothers belong to low socioeconomic groups, the fastest growing population of single mothers is **educated professional women**.
    c. Most single-parent families **are headed by women**.
  3. **Children in single-parent families**
    a. The percentage of children living in single-parent families varies by ethnic group (Table 18.1).
    b. **Children in single-parent families** are at **increased risk** for failure in school, depression, drug abuse, suicide, criminal activity, and divorce.
    c. Even if the noncustodial parent does not provide financial support, **children who continue to have regular contact with that parent** have fewer of these problems than those who have no contact.
  4. **Child custody**
    a. After divorce, the types of **child custody** that may be granted by the courts include joint, split, and sole custody; **fathers are increasingly being granted** joint or sole custody.
    b. **In sole custody,** the child lives with one parent while the other has visitation rights. Until quite recently, sole custody was the most common type of custody arrangement after divorce.
    c. In **joint residential custody**, which has become more popular, the child spends some time living with each parent.
    d. In **split custody**, each parent has custody of at least one child.

## III. CULTURE IN THE UNITED STATES

A. Characteristics
  1. There are approximately **310 million people** in the United States. The population is made up of many **minority subcultures** as well as a **large, white middle class**, which is the major cultural influence.

2. Although many subcultures have formed the American culture, the culture seems to have certain characteristics of its own.
   a. **Financial and personal independence** are valued at all ages and especially in the elderly. Most **elderly Americans** spend their last years **living on their own**; only about 20% live with family members and about 5% live in nursing homes.
   b. Emphasis is placed on **personal hygiene** and cleanliness.
   c. The **nuclear family** with few children is valued.

B. **Culture and illness**
   1. While ethnic groups are not homogeneous (i.e., their members have different backgrounds and different reasons for emigrating), groups often have **characteristic ways of dealing with illness**.
   2. Although the major psychiatric disorders such as schizophrenia and depression are seen to about the same extent in all cultures, **the sorts of behavior considered abnormal may differ** considerably by culture.
   3. While differences in presentation of symptoms may be the result of the individual characteristics of a patient, they may also be caused by the **characteristics of the particular ethnic group**.
   4. A patient's belief system has much to do with adherence and response to management. Physicians must have respect for and work in the context of such beliefs in order to help patients. For example:
      a. In certain ethnic groups, it is believed that illness can be cured by eating certain **foods**. Therefore, if not contraindicated medically, the doctor should attempt to make available the food the ill patient believes can help him or her.
      b. The idea that an **outside influence** (e.g., a hex or a curse imposed by the anger of an acquaintance or relative) can cause illness is seen in some ethnic groups. The doctor should not dismiss the patient's belief, but rather should ask the patient who can help to remove the curse and involve that person in the management plan.
      c. People may seek health care from **folk or religious healers** (e.g., *chamanes, curanderos,* and *espiritistas* among Latinos). Management provided by these healers includes **herbal medicines** and specific changes in diet. The physician should not disparage the use of folk medicine but rather include it, if possible, in the management plan.
      d. A belief in **communication with spirits of the dead** is seen in some cultures (e.g., Latino). Because they are shared by members of a cultural group, such beliefs are not delusional.

C. **Acculturative stress**
   1. The concept of acculturative stress is used as an alternative to the term "culture shock." It is an **emotional response**, involving **psychiatric symptoms** as well as **increased susceptibility to disease**, which is related to geographic relocation and the need to adapt to unfamiliar social and cultural surroundings. Acculturative stress is reduced when groups of immigrants of a particular culture live in the same geographic area.
   2. **Young immigrant men** appear to be at **higher risk for acculturative stress**, including symptoms such as paranoia and depression, than other sex and age groups. This is true in part because
      a. Young men **lose the most status** on leaving their culture of origin.
      b. Unlike others in the group who can stay at home among familiar people, young men often must get out into the new culture and earn a living.

D. **Ethnic disparities in health care**
   1. Racial and ethnic minorities in the United States often face obstacles in obtaining quality mental and physical health care.
   2. Ethnic disparities in health care result in part from
      a. Economic factors, for example, the average **income** of African American families is only about **half that of white families**.
      b. Decreased physical access to health care.
      c. Doctor–patient communication difficulties.
      d. Overt bias and negative racial stereotypes held by majority physicians.
      e. Relative scarcity of minority physicians.

# IV.  AMERICAN SUBCULTURES

## A. African Americans

1. There are approximately **37 million** African Americans (about 12.4% of the total population) in the United States.
2. Compared to white Americans, **African Americans** have
   a. **Shorter life expectancies** (see Figure 3.1).
   b. **Higher rates of** hypertension, heart disease, stroke, infant mortality (see also Table 1.2), obesity, asthma, tuberculosis, diabetes, prostate cancer, and AIDS.
   c. **Higher death rates** from heart disease and from most forms of cancer.
3. **Religion** and **strong extended family networks** play a major role in social and personal support among many African Americans. This may in part explain why the overall **suicide rate is lower** among African Americans than among white Americans.
4. While the overall suicide rate is lower, suicide in African American teenagers, once uncommon, has more than doubled in the last 20 years. It is now the third leading cause of death in this group, with homicide the leading cause, and accidents second. In white teenagers, accidents are the leading cause of death, with homicide second, and suicide third.

## B. Hispanic/Latino Americans

1. **Overview**
   a. With **45 million** people (15% of the population), Hispanic Americans (mainly people from Spanish-speaking regions of Latin America, i.e., Latinos) are now the **largest minority group** in the United States.
   b. As a group, Latinos place great value on the nuclear family and on **nuclear families with many children**.
   c. **Respect for the elderly** is important. Younger people are expected to care for elderly family members, to **protect elderly relatives from negative medical diagnoses**, and, often, to make medical decisions concerning the care of elderly relatives.
   d. Among some Latinos, **"hot" and "cold" influences** are believed to relate to illness.
   e. Latino women are less likely to get mammograms and more likely to have cervical cancer than are white or African American women.
2. Two-thirds of all Latinos, especially those in the Southwest, are of **Mexican** origin.
3. The second largest group of Latinos is of **Puerto Rican** origin (4 million people). Most live in the Northeastern states.
4. Over 1.5 million Latinos are of **Cuban** origin and live primarily in the Southeast, especially in Florida.
5. Although the explanation is elusive, Latinos have longer life expectancies than African-Americans or White Americans (see also Table 3.1).

## C. Asian Americans

1. There are more than **13 million** Asian Americans in the United States. The largest groups are **Chinese, Filipino,** and **Asian Indian**.
2. Other Asian American groups include the **Vietnamese, Korean,** and **Japanese**.
3. Although **many groups are assimilated**, ethnic differences may still result in different responses to illness among Asian American groups.
4. Characteristics of these cultures include the following:
   a. As in Latino cultures, adult Asian American children **show strong respect for** and **are expected to care for their elderly parents**, protect elderly relatives from negative medical diagnoses, and make medical decisions about elderly relatives' care.
   b. Patients may express emotional pain as physical illness.
   c. In some Asian American groups, the **abdominal-thoracic area**, rather than the brain, is often thought to be the **spiritual core** of the person. Thus, the concept of brain death and resulting organ transplant are generally not well accepted.
   d. **Folk remedies** include **coining** (a coin is rubbed on the affected area pressing a medicated oil into the skin); Injuries occurring as a result of use of such remedies may be mistaken by medical personnel for abuse (see Chapter 20).

e. Certain disorders, **for example, gastric cancer** are more common in Asians living in their native countries than in Asians living in the United States. For example, rates of gastric cancer are four times higher in Japanese people living in Japan than in Japanese Americans living in Los Angeles. Culture-related dietary factors (e.g., more nitrate-rich foods in Japan) may help explain this difference.

D. **Native Americans: American Indians and Eskimos**
1. There are about **2.4 million Native Americans** in the United States.
2. Native Americans have their own program of medical care under the direction of the **Indian Health Service** of the federal government.
3. The distinction between mental and physical illness may be blurred; engaging in forbidden behavior and witchcraft are thought to result in illness.
4. In general, Native Americans have low incomes and **high rates of alcoholism** and **suicide, particularly among teenagers**.

E. **Americans of Middle Eastern/North African descent**
1. People of Middle Eastern or North African origin (about **1.2 million**), who speak dialects of the **Arabic language** (e.g., Saudi Arabia, Kuwait, Bahrain, Iraq, Oman, Qatar, Syria, Jordan, Lebanon, and Egypt), are often referred to as Arabs. Other Middle Eastern groups include people from Iran, Afghanistan, and Pakistan.
2. Some Middle Eastern people are Christian (e.g., Coptic Christian) or Jewish; most follow the **Muslim** religion.
3. People who follow the Muslim religion **value female modesty** and purity. Female patients may wish to remain as covered as possible in the examining room (e.g., head and face covered by a scarf). They often prefer to have a female physician or, if examined by a male physician, may wish to have their husband or mother present. Physicians should make every effort to honor such wishes.

F. **Americans of European descent**
1. **Anglo Americans** are those originating in English-speaking European countries, mostly from Ireland.
2. Anglo Americans in general are less emotional, more stoic, and less vocal about pain and illness than members of groups of **Mediterranean origin** (e.g., Jewish, Greek, and Italian people).
3. Therefore, Anglo Americans may become very ill before seeking treatment, while people of Mediterranean origin may be considered complainers and ignored when they are, in fact, quite ill.

# Review Test

**Directions:** Each of the numbered items or incomplete statements in this section is followed by answers or by completions of the statement. Select the **one** lettered answer or completion that is **best** in each case.

**1.** A 24-year-old married Muslim woman, who is experiencing severe pelvic pain, is brought to the emergency room by her husband. When instructed to disrobe and put on a hospital gown, she refuses unless she can be assured that she will be seen by a female physician. The most appropriate statement the male emergency room physician can make at this time is

**(A)** "I will try to locate a female physician but if I cannot do so, I must examine you."
**(B)** "I am a board-certified physician and am as qualified as a female doctor to examine and treat you."
**(C)** "I will try to locate a female physician; if I cannot do so, how can I help you be more comfortable with me as your doctor?"
**(D)** "I cannot help you if you will not cooperate."
**(E)** "Severe pelvic pain is sometimes life threatening. I must examine you immediately."

### Questions 2–4

An elementary school in Texas includes children from many cultures. In fact, the principal has discovered that the population of the school directly mirrors that of the US population.

**2.** If the school's principal is trying to estimate how many of the school's students live in a "traditional" family situation, her best guess is

**(A)** <10%
**(B)** 11%–19%
**(C)** 20%–30%
**(D)** 35%–45%
**(E)** 55%–65%

**3.** Similarly, the principal's best guess about the percentage of Latino students who live with a single mother is

**(A)** <10%
**(B)** 11%–19%
**(C)** 20%–30%
**(D)** 35%–45%
**(E)** 55%–65%

**4.** The principal's best guess about the percentage of students who are Native American is

**(A)** <10%
**(B)** 11%–19%
**(C)** 20%–30%
**(D)** 35%–45%
**(E)** 55%–65%

**5.** A large extended family immigrates to the United States. The person in the family who is at highest risk for psychiatric symptoms after the move is the

**(A)** 84-year-old great-grandfather
**(B)** 28-year-old uncle
**(C)** 36-year-old aunt
**(D)** 10-year-old sister
**(E)** 55-year-old grandmother

**6.** A 12-year-old child is told to write a report about his "nuclear family." To do this task correctly, the report must contain information on his

**(A)** 84-year-old great-grandfather
**(B)** 28-year-old uncle
**(C)** 36-year-old aunt
**(D)** 10-year-old sister
**(E)** 55-year-old grandmother

### Questions 7 and 8

In the United States, independence is valued at all ages. However, many elderly people require care by others when they become incapacitated. Nursing home care is one option for such care.

**7.** What percentage of elderly Americans spend their last years living in a nursing home?

**(A)** <10%
**(B)** 11%–19%
**(C)** 20%–25%
**(D)** 35%–45%
**(E)** 55%–65%

**8.** Which of these patients is most likely to spend the last years of her life in a nursing home?

**(A)** An 80-year-old Anglo American woman
**(B)** An 80-year-old Puerto Rican American woman
**(C)** An 80-year-old Japanese American woman
**(D)** An 80-year-old Mexican American woman
**(E)** An 80-year-old Vietnamese American woman

**9.** A physician has two 56-year-old male patients. One of them is African American and one is white. Statistically, the African American patient has a lower likelihood of

**(A)** stroke
**(B)** asthma
**(C)** hypertension
**(D)** suicide
**(E)** prostate cancer

**10.** Which of the following living situations is most common in the United States?

**(A)** A 34-year-old medical resident living with his parents
**(B)** A 46-year-old divorced man living with his 10-year-old son
**(C)** A 65-year-old man living with his daughter and her husband
**(D)** A 46-year-old single man living alone
**(E)** A 46-year-old man living with his wife and children

**11.** A 26-year-old woman and a 29-year-old man get married after a 2-year engagement. They are both Episcopalian and are both from middle-class families. Both sets of their parents are divorced. Which of the following factors puts this couple at highest risk for divorce?

**(A)** Their ages
**(B)** The length of their engagement
**(C)** Their parents' marital histories
**(D)** Their socioeconomic backgrounds
**(E)** Their religious backgrounds

**12.** The daughter of a 65-year-old Vietnamese woman brings her mother in for management of a serious medical condition. The older woman, who lives with her daughter, is alert and oriented. The necessary management regimen is quite complex and the older woman does not speak English. To best convey the needed information to this patient, the physician should

**(A)** write the instructions down in English to be translated later
**(B)** explain the instructions to the daughter and have her monitor her mother's treatment
**(C)** call in a translator to explain the instructions to the mother
**(D)** ask the daughter to translate the instructions to the mother
**(E)** refer the patient to a doctor who speaks Vietnamese

**13.** A 40-year-old Mexican American man who has been diagnosed with hypertension tells the physician that a healer, used by many members of his community, told him that eating corn every day will lower his blood pressure. He explains that the healer told him hypertension is a "hot" illness and corn is a "cold" food. If eating corn poses no danger to this patient, what is the doctor's most appropriate next statement?

**(A)** "There is no medical evidence that corn is helpful for lowering blood pressure."
**(B)** "I cannot treat you until you stop going to the healer."
**(C)** "Is the healer trained in modern medicine?"
**(D)** "There are medical treatments for high blood pressure that you can use along with eating corn."
**(E)** "Try the corn for a month and if your blood pressure is still high, I will give you medication to lower it."

**14.** A 70-year-old Mexican American woman, whose husband died 4 months ago, calmly tells her physician that she and her husband still communicate with each other. The patient shows no evidence of a thought disorder and her physical examination is unremarkable. Which of the following is the most appropriate question or statement from the physician at this time?

**(A)** "Do you believe that your husband is still alive?"

**(B)** "Do other people in the Mexican American community believe that the living and the dead communicate with each other?"

**(C)** "I would like you to take a medication called risperidone for the next few months."

**(D)** "Most people do not think that they can communicate with the dead."

**(E)** "How do you feel when your husband communicates with you?"

# Answers and Explanations

**Typical Board Question**

**The answer is B.** The most likely explanation for this difference between the twins (e.g., the one in Japan has and the one in the United States has not been diagnosed with gastric cancer) is that environmental factors are likely to play a role in the development of gastric cancer. If only genetic factors were involved, both women would be likely to have the disease. A diet high in nitrates such as that eaten in Japan is a risk factor for gastric cancer but it is not clear that this is the only environmental factor to which the two women are differentially exposed. There is no reason to believe that testing techniques for gastric cancer are better in Japan than in the United States or that exercise can prevent gastric cancer.

1. **The answer is C.** Muslim women often prefer to have a female physician, particularly for gynecological or obstetrical problems. In this case, the physician should try to honor the patient's wishes. If this is not possible, the patient should be consulted for alternative acceptable strategies, for example, she may suggest having her husband or other family member (e.g., her mother) present when she is examined by the male physician. Trying to impress the patient with one's credentials or frighten her into adherence are not appropriate or useful strategies (see Chapter 21).

2. **The answer is C.** Approximately 25% of American children live in a "traditional" family situation (the mother stays home and the father works).

3. **The answer is C.** Approximately 26% of Latino children live with a single mother.

4. **The answer is A.** Native Americans (2.4 million) make up less than 1% of all Americans (310 million).

5. **The answer is B.** Young immigrant men, such as the 28-year-old uncle, are at higher risk for psychiatric symptoms when entering a new culture than are any other gender or age group. This is because they lose the most status on leaving their old culture and because, unlike other groups that can stay at home among their families, young men often must get out into the new culture and make a living.

6. **The answer is D.** The "nuclear family" consists of parents and dependent children (e.g., the boy's sister) living in one household. The great-grandfather, uncle, aunt, and grandmother usually are part of the "extended family."

7. **The answer is A. 8. The answer is A.** About 5% of elderly Americans spend their last years living in a nursing home. Elderly Asian American and Hispanic American people are more likely than Anglo Americans to be cared for by their adult children rather than placed in a nursing home.

9. **The answer is D.** Statistically, a middle-aged African American patient has a lower likelihood of suicide than a white patient of the same age. However, when compared to white patients, African American patients have a higher likelihood of stroke, asthma, hypertension, and prostate cancer as well as heart disease, tuberculosis, diabetes, and AIDS.

10. **The answer is E.** Of the listed choices, a 46-year-old man living with his wife and children is the most common living situation in the United States. While the divorce rate is high, most people in their 40s are married, not single or divorced. It is relatively uncommon to see a self-supporting adult, such as the 34-year-old medical resident, living with his parents. It is also relatively uncommon to see a 65-year-old man living with his children.

11. **The answer is C.** Of the listed factors, their parents' histories of divorce are a risk factor for divorce for this couple. Teenage marriages, short courtship, and differences in socioeconomic and religious backgrounds also put couples at risk for divorce.

12. **The answer is C.** When the management regimen is complex and the patient does not speak English, the physician's best choice is to call in a translator so that he can explain the instructions directly to his patient (in this case, the elderly woman). Communicating as directly as possible with the patient is particularly important in cultures in which adult children may protect an elderly relative from a negative medical diagnosis (e.g., Asian and Hispanic cultures). Thus, in translating the information, or monitoring the treatment, the daughter may not relay the complete picture to the elderly patient. Writing the instructions down in English to be translated later is not appropriate because it is uncertain how and when the translation will be done. Since the doctor can call in a translator, there is no reason to refer the patient to another doctor. Patients expect to receive care when they visit a physician, and referrals should be made only for medical reasons.

13. **The answer is D.** As long as the treatment will not harm the patient, the physician should try to work in conjunction with the healer. Since in this case the folk remedy is innocuous, the patient can continue using it along with traditional medical management (e.g., an antihypertensive agent). The physician should not try to separate the patient from his cultural beliefs by refusing to treat him until he stops using the folk healer, questioning the healer's training in modern medicine, or doubting the value of the recommended remedy. It could be dangerous to delay the patient's treatment for a month to prove to him that eating corn will not help his condition.

14. **The answer is B.** This Mexican American patient who reports that she communicates with her dead husband is probably not experiencing a delusion (i.e., a false belief not shared by others [see Table 11.1]). Rather, she is most likely to be reporting a cultural phenomenon based on the belief, in some Latino cultures, that the line between the dead and the living is blurred. As further evidence that this is not a delusion the patient shows no evidence of a thought disorder. Thus, she does not need to take an antipsychotic such as risperidone. There is no evidence that she either believes her husband is alive or that she is disturbed by these experiences.

# chapter 19 Sexuality

**Typical Board Question**

Concerned parents tell their doctor that their 8-year-old son only wants to play with girls, likes to dress up like a girl, and insists on urinating sitting down. He also says that boys are dirty and that girls have better stuff, and that he wants to be called by a girl's name. What is the most appropriate intervention by the physician at this time?

**(A)** Tell the parents to give the child a time-out whenever they see him playing with girls.
**(B)** Tell the parents to give the child only masculine toys such as trucks and action figures to play with.
**(C)** Teach the parents that it is OK for the child to have these interests and help them accept the child as he is.
**(D)** Inform the parents that it is likely that the child will have a homosexual orientation.
**(E)** Reassure the parents that cross-gender behavior is common and will disappear in time.
**(F)** Tell the parents that they should consider sex reassignment surgery for the child.

*(See "Answers and Explanations" at end of chapter.)*

## I. SEXUAL DEVELOPMENT

A. **Prenatal physical sexual development**
   1. Differentiation of the **gonads** is dependent on the presence or absence of the **Y chromosome**, which contains the testis-determining factor gene.
   2. The androgenic secretions of the fetal **testes** direct the differentiation of **male** internal and external genitalia.
      a. **In the absence of androgens** during prenatal life, internal and external **genitalia are female**.
      b. In **androgen insensitivity syndrome** (formerly testicular feminization), despite an **XY genotype** and testes that secrete androgen, a genetic defect prevents the body cells from responding to androgen, resulting in a female phenotype. At puberty, the descending testes may appear as labial or inguinal masses.
      c. In the presence of excessive adrenal androgen secretion prenatally **(congenital virilizing adrenal hyperplasia, formerly adrenogenital syndrome)**, the genitalia of a genetic female are masculinized and the child may be visually identified initially as male.

B. **Prenatal psychological sexual development**
   1. Differential exposure to gonadal hormones during prenatal life also results in **gender differences in certain brain areas** (e.g., the hypothalamus, anterior commissure, corpus callosum, and thalamus).

| table **19.1** | Gender Identity, Gender Role, and Sexual Orientation | | |
|---|---|---|---|
| **Term** | **Definition** | **Presumed Etiology** | **Comments** |
| Gender identity | Sense of self as being male or female | Differential exposure to prenatal sex hormones | May not agree with physiological sex (i.e., gender identity disorder) |
| Gender role | Expression of one's gender identity in society | Societal pressure to conform to sexual norms | May not agree with gender identity or physiological sex (e.g., choice of opposite gender's clothing) |
| Sexual orientation | Persistent and unchanging preference for people of the same sex (homosexual) or the opposite sex (heterosexual) for love and sexual expression | Differential exposure to prenatal sex hormones Genetic influences | True bisexuality is uncommon; most people have a sexual preference Homosexuality is considered a normal variant of sexual expression |

2. **Gender identity, gender role**, and **sexual orientation** (Table 19.1) also may be affected by prenatal exposure to gonadal hormones.
   a. Individuals with **gender identity disorder** (transsexual or transgender individuals) have a pervasive psychological feeling of being born into the body of the wrong sex despite a body form typical of their physiological sex.
   b. School-age children with gender identity disorder prefer to dress like and have playmates of the opposite sex. Since **gender identity is permanent**, the most effective management of this situation is to help parents accept the child as he or she is.
   c. In adulthood, these individuals commonly take the hormones of their preferred sex in order to better assume that gender role and may seek surgery to change their genital sex.

# II. THE BIOLOGY OF SEXUALITY IN ADULTS

In adults, alterations in circulating levels of gonadal hormones (estrogen, progesterone, and testosterone) can affect sexual interest and expression.

A. **Hormones and behavior in women**
   1. Because estrogen is only minimally involved in libido, **menopause (i.e., cessation of ovarian estrogen production)** and **aging do not reduce sex drive** if a woman's general health is good (see Chapter 2).
   2. **Testosterone** is secreted by the adrenal glands (as well as the ovaries and testes) throughout adult life and is believed to play an important role in **sex drive in both men and women.**

B. **Hormones and behavior in men**
   1. Testosterone levels in men generally **are higher than necessary** to maintain normal sexual functioning; low testosterone levels are less likely than relationship problems, age, alcohol use, or unidentified illness to cause sexual dysfunction.
   2. Psychological and physical **stress may decrease testosterone** levels.
   3. Medical treatment with **estrogens, progesterone**, or **antiandrogens** (e.g., to treat prostate cancer) can decrease testosterone availability via hypothalamic feedback mechanisms, resulting in **decreased sexual interest and behavior**.

C. **Homosexuality (i.e., gay or lesbian sexual orientation; see Table 19.1)**
   1. **Etiology**
      a. The etiology of homosexuality is believed to be related to **alterations in levels of prenatal sex hormones** (e.g., increased androgens in females and decreased androgens in males) resulting in anatomic changes in some hypothalamic nuclei; sex hormone levels in adulthood are indistinguishable from those of heterosexual people of the same biological sex.

| table   **19.2**   Characteristics of the Stages of Sexual Response Cycles in Men and Women | | |
|---|---|---|
| **Men** | **Women** | **Both Men and Women** |
| *Excitement Stage* | | |
| Penile erection | Clitoral erection<br>Labial swelling<br>Vaginal lubrication<br>Tenting effect (rising of the uterus in the pelvic cavity) | Increased pulse, blood pressure, and respiration<br>Nipple erection |
| *Plateau Stage* | | |
| Increased size and upward movement of the testes<br>Secretion of a few drops of sperm-containing fluid | Contraction of the outer third of the vagina, forming the orgasmic platform (enlargement of the upper third of the vagina) | Further increase in pulse, blood pressure, and respiration<br>Flushing of the chest and face (the "sex flush") |
| *Orgasm Stage* | | |
| Forcible expulsion of seminal fluid | Contractions of the uterus and vagina | Contractions of the anal sphincter<br>Further increase in pulse, blood pressure, and respiration |
| *Resolution Stage* | | |
| Refractory, or resting, period (length varies by age and physical condition) when restimulation is not possible | Little or no refractory period | Muscle relaxation<br>Return of the sexual, muscular, and cardiovascular systems to the prestimulated state over 10–15 min |

    **b.** Evidence for involvement of **genetic factors** includes markers on the X chromosome and higher concordance rate in monozygotic than in dizygotic twins.

    **c.** **Social factors**, such as early sexual experiences, **are not associated with the etiology** of homosexuality.

    **d.** Homosexuality is a normal variant of sexual expression. Because it is not a dysfunction, **no treatment is needed**. People who are uncomfortable with their sexual orientation may benefit from psychological intervention to help them become more comfortable.

  **2. Occurrence**

    **a.** By most estimates, at least **5%–10% of the population** has an exclusively homosexual sexual orientation; many more people have had at least one sexual encounter leading to arousal with a person of the same sex.

    **b.** There are **no significant ethnic differences** in the occurrence of homosexuality.

    **c.** Many people with gay and lesbian sexual orientations have experienced heterosexual sex and have had children.

**D. The sexual response cycle**

  **1.** Masters and Johnson devised a **four-stage model** for sexual response in both men and women, including the **excitement, plateau, orgasm**, and **resolution** stages (Table 19.2).

  **2.** Sexual dysfunctions involve difficulty with one or more aspects of the sexual response cycle.

# III. SEXUAL DYSFUNCTION

**A. Characteristics**

  **1.** Sexual dysfunction can result from biological, psychological, or interpersonal causes, or from a combination of causes.

    **a.** **Biological causes** include an unidentified general medical condition (e.g., **diabetes** can cause erectile dysfunction; **pelvic adhesions** can cause dyspareunia), **side effects of medication** (e.g., selective serotonin reuptake inhibitors [SSRIs] can cause delayed orgasm), **substance abuse** (e.g., alcohol use can cause erectile dysfunction), and **hormonal** or **neurotransmitter alterations**.

b. **Psychological causes** include current relationship problems, stress, depression, and anxiety (e.g., guilt, performance pressure). In men with erectile disorder, the presence of morning erections, erections during masturbation, or erections during rapid eye movement (REM) sleep suggests a psychological rather than a physical cause.

2. Dysfunctions may always have been present (**primary sexual dysfunctions**), or, more commonly, they occur after an interval when function has been normal (**secondary sexual dysfunctions**).

B. *Diagnostic and Statistical Manual of Mental Disorders, Fourth Edition, Text Revision (DSM-IV-TR)* classifications of sexual dysfunctions

1. The sexual desire disorders are **hypoactive sexual desire** disorder and **sexual aversion** disorder (disorders of the excitement phase).

2. The sexual arousal disorders are **female sexual arousal disorder** and **male erectile disorder** (disorders of the excitement and plateau phases).

3. The orgasmic disorders are **male orgasmic disorder, female orgasmic disorder**, and **premature ejaculation** (disorders of the orgasm phase).

4. The sexual pain disorders are **dyspareunia** and **vaginismus** (not caused by a general medical condition).

5. **Table 19.3** shows characteristics of the sexual dysfunctions.

C. **Management**

1. The physician must **understand** the patient's sexual problem before proceeding with treatment (e.g., clarify what a patient means when he says, "I have a problem with sex.").

2. The physician should **not assume anything** about a patient's sexuality (e.g., a middle-aged married male patient may be having an extramarital homosexual relationship).

3. There is a growing tendency for physicians to **manage the sexual problems of heterosexual and homosexual patients** rather than to refer these patients to sex therapists.

4. Management of sexual problems may be behavioral, medical, or surgical.

t a b l e   **19.3**   Characteristics of the *DSM-IV-TR* Sexual Dysfunctions

| Disorder | Characteristics |
| --- | --- |
| Hypoactive sexual desire disorder | Decreased interest in sexual activity |
| Sexual aversion disorder | Aversion to and avoidance of sexual activity |
| Female sexual arousal disorder | Inability to maintain vaginal lubrication until the sex act is completed, despite adequate physical stimulation (reported in as many as 20% of women) |
| Male erectile disorder (commonly called "impotence") | Lifelong or primary (rare): Has never had an erection sufficient for penetration<br>Acquired or secondary (the most common male sexual disorder): Is currently unable to maintain erections despite normal erections in the past<br>Situational (common): Has difficulty maintaining erections in some sexual situations, but not in others |
| Orgasmic disorder (male and female) | Lifelong: Has never had an orgasm<br>Acquired: Is currently unable to achieve orgasm despite adequate genital stimulation and normal orgasms in the past<br>Reported more often in women than in men |
| Premature ejaculation | Ejaculation before the man would like it to occur<br>Plateau phase of the sexual response cycle is short or absent<br>Is usually accompanied by anxiety<br>Is the second most common male sexual disorder |
| Vaginismus | Painful spasms occur in the outer third of the vagina, which make intercourse or pelvic examination difficult without pelvic pathology |
| Dyspareunia | Persistent pain occurs in association with sexual intercourse without pelvic pathology<br>Can also be caused by pelvic pathology, e.g., pelvic inflammatory disease (PID) caused by chlamydia infection (most common) or gonorrhea (most serious)<br>Occurs much more commonly in women; can occur in men |

5. **Behavioral management techniques**
   a. In **sensate-focus exercises** (used to manage sexual desire, arousal, and orgasmic disorders), the individual's awareness of touch, sight, smell, and sound stimuli are increased during sexual activity, and psychological pressure to achieve an erection or orgasm is decreased.
   b. In the **squeeze technique**, which is used to manage **premature ejaculation**, the man is taught to identify the sensation that occurs just before the emission of semen. At this moment, the man asks his partner to exert pressure on the coronal ridge of the glans on both sides of the penis until the erection subsides, thereby delaying ejaculation.
   c. **Relaxation techniques, hypnosis**, and **systematic desensitization** (see Chapter 17) are used to reduce anxiety associated with sexual performance.
   d. **Masturbation** may be recommended to help the person learn what stimuli are most effective for achieving arousal and orgasm.
6. **Medical and surgical management**
   a. Because they delay orgasm, **SSRIs** (e.g., fluoxetine) are used to manage **premature ejaculation**.
   b. **Systemic administration of opioid antagonists** (e.g., naltrexone) and vasodilators (e.g., yohimbine) have been used to manage erectile disorder.
   c. In erectile disorder, **sildenafil citrate** (Viagra) and related agents work by inhibiting an enzyme (phosphodiesterase-5 [PDE5]) that destroys cyclic guanosine monophosphate (cGMP), a vasodilator secreted in the penis with sexual stimulation. Thus, degradation of cGMP is slowed and the erection persists. Side effects include blue vision, and it is contraindicated in men who take nitrates. Newer PDE5 inhibitors with greater potency and selectivity than sildenafil include **vardenafil** (Levitra, Nuviva) and **tadalafil** (Cialis).
   d. **Intracorporeal injection of vasodilators** (e.g., papaverine, phentolamine) or implantation of **prosthetic devices** are also used to manage **erectile dysfunction**.
   e. **Apomorphine hydrochloride** (Uprima) increases sexual interest and erectile function by increasing dopamine availability in the brain. It is dissolved sublingually and its side effects include postural hypotension and syncope (fainting).

# IV. PARAPHILIAS

A. **Definition.** Paraphilias involve the preferential use of **unusual objects** of sexual desire or engagement **in unusual sexual activity (Table 19.4)**. To fit *DSM-IV-TR* criteria, the behavior must continue over a period of at least 6 months and cause impairment in occupational or social functioning.

| table **19.4** | Sexual Paraphilias |
|---|---|
| **Paraphilia** | **The Preferential Means of Obtaining Sexual Pleasure is By** |
| Exhibitionism | Revealing one's genitals to unsuspecting women so that they will be shocked |
| Fetishism | Contact with inanimate objects (e.g., women's shoes, rubber sheets) |
| Transvestic fetishism | Wearing women's clothing, particularly underclothing (exclusive to heterosexual men) |
| Frotteurism | Rubbing the penis against a clothed woman who is not consenting and not aware (e.g., on a crowded train) |
| Necrophilia | Engaging in sexual activity with corpses |
| Pedophilia | Engaging in fantasies or actual behaviors with children under age 14 yrs, of the opposite or same sex; is the most common paraphilia |
| Sexual masochism | Receiving physical pain or humiliation |
| Sexual sadism | Giving physical pain or humiliation |
| Telephone scatologia | Engaging unsuspecting women in telephone conversations of a sexual nature (obscene phone calls) |
| Voyeurism | Secretly watching other people (often by using binoculars or cameras) undressing or engaging in sexual activity |
| Zoophilia | Engaging in sexual activity with animals |

B. Occurrence and management
1. Paraphilias occur **almost exclusively in men**.
2. **Pharmacologic management** includes **antiandrogens** and **female sex hormones** for paraphilias that are characterized by hypersexuality.

# V. ILLNESS, INJURY, AND SEXUALITY

A. Heart disease and myocardial infarction (MI)
1. Men who have a history of MI often have **erectile dysfunction**. Both men and women who have a history of MI may have **decreased libido** because of the side effects of cardiac medications and the **fear that sexual activity will cause another heart attack**.
2. Generally, if exercise that raises the heart rate to **110–130 bpm** (e.g., exertion equal to climbing two flights of stairs) can be tolerated without severe shortness of breath or chest pain, sexual activity can be resumed after a heart attack.
3. **Sexual positions** that produce the least exertion in the patient (e.g., the **partner in the superior position**) are the safest after MI.

B. Diabetes
1. One-quarter to one-half of diabetic men (more commonly older patients) have **erectile dysfunction**. Orgasm and ejaculation are less likely to be affected.
2. The major causes of erectile dysfunction in men with diabetes are **vascular changes** and **diabetic neuropathy** caused by damage to blood vessels and nerve tissue in the penis as a result of **hyperglycemia**.
   a. Erectile problems generally occur several years after diabetes is diagnosed but **may be the first symptom** of the disease.
   b. **Poor metabolic control** of diabetes is related to increased incidence of sexual problems.
   c. Sildenafil citrate and related agents often are effective in diabetes-related erectile disorders.
   d. Although physiologic causes are most important, **psychological factors** also may influence erectile problems associated with diabetes.

C. Spinal cord injury
1. Spinal cord injuries in **men** cause erectile and orgasmic dysfunction, retrograde ejaculation (into the bladder), reduced testosterone levels, and decreased fertility.
2. Spinal cord injuries in **women** cause problems with vaginal lubrication, pelvic vasocongestion, and orgasm. Fertility is usually not adversely affected.

# VI. AGING AND SEXUALITY

A. Physical changes. Alterations in sexual functioning normally occur with the aging process.
1. **In men**, these changes include **slower erection, diminished intensity of ejaculation, longer refractory period**, and **need for more direct stimulation**.
2. In **women**, these changes include **vaginal thinning, shortening of vaginal length**, and **vaginal dryness**.
3. Hormone replacement therapy, which can reverse these vaginal changes, is used less frequently now than in the past (see Chapter 2). However, local application of a moisturizing agent to the vagina can be helpful.

B. Sexual interest and activity
1. In spite of physical changes, societal attitudes, and loss of the sexual partner because of illness or death, **sexual interest usually does not change significantly with increasing age**.
2. Continued sexual activity is associated with good health. Prolonged abstinence from sex leads to faster physical atrophy of the genital organs in old age ("**use it or lose it**").

| t a b l e    **19.5** The Effects of Some Prescription Drugs on Sexuality | | |
| --- | --- | --- |
| **Effect** | **Drug Type (Representative Agent)** | **Associated Neurotransmitter ($\uparrow$ [Increased] or $\downarrow$ [Decreased] Availability)** |
| Reduced libido | Antidepressant (fluoxetine)<br>Antihypertensive (propranolol)<br>Antihypertensive (methyldopa) | $\uparrow$Serotonin<br>$\downarrow$Norepinephrine $\beta$<br>$\uparrow$Central norepinephrine $\alpha$ |
| Increased libido | Antiparkinsonian (levodopa [L-dopa]) | $\uparrow$Dopamine |
| Erectile dysfunction | Antihypertensive (propranolol)<br>Antihypertensive (methyldopa)<br>Antidepressant (fluoxetine)<br>Antipsychotic (thioridazine) | $\downarrow$Norepinephrine $\beta$<br>$\uparrow$Central norepinephrine $\alpha$<br>$\uparrow$Serotonin<br>$\downarrow$Dopamine |
| Vaginal dryness | Antihistamine (diphenhydramine)<br>Anticholinergic (atropine) | $\downarrow$Histamine<br>$\downarrow$Acetylcholine |
| Inhibited orgasm (in men and women) | Antidepressant (fluoxetine) | $\uparrow$Serotonin |
| Priapism (persistent erection) | Antidepressant (trazodone) | $\uparrow$Serotonin |
| Inhibited ejaculation | Antidepressant (fluoxetine)<br>Antipsychotic (thioridazine) | $\uparrow$Serotonin<br>$\downarrow$Dopamine |

# VII. DRUGS AND SEXUALITY

A. **Prescription drugs** can affect libido, erection, orgasm, ejaculation, and other sexual functions, often as a result of their effects on neurotransmitter systems (Table 19.5).

B. Prescription drugs that lead to **decreased sexual function** include
   1. **Antihypertensives**, particularly $\alpha$-adrenergic agonists (e.g., methyldopa) and $\beta$-adrenergic blockers (e.g., propranolol); the fewest sexual problems are found with the use of angiotensin-converting enzyme (ACE) inhibitors (e.g., captopril).
   2. **Antidepressants**, particularly SSRIs, since serotonin may depress sexuality and delay orgasm.
   3. **Antipsychotics**, particularly dopamine-2 ($D_2$) receptor blockers
      a. Dopamine may enhance sexuality; its blockade may decrease sexual functioning.
      b. Prolactin levels increase as a result of dopamine blockade; this may in turn depress sexuality.

C. Drugs of abuse
   1. **Alcohol and marijuana** increase sexuality in the short term by decreasing psychological inhibitions.
      a. With long-term use, **alcohol may cause liver dysfunction**, resulting in increased estrogen availability and sexual dysfunction in men.
      b. Chronic use of **marijuana may reduce testosterone levels** in men and **pituitary gonadotropin** levels in women.
   2. **Amphetamines** and **cocaine** increase sexuality by stimulating dopaminergic systems.
   3. **Heroin** and, to a lesser extent, **methadone** are associated with suppressed libido, retarded ejaculation, and failure to ejaculate.

# VIII. THE HUMAN IMMUNODEFICIENCY VIRUS AND SEXUALITY

A. Occurrence of human immunodeficiency virus (HIV)
   1. More than **33 million people in the world** are infected with HIV.
      a. Most HIV-infected people live in Africa, Asia, and Eastern Europe.

| table **19.6** Route of Contact and Chance of Contracting HIV | |
| --- | --- |
| **Infection Route** | **Approximate Chance of Contracting HIV** |
| *Sexual Activity with an HIV-Infected Person* | |
| Anal intercourse | 1 in 10 to 1,600 |
| Vaginal intercourse with an infected man | 1 in 200 to 2,000 |
| Vaginal intercourse with an infected woman | 1 in 700 to 3,000 |
| *Direct Contact with Blood of an HIV-Infected Person* | |
| Transfusion | 1 in 1.05 (95 in 100) |
| Needle sharing | 1 in 150 |
| Needle stick | 1 in 200 |
| *HIV-Positive Mother to Fetus* | |
| Mother to fetus (mother not taking AZT) | 1 in 4 |
| Mother to fetus (mother taking AZT) | <1 in 10 |

AZT, zidovudine.

    **b.** Fewer than 1 million infected people live in North America.

    **c.** Fewer than 2 million infected people live in Latin America and the Caribbean; about 0.5 million live in Western and Central Europe.

  **2.** There is a **sex difference** in the HIV viral load and the symptoms of AIDS; a woman with the same HIV viral load as a man is likely to develop AIDS sooner than the man.

**B. Transmission of HIV**

  **1.** Because of the likelihood of tissue tearing leading to contact with the blood supply, **anal intercourse** is the sexual behavior that is riskiest for transmitting HIV (Table 19.6).

  **2.** Patients who are HIV-positive must protect their sexual partners from infection. If they fail to do so (e.g., do not use a condom) and the physician has knowledge of such failure, the physician must ensure that the threatened partner is informed (see Chapter 23).

  **3.** Prenatal treatment with **zidovudine (AZT)** or **nevirapine (Viramune)** can reduce the risk of transmission of HIV from mother to fetus. However, high-risk pregnant women cannot be compelled to be tested or treated (see Chapter 23).

# Review Test

**Directions:** Each of the numbered items or incomplete statements in this section is followed by answers or by completions of the statement. Select the **one** lettered answer or completion that is **best** in each case.

**1.** A 45-year-old physician states that he has been living with another man in a stable, sexual, love relationship for the past 10 years. This physician is most likely to have a history in adolescence of

(A) seduction by an older man
(B) mental illness
(C) sexual fantasies about men
(D) choosing to spend time alone
(E) wanting sex change surgery

**2.** A 32-year-old man who was recently diagnosed with HIV states that he is sure he got the infection from a sexual encounter he had while he was on vacation. Which of the following is the most appropriate question to ask the patient in order to determine his sexual orientation?

(A) "Would you describe yourself as homosexual?"
(B) "Are you mainly gay or mainly straight?"
(C) "Are you exclusively gay or exclusively straight?"
(D) "Do you prefer to have sex with men, women, or both men and women?"
(E) "Do you think you are heterosexual or homosexual?"

**3.** A 29-year-old woman says that she has always felt as if she were "a man in the body of a woman." Physical and pelvic examinations are normal. She is sexually attracted to heterosexual women and wants to wear men's clothes, take male hormones, and undergo a mastectomy and surgical sex reversal so that she can live as a man. The best way to describe this patient is that she has

(A) congenital virilizing adrenal hyperplasia
(B) androgen insensitivity syndrome
(C) gender identity disorder
(D) transvestic fetishism
(E) a lesbian sexual orientation

**4.** A 17-year-old woman comes to the doctor because she has never menstruated and because she has discovered labial masses. Initial examination reveals a tall, thin female with normal external genitalia and breast development. A pelvic examination is not performed. There are no Barr bodies in the buccal smear. The best way to describe this patient is that she has

(A) congenital virilizing adrenal hyperplasia
(B) androgen insensitivity syndrome
(C) gender identity disorder
(D) transvestic fetishism
(E) a lesbian sexual orientation

**5.** A 35-year-old man must wear women's high heels and lingerie to become aroused whenever he has sexual intercourse with a woman. He denies having sexual interest in men. The best way to describe this patient is that he has

(A) congenital virilizing adrenal hyperplasia
(B) androgen insensitivity syndrome
(C) gender identity disorder
(D) transvestic fetishism
(E) a gay sexual orientation

**6.** The best estimate of the occurrence of homosexuality in men is

(A) 0.5%–1%
(B) 2%–3%
(C) 5%–10%
(D) 20%–25%
(E) 30%–35%

**7.** A 50-year-old man shows breast enlargement after years of abusing a substance. The substance he is most likely to have abused is

(A) alcohol
(B) marijuana
(C) heroin
(D) amphetamine
(E) amyl nitrite

## Questions 8 and 9

A 34-year-old man has been taking fluoxetine for treatment of depression for the past 4 months. His mood is now normal but he reports that he is having sexual problems.

**8.** Which of the following sexual dysfunctions is this man most likely to report?

(A) Primary erectile disorder
(B) Secondary erectile disorder
(C) Premature ejaculation
(D) Delayed orgasm
(E) Dyspareunia

**9.** The neurotransmitter alteration most likely to be associated with this man's sexual problem is

(A) increased dopamine
(B) decreased dopamine
(C) increased serotonin
(D) decreased serotonin
(E) decreased norepinephrine

**10.** A 30-year-old male patient who is HIV positive asks the doctor what type of sexual behavior poses the most risk for transmitting HIV to his partner. The doctor's best response is

(A) anal intercourse
(B) oral-penis contact (fellatio)
(C) oral-vulva contact (cunnilingus)
(D) vaginal intercourse
(E) kissing

**11.** A husband and wife in their mid-30s state that they are having sexual problems. During the interview the doctor discovers that while their sex life had been good, the last time they tried to have intercourse (4 weeks previously), the husband could not maintain an erection. Which of the following agents is most likely to have caused this |sexual problem?

(A) Cocaine
(B) Propranolol
(C) Levodopa (L-dopa)
(D) Amyl nitrite
(E) Dextroamphetamine

**12.** A 65-year-old married couple complains to the doctor that their sex life is not what it used to be. Which of the following problems is the couple most likely to report?

(A) Premature ejaculation
(B) Vaginal dryness
(C) Shorter refractory period
(D) Decreased sexual interest
(E) Vaginismus

**13.** A 32-year-old man complains that he has no problem with erection, but that he usually has an orgasm and ejaculates before he achieves vaginal penetration. This man's complaint

(A) is uncommon
(B) is associated with depression
(C) is associated with an absent excitement phase
(D) can be effectively managed with intensive psychotherapy
(E) can be effectively managed with the squeeze technique

## Questions 14 and 15

A 62-year-old patient tells the physician that he is having difficulty maintaining an erection when he has intercourse with his wife.

**14.** Which of the following illnesses is most likely to be associated with this man's problem?

(A) Alzheimer disease
(B) Untreated hypertension
(C) Untreated diabetes
(D) Myocardial infarction
(E) Untreated schizophrenia

**15.** The physician recommends that the patient take sildenafil citrate (Viagra) prior to having intercourse. The major action of this agent in the management of erectile disorder is to

(A) increase the concentration of cGMP
(B) decrease the concentration of cGMP
(C) increase the degradation of cGMP
(D) increase the concentration of phosphodiesterase 5 (PDE5)
(E) decrease the degradation of prostaglandin E

**16.** A 25-year-old man masturbates by rubbing against unsuspecting women in crowded buses. This man is showing which of the following paraphilias?

**(A)** Fetishism
**(B)** Exhibitionism
**(C)** Frotteurism
**(D)** Voyeurism
**(E)** Sexual masochism

**17.** A 55-year-old married patient complains of erectile dysfunction. The man has Parkinson disease that is well controlled with l-dopa and he is able to work full time. He also has a part-time job that causes him to work late most evenings. The patient also relates that he drinks two martinis each evening, smokes two packs of cigarettes a day, and sometimes uses cocaine. His sexual dysfunction is most likely to be associated with his

**(A)** work schedule
**(B)** cocaine use
**(C)** L-dopa use
**(D)** alcohol drinking
**(E)** cigarette smoking

**18.** The tenting effect is most likely to begin in which stage of the sexual response cycle and in men only, women only, or both men and women?

**(A)** Excitement phase: Men only
**(B)** Plateau phase: Men only
**(C)** Orgasm phase: Men only
**(D)** Excitement phase: Men and women
**(E)** Plateau phase: Men and women
**(F)** Orgasm phase: Men and women
**(G)** Excitement phase: Women only
**(H)** Plateau phase: Women only
**(I)** Orgasm phase: Women only

**19.** The sex flush is most likely to begin in which stage of the sexual response cycle and in men only, women only, or both men and women?

**(A)** Excitement phase: Men only
**(B)** Plateau phase: Men only
**(C)** Orgasm phase: Men only
**(D)** Excitement phase: Men and women
**(E)** Plateau phase: Men and women
**(F)** Orgasm phase: Men and women
**(G)** Excitement phase: Women only
**(H)** Plateau phase: Women only
**(I)** Orgasm phase: Women only

**20.** Which stage of the sexual response cycle shows the greatest difference between men and women?

**(A)** Excitement
**(B)** Plateau
**(C)** Orgasm
**(D)** Resolution

**21.** Uterine contractions mainly occur in which stage of the sexual response cycle?

**(A)** Excitement
**(B)** Plateau
**(C)** Orgasm
**(D)** Resolution

**22.** The most common cause of pelvic inflammatory disease (PID) in women is

**(A)** gonorrhea
**(B)** syphilis
**(C)** trichomoniasis
**(D)** chlamydial infection
**(E)** candidiasis

**23.** A man and woman in their mid 20s who have been married for 3 years come to a physician for evaluation of infertility. During the interview the wife states, "I cannot understand why I cannot get pregnant. We have had sexual relations two to three times per week for the past year." What is the most appropriate next step for the physician to take?

**(A)** Refer the couple for marital counseling
**(B)** Perform a gynecological exam on the wife
**(C)** Perform a testicular exam on the husband
**(D)** Suggest that the husband undergo a fertility evaluation
**(E)** Suggest that the wife undergo a fertility evaluation
**(F)** Ask the couple what they mean by "sexual relations"

**24.** Concerned parents tell the doctor that last week their 6-year-old daughter walked in on them while they were having intercourse. This week they found their daughter with another 6-year-old girl playing the male role in what looked like a simulation of sexual intercourse. Physical exam is normal. The next step for the doctor to take is to

**(A)** Reassure the parents that this behavior is typical in children of this age
**(B)** Tell the parents that the child is likely to have a lesbian sexual orientation in adulthood
**(C)** Refer the family to a child psychiatrist
**(D)** Evaluate the child's sex hormone levels
**(E)** Advise the parents that the child probably has been sexually abused

# Answers and Explanations

## Typical Board Question

**The answer is C.** This 8-year-old boy, who has adopted the play, dress, and social preferences typical of a school-age girl, is showing evidence of gender identity disorder. Gender identity is related to early exposure of the brain to sex hormones and is unchangeable. The most effective strategy in dealing with parents of children with this disorder is to teach them that it is OK for the child to have these interests and help them accept the child as he or she is. Presenting only masculine toys or preventing use of feminine toys will not be effective in changing this child's behavior (see also answer to Question 3 below). When the child is an adult, he can decide whether or not to pursue sex reassignment surgery. Unlike this child, homosexual individuals are comfortable with their biological sex but prefer to have romantic and sexual relationships with people of their own sex.

1. **The answer is C.** Like other men with a homosexual sexual orientation, this physician is likely to have a history of sexual fantasies about men (heterosexual men commonly have a history of sexual fantasies about women). Homosexuality is a normal variant of sexual expression and is biologically based. There is no evidence that it is associated with a history in adolescence of seduction by an older man, mental illness, or a preference for being alone. While people with gender identity disorder (feeling of being born into the wrong body) may seek sex reassignment surgery, in homosexuality there is no desire to change biological sex.

2. **The answer is D.** The most appropriate question to ask this patient is a straightforward one, for example, "Do you prefer to have sex with men, women, or both men and women?" Using descriptors such as homosexual, heterosexual, gay, and straight is less likely to clarify the patient's sexual orientation and behavior.

3. **The answer is C.** This patient, who has always felt as if she were "a man in the body of a woman" in the presence of a normal female body, has gender identity disorder. Females with congenital virilizing adrenal hyperplasia have masculinized genitalia, and transvestic fetishists are always male. People with androgen insensitivity syndrome are genetic males with female bodies (with which they are content); they usually have sexual interest in men. Lesbian women have sexual interest in women but have a female gender identity and no desire to change their physical sex. (See also answers to Questions 4 and 5.)

4. **The answer is B.** This patient, who has a female phenotype despite a male genotype (e.g., no Barr bodies in the buccal smear), has androgen insensitivity syndrome. In this genetic defect, body cells do not respond to the androgen being produced by the testes, resulting in failure of physical masculinization. The masses noted by the patient are testes, which have descended into the labia. People with androgen insensitivity syndrome are generally heterosexual with respect to phenotypic sex (i.e., women with sexual interest in men). (See also answers to Questions 3 and 5.)

5. **The answer is D.** This patient, who must wear women's clothes to become sexually aroused, is showing transvestic fetishism. (See also answers to Questions 3 and 4.)

6. **The answer is C.** The best estimate of the occurrence of homosexuality in men is 5%–10%.

7. **The answer is A.** The substance that this 50-year-old man with breast enlargement is most likely to have abused is alcohol. Long-term use of alcohol damages the liver, resulting in accumulation of estrogens and feminization of the body. Marijuana, heroin, amphetamine, and amyl nitrite are much less likely to cause estrogen accumulation.

8. **The answer is D. 9. The answer is C.** While they may be associated with loss of libido and erectile disorder, fluoxetine and other selective serotonin reuptake inhibitors (SSRIs) are more likely to cause delayed or absent orgasm (orgasmic disorder). That is why the SSRIs are useful in managing premature ejaculation. Dyspareunia is not associated specifically with SSRI treatment. The neurotransmitter alteration most likely to be associated with delayed or absent orgasm is increased serotonin resulting from treatment with fluoxetine. Increased dopamine tends to increase sexual interest and performance. Decreased dopamine, decreased serotonin, and decreased norepinephrine are less likely to be associated with delayed orgasm than is increased serotonin.

10. **The answer is A.** Because tissue tears providing access to the blood supply are more likely to occur in anal intercourse, this is the type of sexual behavior that poses the most risk for transmitting HIV. While it is possible to transmit HIV by other sexual behaviors (e.g., fellatio [oral-penile contact], cunnilingus [oral-vulval contact], vaginal intercourse, and kissing), such transmission is much less likely than with anal intercourse.

11. **The answer is B.** Of the listed agents, the one most likely to have caused erectile disorder is propranolol, an antihypertensive medication (b-blocker). Cocaine, amphetamines, and L-dopa tend to increase sexual interest and performance by elevating dopamine availability. Amyl nitrite (a vasodilator) is used to enhance the sensation of orgasm.

12. **The answer is B.** This 65-year-old married couple is most likely to be having sexual problems because of vaginal dryness due to lack of estrogen after menopause. Aging is also characterized by a longer refractory period and delayed ejaculation in men and decreased intensity of orgasm in men and women. Although sexual behavior may decrease with aging because of these problems, sexual interest remains about the same. Vaginismus is not particularly associated with aging.

13. **The answer is E.** This man is describing premature ejaculation, a common sexual dysfunction, which can be effectively managed with the squeeze technique (not psychotherapy). Premature ejaculation is associated with an absent plateau phase of the sexual response cycle and is not specifically associated with depression.

14. **The answer is C. 15. The answer is A.** Untreated diabetes is most likely to be associated with erectile dysfunction. Although the medications used to manage these conditions are associated with erectile dysfunction, untreated cardiac problems, hypertension, and schizophrenia are not associated with erectile dysfunction. Alzheimer disease is not associated with erectile dysfunction. In fact, sexual expression may be the last form of communication between a couple in which one partner has Alzheimer disease. Sildenafil citrate (Viagra) works by increasing the concentration of cGMP, a vasodilator, in the penis which causes erection to persist.

16. **The answer is C.** This man who masturbates by rubbing against women in crowded buses is exhibiting frotteurism. Exhibitionism involves a sexual preference for revealing one's genitals to unsuspecting persons so that they will be shocked. Fetishism is a sexual preference for inanimate objects. Sexual masochism is a preference for receiving physical pain or humiliation. Voyeurism is a preference for secretly watching people undressing or engaging in sexual activity.

17. **The answer is D.** This patient's erectile problems are most likely to be associated with his alcohol drinking. Cigarette smoking is less likely than alcohol to affect sexual function. L-dopa and cocaine tend to increase rather than decrease sexual interest and performance by elevating dopamine availability. The man's work schedule, while stressful, is less likely than alcohol to affect his sexual functioning.

18. **The answer is G.** The tenting effect, elevation of the uterus in the pelvic cavity, begins during the excitement phase of the sexual response cycle in women.

19. **The answer is E.** The sex flush first appears during the plateau phase of the sexual response cycle in both men and women.

20. **The answer is D.** Resolution shows the greatest difference between men and women. Men have a resting (refractory) period after orgasm when restimulation is not possible. Women are less likely than men to have a refractory period.

21. **The answer is C.** Uterine contractions occur mainly during the orgasm phase of the sexual response cycle.

22. **The answer is D.** The most common cause of pelvic inflammatory disease (PID) in women is chlamydial infection; it may account for as many as 50% of the cases. Other sexually transmitted diseases can also cause PID, but are less common in the population than chlamydial infection.

23. **The answer is F.** The most appropriate next step for the physician to take is to clarify what the couple means by "sexual relations." Sexually inexperienced people may not know that some forms of sexual expression (e.g., fellatio, intercourse without ejaculation) cannot result in pregnancy. It is inappropriate to conduct physical or laboratory examinations for the cause of infertility until the physician is assured that the couple is having sexual intercourse involving vaginal penetration and ejaculation.

24. **The answer is A.** The next step for the doctor to take is to reassure the parents that curiosity about sexual behavior is typical for children of this age. Although the parents should speak to the child to be sure that she has not been sexually abused by an adult, her behavior with the other girl can be explained as an attempt to replicate the behavior of her parents. Since sexual orientation is primarily biological, there is no reason to believe that observing sexual behavior or playing the male role in a sexual game will result in the child's having a lesbian sexual orientation. Since physical examination is unremarkable, the child's sex hormone levels are likely to be normal.

# chapter **20**   Aggression and Abuse

## Typical Board Question

The concerned mother of an 11-year-old boy brings her son to the doctor after discovering him in bed with and sexually fondling his 4-year-old male cousin. The mother notes that at a recent meeting, the 11-year-old's teacher reported that, while he had been doing well in school and with friends, his grades recently have been slacking and he has stopped socializing with the other children in class. Physical examination is unremarkable. Which of the following should the doctor consider first to explain the boy's problematic behavior?

(A) He has conduct disorder
(B) He has been sexually abused by an adult
(C) He is showing normal pre-adolescent behavior
(D) He has oppositional defiant disorder
(E) He is experiencing the emergence of a homosexual orientation

*(See "Answers and Explanations" at end of chapter.)*

## I. AGGRESSION

A. **Social determinants of aggression**
   1. Factors associated with increased aggression include poverty, frustration, physical pain, and exposure to aggression in the media (e.g., **violence on television**).
   2. Children at risk for showing aggressive behavior in adulthood have frequently moved and changed schools repeatedly, have been **physically** and/or **sexually abused, mistreat animals** and younger or weaker children, and cannot defer gratification. Their parents frequently display criminal behavior, and abuse drugs and alcohol.
   3. Homicide occurs more often in **low socioeconomic populations** and its incidence is increasing. At least half of the homicides result from **guns**.
   4. In African American and white **males 15–24 years of age**, homicide is the **leading** and **second leading cause of death** respectively; Accidents are the second and first leading cause of death in African American and white males respectively in this age group.

B. **Biological determinants of aggression**
   1. **Hormones**
      a. **Androgens** are closely associated with aggression. In most animal species and human societies, males are more aggressive than females; **homicide** involving strangers is **committed** almost exclusively by **men**.
      b. **Androgenic** or **anabolic steroids**, often taken by bodybuilders to increase muscle mass, can result in **high levels of aggression** and even psychosis. Severe depression frequently occurs in withdrawal from these hormones.

   c. **Estrogen, progesterone**, and **antiandrogens** therefore can be useful in treating male sex offenders (see Chapter 19).
2. **Substances of abuse and their effects on aggression**
   a. Low doses of **alcohol** and **barbiturates** inhibit aggression, while high doses facilitate it.
   b. While intoxicated heroin users show little aggression, increased aggression is associated with the use of **cocaine, amphetamines**, and **phencyclidine (PCP)**.
3. **Neural bases of aggression**
   a. **Serotonin** and g-aminobutyric acid (GABA) inhibit aggression, and dopamine and norepinephrine facilitate it; low levels of the serotonin metabolite 5-hydroxyindoleacetic acid (5-HIAA) are seen in people who show impulsive aggression (see Chapter 4).
   b. **Drugs** used to treat inappropriate aggressiveness include antidepressants, benzodiazepines, antipsychotics (particularly atypical agents), and mood stabilizers (e.g., lithium).
   c. **Abnormalities of the brain** (e.g., abnormal activity in the **amygdala** and prepiriform area, and psychomotor and temporal lobe epilepsy) and lesions of the temporal lobes, frontal lobes, and hypothalamus are associated with increased aggression.
   d. **Violent people** often have a history of **head injury** or show abnormal electroencephalogram (EEG) readings.

## II.  ABUSE AND NEGLECT OF CHILDREN AND THE ELDERLY

A. **Overview**
1. Types of child (persons under age 18) and elder (persons aged 65 and over) abuse include **physical abuse, emotional** or **physical neglect**, and **sexual abuse**. The elderly may also be exploited for monetary gain.
2. **Abuse-related injuries** must be differentiated from injuries obtained during normal activity. Examples of **accidental** (i.e., non-abuse) **injuries** in children include bruises and scrapes on bony prominences (e.g., chin, forehead, knees, elbows) or, in the elderly, bruising on extensor surfaces of the limbs.
3. Occurrence of abuse and characteristics and signs that indicate neglect and abuse are shown in Table 20.1.

B. **Sequelae of child abuse**
1. Children who are being abused often seem **sad**, show **behavioral changes** (e.g., are no longer outgoing and friendly), and **do poorly in school**.
2. Adults who were abused as children are more likely to
   a. have **dissociative disorders (e.g., dissociative identity disorder)** and **borderline personality disorder** (see Chapter 14)
   b. have **posttraumatic stress disorder** and other anxiety disorders (see Chapter 13)
   c. have **depression** and **substance abuse** disorders (see Chapters 12 and 9, respectively)
   d. **abuse** their own children

C. **Sexual abuse of children**
1. **Signs**
   a. **Sexually transmitted diseases (STDs)** in children are signs of sexual abuse; children do not contract STDs through casual contact with an infected person or with their bedclothes, towels, or toilet seats.
   b. **Genital** or **anal trauma** is also a sign of sexual abuse.
   c. Young children have only a vague knowledge about sexual activities; specific **knowledge about sexual acts** (e.g., fellatio) in a young child often indicates that the child has been sexually abused.
   d. Recurrent **urinary tract infections** and excessive **initiation of sexual activity** with friends or with younger children, also are signs of sexual abuse.

| t a b l e **20.1** Physical Abuse of Children and Elders |
| --- |

| Category | Features of Child Physical Abuse | Features of Elder Physical Abuse |
| --- | --- | --- |
| *Occurrence* | | |
| Annual occurrence | At least 1 million cases are reported<br>Most cases are not reported | At least 1 million cases are reported<br>Most cases are not reported |
| Most likely abuser | The closest family member (e.g., the mother) | The closest family member (e.g., spouse, daughter, son, or other relative) with whom the person lives (and who is often supported financially by the elder) |
| *Characteristics of the Abused and the Abuser* | | |
| Characteristics of the abused | Hyperactivity or mild physical handicap; child is perceived as slow or different<br>Premature, low-birth-weight infant<br>Colicky or "fussy" infant<br>Physical resemblance to the abuser's absent, rejecting, or abusive partner<br>In one-third of cases, victims are younger than 5 yr of age; in one-fourth of cases, victims are 5–9 yr of age | Some degree of worsening cognitive impairment (e.g., Alzheimer disease)<br>Physical dependence on others<br>Incontinence<br>Does not report the abuse, but instead says that he fell and injured himself |
| Characteristics of the abuser | Substance abuse<br>Poverty<br>Social isolation<br>Delays seeking treatment for the victim<br>Personal history of abuse by caretaker or spouse | Substance abuse<br>Poverty<br>Social isolation<br>Delays seeking treatment for the victim |
| *Signs of Abuse* | | |
| Neglect | Poor personal care and hygiene (e.g., diaper rash, dirty hair)<br><br>Lack of needed nutrition | Poor personal care and hygiene (e.g., urine odor in incontinent person), lack of medication or health aids such as eyeglasses, or dentures<br>Lack of needed nutrition |
| Bruises | Particularly in the areas not likely to be injured during normal play, such as buttocks or lower back, or not over bony prominences<br>Belt or belt-buckle marks | Often on the inner (flexor) surfaces of arms from being grabbed |
| Fractures and burns | Fractures at different stages of healing<br>Spiral fractures caused by twisting the limbs<br>Cigarette and other burns<br>Wrist or ankle rope burns caused by tying to a bed or chair<br>Burns on the feet or buttocks caused by immersion in hot water | Fractures at different stages of healing<br>Spiral fractures caused by twisting the limbs<br>Cigarette and other burns<br>Wrist or ankle rope burns caused by tying to a bed or chair |
| Other signs | Internal abdominal injuries (e.g., ruptured spleen)<br>"Shaken baby" syndrome (i.e., retinal detachment or hemorrhage, and subdural hematoma caused by shaking the infant to stop it from crying)<br>Injuries of the mouth caused by forced feeding | Internal abdominal injuries (e.g., ruptured spleen)<br>Evidence of depleted personal finances (the elder's money was spent by the abuser and other family members)<br>Injuries of the mouth caused by forced feeding |

2. **Occurrence**
   a. An estimated 500,000 American children are sexually abused per year.
   b. Most sexually abused children are **8–13 years of age**, and 25% are younger than 8 years old.
   c. Approximately 20% of women and 5%–10% of men report sexual abuse at some time during their childhood and adolescence.
3. **Characteristics of the sexual abuser**
   a. Seventy percent to ninety percent of sexual abusers are **known to the child** and 90% of these are men. About 50% of these men are relatives (e.g., uncle, father, stepfather), and 50% are family acquaintances (e.g., mother's boyfriend, neighbor).
   b. **Alcohol** and **drugs** are commonly used by the abuser.

**c.** The abuser typically has **marital problems** and **no appropriate alternate sexual partner**; occasionally, he is a pedophile (i.e., he prefers children to appropriate sexual partners) (see Chapter 19).

## III.  PHYSICAL AND SEXUAL ABUSE OF DOMESTIC PARTNERS

**A.  Occurrence**
  **1.** Domestic partners are **couples who live together** and share living expenses and household responsibilities.
    **a.** Abuse occurs when one partner has **power** (e.g., physical, financial, psychological) over the other.
    **b.** Domestic abuse occurs between married couples (spousal abuse) but also between unmarried heterosexual or homosexual couples, adult siblings, or couples in other domestic arrangements.
  **2. Domestic abuse** is a common reason women come to a hospital emergency room. The abuse may be physical or sexual and the abuser is almost always male.
  **3.** The abused person **may not report to the police** or **leave the abuser** because he or she has nowhere to go and because the abuser has **threatened to harm the abused** if he or she reports or leaves him. (In fact, a woman has a greatly increased risk of being killed by her abusive partner if she leaves.)

**B.  Evidence of domestic abuse**
  **1.** The victim commonly has **bruises** (e.g., blackened eyes) and broken bones.
  **2.** In **pregnant women** (who have a higher risk of being abused), the **injuries** are often in the **"baby zone"** (i.e., the breasts and abdomen).
  **3.** An **irrational explanation** of how the injury occurred, **delay** in seeking treatment, and appearance of **sadness** in the victim are other indications of domestic abuse.

**C.** The **cycle of abuse** includes three phases
  **1. Buildup of tension** in the abuser
  **2.** Abusive behavior (battering)
  **3. Apologetic** and **loving behavior** by the abuser toward the victim.

**D. Characteristics** of domestic abusers and their abused partners can be found in Table 20.2.

| t a b l e      **20.2**      Physical and Sexual Abuse of Domestic Partners |
| --- |
| *Characteristics of the Abuser* |
| • Is almost always male |
| • Often uses alcohol or drugs |
| • Is impulsive and angry |
| • Has a low tolerance for frustration |
| • Has threatened to harm the abused if he or she reports or leaves him |
| • Shows apologetic and loving behavior after the abuse |
| • Has low self-esteem |
| *Characteristics of the Abused* |
| • Has been raised in a home in which there was domestic abuse |
| • Is financially or emotionally dependent on the abuser |
| • Can be male or female |
| • Blames him- or herself for the abuse |
| • May neither report to the police nor leave the abuser |
| • Has low self-esteem |

## IV. THE ROLE OF THE PHYSICIAN IN SUSPECTED CHILD, ELDER, AND DOMESTIC PARTNER ABUSE

**A. Child and elder abuse**
1. According to the law in every state, **physicians must report** suspected **physical** or **sexual abuse of a child** or **elderly person**, or of an adult who appears to be physically or mentally impaired, to the appropriate family social service agency (e.g., state child-protective service or state adult-protective service) **before** or **in conjunction with treatment** of the patient.
2. The physician is **not required to tell the suspected abuser of the child** or **impaired elder** that he or she suspects abuse.
3. The physician **does not need family consent** to hospitalize the abused child or elderly person for protection or treatment.
4. Even if there was no intention to injure, if a **cultural remedy** such as "coining" (see Chapter 20) injures a child or elderly person, such injury also **must be reported** to the appropriate agency.

**B. Domestic partner abuse**
1. **Direct reporting by the physician of domestic partner abuse is not appropriate** because the victim is usually a competent adult between the ages of 18 and 64.
2. A physician who suspects **domestic partner abuse** should
   a. Document the abuse.
   b. Ensure the safety of the abused person.
   c. Develop an **emergency escape plan** for the abused person.
   d. Provide **emotional support** to the abused person.
   e. Refer the abused person to an **appropriate shelter or program**.
   f. Encourage the abused person to report the case to law-enforcement officials.

## V. SEXUAL AGGRESSION: RAPE AND RELATED CRIMES

**A. Definitions. Rape** is a crime of violence, not of passion, and is known legally as "**sexual assault**," or "aggravated sexual assault."
1. Rape involves **sexual contact without consent**.
2. Vaginal penetration by a penis, finger, or other object may occur.
3. Erection and ejaculation do not have to occur.
4. **Sodomy** is defined as the insertion of the penis into the **oral** or **anal orifice**. The victim may be male or female.

**B. Legal considerations**
1. Because **rapists may use condoms** to avoid contracting HIV or to avoid DNA identification, or because they may have difficulty with erection or ejaculation, semen may not be present in the vagina of a rape victim.
2. A victim is **not required to prove that she resisted the rapist** for him to be convicted. A rapist can be convicted even though the victim asks him to use a condom or other form of sexual protection.
3. Certain information about the victim (e.g., previous sexual activity, "seductive" clothing worn at the time of the attack) is generally not admissible as evidence in rape trials.
4. **Husbands can be prosecuted** for forcing their wives to have intercourse. It is illegal to force anyone to engage in sexual activity.
5. Even if a woman consents to go on a date with a man and consents to sexual activity not involving intercourse, a man can be prosecuted for rape ("**date rape**").
6. Consensual sex may be considered rape ("**statutory rape**") if the victim is younger than 16 or 18 years old (depending on state law) or is older than this but is **physically** or **mentally impaired**.

C. **Characteristics of the rapist and victim**
1. **The rapist**
   a. **Rapists** are usually younger than 25 years of age.
   b. They are usually the **same race** as the victim.
   c. They are usually **known to the victim**.
   d. They often use **alcohol**.
2. **The victim**
   a. Rape victims are most typically between **16–24** years of age.
   b. Rape most commonly occurs **inside the victim's home**.
   c. **Vaginal injuries may be absent**, particularly in parous women (those who have had children).

D. **The sequelae of rape**
1. For a variety of reasons, including shame, fear of retaliation, and the difficulties involved in substantiating rape charges, **only 25% of all rapes are reported to the police.**
2. Others may commonly **blame the victim** in rape cases.
3. The length of the emotional recovery period after rape varies, but is commonly **at least 1 year. Posttraumatic stress disorder** sometimes occurs after rape (see Chapter 14).
4. The most effective type of counseling is group therapy with other rape victims.

E. **The role of the physician in rape cases**
1. **Immediately after the rape**, the physician should
   a. Take the patient's history in a supportive manner, and not question the patient's veracity or judgment.
   b. Perform a general **physical examination** and conduct **laboratory tests** (e.g., cultures for sexually transmitted diseases from the vagina, anus, and pharynx; test for presence of semen).
   c. Prescribe prophylactic **antibiotics** and postcoital **contraceptive measures** (e.g., levonorgestrel ["Plan B"]) if appropriate.
   d. **Encourage** the patient to notify the police. The doctor is not required to notify the police if the woman is a competent adult.
2. **Up to 6 weeks after the rape**
   a. Discuss with the patient the **emotional** and **physical sequelae** of the rape (e.g., suicidal thoughts, vaginal bleeding) and, if needed, refer her for long-term counseling or a support group.
   b. Do a **pregnancy test** and repeat other laboratory tests if appropriate.

# Review Test

**Directions:** Each of the numbered items or incomplete statements in this section is followed by answers or by completions of the statement. Select the **one** lettered answer or completion that is **best** in each case.

**1.** At a postpartum examination 3 weeks after a normal delivery, a physician notices that the patient has a torn vaginal orifice. When asked, the patient tells the doctor that her husband forced her to resume sexual intercourse 10 days after giving birth even though she told him "No." What is the most appropriate thing for the doctor to say to the patient at this time?

(A) "Have you been abused like this in the past?"
(B) "Tearing of the vaginal orifice is a normal complication of intercourse after vaginal delivery"
(C) "I am sorry for your experience, no one deserves that kind of treatment"
(D) "I must call the police and report that you have been sexually abused"
(E) "Please tell me more about your relationship with your husband"

**2.** A 3-month-old infant is brought to the emergency department unconscious. While no external injuries are seen, physical examination reveals a subdural hematoma and retinal hemorrhages. The parents tell the physician that the child fell off his changing table the previous day. After stabilizing the child, the emergency department physician should

(A) contact the state child-protective service agency
(B) question the parents to determine if they have abused the child
(C) inform the parents that he suspects that they have abused the child
(D) obtain the parents' permission to hospitalize the child
(E) obtain the parents' permission to call a pediatric neurologist

## Questions 3 and 4

A 4-year-old girl tells the physician that her father asked her to touch his penis. Physical examination of the child is unremarkable.

**3.** The most appropriate next step for the physician to take is to

(A) contact the state child-protective service agency
(B) ask the mother's permission to consult with a child psychiatrist
(C) question the father about the child's remark
(D) question the child further to determine if she is telling the truth
(E) contact a child psychiatrist to determine if the child is telling the truth
(F) contact a pediatric gynecologist to determine if sexual abuse has occurred

**4.** In evaluating the risk of leaving this child with her parents, which of the following is most closely associated with an increased risk that the child will be abused again?

(A) The child has a quiet, passive personality
(B) The parents are involved in marital therapy
(C) The parents are mentally retarded
(D) There is a history of abuse in the parents' own childhoods
(E) The parents are employed in law enforcement

**5.** Which of the following injuries in a 4-year-old child is most likely to be the result of physical abuse?

(A) Cut chin
(B) Bilateral bruises on the knees
(C) Scraped forehead
(D) Cut elbow
(E) Ruptured spleen

**6.** A 40-year-old woman comes to the emergency room with bruises on her right cheek and a deep laceration above her right eye. The woman, who notes that she has had "a problem with alcohol" for more than 10 years, states that her husband hit her because she did not have dinner on the table when he came home from work. After treating her injuries, the most appropriate question for the physician to ask is

**(A)** "Would you describe yourself as an alcoholic?"
**(B)** "Why do you think your husband abuses you?"
**(C)** "Do you think it is safe for you to return home to your husband?"
**(D)** "Would you like to talk about your problem with alcohol?"
**(E)** "Did your father abuse your mother?"
**(F)** "Do you think your drinking has had a negative effect on your marriage?"
**(G)** "Would you like some information on Alcoholics Anonymous?"

**7.** An 18-year-old **retarded** woman with mental retardation and an IQ of 50 agrees to have sexual intercourse with the 18-year-old president of the high school senior class. Sexual intercourse between these two people is best described as

**(A)** consensual sex
**(B)** statutory rape
**(C)** sodomy
**(D)** child abuse
**(E)** sexual abuse

**8.** A 33-year-old single woman who has a 4-year-old child comes to the emergency room and reports that she was raped by a man she was on a date with 2 days ago. The physical examination shows no physical evidence of rape (e.g., no injuries, no semen). She appears anxious, disheveled, and "spacey." It is most likely that this woman

**(A)** is delusional
**(B)** is malingering
**(C)** has hypochondriasis
**(D)** has conversion disorder
**(E)** has been raped and the rapist used a condom

**9.** A 7-year-old child and her mother both have chlamydia. The child's infection is most likely to be the result of

**(A)** sleeping in the same bed as the mother
**(B)** sexual abuse
**(C)** masturbation
**(D)** using the mother's towel
**(E)** bathing in the mother's bathtub

**10.** On at least three occasions, a 10-year-old boy is found taking lunch money from the other children in his class. The boy is underweight, has dirty clothes and hair, and lives in a motel room with his single mother and four siblings. This picture most closely suggests

**(A)** attention deficit/hyperactivity disorder (ADHD)
**(B)** Tourette disorder
**(C)** conduct disorder
**(D)** oppositional defiant disorder
**(E)** child neglect

**11.** A mother brings her 9-year-old daughter to the physician who has been caring for the family for the past 10 years. The mother reports that over the past 2 weeks, the child has been urinating frequently and complaining of pain on urination. She notes that 2 months ago, the child showed the same symptoms. The physician observes that, while formerly friendly and outgoing, the child now seems sad and does not make eye contact with him. The mother also states that since she remarried 5 months ago, the child has been doing poorly in school. The most likely explanation for this clinical picture is that the child

**(A)** is angry that her mother remarried
**(B)** is complaining to gain attention from her mother
**(C)** is being sexually abused by the mother's new husband
**(D)** is complaining to avoid school
**(E)** is complaining to explain her school problems

**12.** A 93-year-old mildly demented woman, who is occasionally incontinent, lives with her daughter. She attends a day care program from 9 AM to 1 PM. From 1 PM to 4 PM, a neighbor (who has an alcoholic son and an unemployed son) takes care of the elderly woman. The woman is brought to the emergency room by her daughter with injuries that suggest physical abuse. The person most likely to have abused this woman is

**(A)** a day care program worker
**(B)** the neighbor's alcoholic son
**(C)** the neighbor
**(D)** the elderly woman's daughter
**(E)** the neighbor's unemployed son

# Answers and Explanations

## Typical Board Question

**The answer is B.** While heterosexual and homosexual play between children of about the same age is typically normal (see Chapters 2 and 19), sexual play between children who vary in age (no matter what their sex) is of concern. In this case, the behavior by the older child suggests that recently he has been sexually abused by an adult and is replicating what has been done to him with his 4-year-old cousin. His slacking grades and unsociable behavior give further evidence that the 11-year-old boy has been abused. Conduct disorder and oppositional defiant disorder are unlikely since the child has no previous history of behavior problems.

1. **The answer is E.** No one has the right to force another person to have sexual activity, and tearing of the vaginal orifice, while not a normal complication of intercourse after vaginal delivery, can occur if intercourse is resumed too soon after childbirth. However, because this woman is a competent adult, if she wants to file charges against her husband, she must report the abuse to the police herself. Certainly no one deserves that kind of treatment, but in order to get more information about the patient's marital relationship, the most appropriate thing for the doctor to say to the patient at this time is "Please tell me more about your relationship with your husband."

2. **The answer is A.** After stabilizing the infant, the emergency department physician should contact the state child-protective service agency to report suspected child abuse. Subdural hematoma, retinal hemorrhage, and retinal detachment are signs of the shaken baby syndrome, a form of child abuse in which an adult shakes a child to stop its crying. The shaken child may have no external injuries. Child abusers, such as these parents, commonly delay seeking treatment and make up some explanation for the injuries such as "the child fell." The physician must report any suspicion of abuse to the appropriate authority, but does not have to question the parents or inform them of this suspicion. Similarly, when a physician suspects child physical or sexual abuse, he or she does not need a parent's permission to examine, hospitalize, or treat the child or to consult with a specialist.

3. **The answer is A. 4. The answer is D.** When a child of any age reports inappropriate sexual touching, the physician must contact the state child-protective service agency. This example demonstrates that a child may show no physical signs of sexual abuse. The physician must assume that patients (even young ones) are telling the truth. The physician does not need to talk to the child further, consult a child psychiatrist, contact a pediatric gynecologist, or talk to the father to confirm the story. The state agency will handle these matters. In evaluating the risk of leaving abused children with their parents, a history of abuse in the parents' own childhoods is associated with an increased risk that the child will be abused again. Intelligence of the parents, employment of the parents in law enforcement, and whether the parents are involved in marital therapy are not specifically associated with the risk of child abuse.

5. **The answer is E.** An internal injury, such as a ruptured spleen, is most likely to be the result of abuse in a 4-year-old child. Chin, knee, forehead, and elbow injuries are more likely to have been obtained during normal play.

6. **The answer is C.** The most important thing for the physician to do is to ensure the safety of this abused patient. Therefore, questioning the woman about whether it is safe for her to return home should be the initial intervention. Implying that her drinking (e.g., "Do you think your drinking has had a negative effect on your marriage?" "Would you describe yourself as an alcoholic?" or "Why do you think that your husband abuses you?") or her father's behavior (e.g., "Did your father abuse your mother?") is related to the abuse seems to blame the victim and is not appropriate. Treatment (e.g., "Would you like to talk about your problem with alcohol?" or "Would you like some information on Alcoholics Anonymous?") can wait until the immediate problem, ensuring her safety, is resolved.

7. **The answer is B.** Even though both are legally of adult age, sexual intercourse between this person with mental retardation and a non-impaired person is best described as statutory rape. Because the woman has impaired mental functioning (i.e., a mental age of 7.5 years, per Chapter 2), she may not fully understand the meaning of her consent in this context. Consensual sex implies that both people have the ability to decide to interact. Sodomy is oral-penile or anal-penile contact. Child abuse and sexual abuse are not the best identifiers for the behavior described here.

8. **The answer is E.** It is most likely that this woman has been raped by the man she went out with ("date rape"). Because there is no semen, the rapist may have used a condom. Parous women such as this patient may show no physical signs of rape. Rape victims may appear anxious, disheveled, and "spacey" (e.g., use of dissociation as a defense mechanism). Patients rarely lie to doctors. There is no indication that this woman is lying for obvious gain (malingering), is delusional, or has hypochondriasis or conversion disorder.

9. **The answer is B.** The child's chlamydia infection is most likely to be the result of sexual abuse. Sexually transmitted diseases are rarely if ever contracted by masturbation or by sleeping in the same bed, using the same towel, or bathing in the same bathtub as an infected person.

10. **The answer is E.** The most likely explanation for this child's stealing behavior is that he is being neglected and is taking money to buy food. Evidence for neglect includes the fact that he is underweight, has dirty clothes and hair, and lives in a crowded situation. It is less likely that he has one of the behavior disruptive disorders, and there is no evidence of ADHD or the tics of Tourette disorder.

11. **The answer is C.** The most likely explanation for this clinical picture is that this 9-year-old girl is being sexually abused by her mother's new husband. Signs of sexual abuse include urinary tract infections and personality changes, e.g., sadness and withdrawal, as well as school problems. It is much less likely that the child's signs and symptoms are because of anger at her mother, or represent an attempt to gain attention or avoid school. Rather, the abuse may help explain the child's recent difficulties in school.

12. **The answer is D.** A close relative who cares for the person (e.g., the daughter) is most likely to have abused this elderly demented woman. Although no excuse for abuse, this may be a result, in part, of the stresses associated with caring for a demented, incontinent elderly person. Unrelated people such as caretakers (even if alcoholic or unemployed) are much less likely than a close relative to abuse an elderly person.

# chapter 21

# The Physician–Patient Relationship

**Typical Board Question**

A 22-year-old man with schizophrenia is brought to the emergency department from an inpatient psychiatric facility a half hour after accidentally cutting himself while slicing bread. The patient has a 5 cm cut on his hand which requires suturing. He refuses treatment for the cut and states "I know I have a thought problem I take medication for, but I never know who to trust. I want to wait until my parents get here. I know my hand can get infected if I wait too long, but I don't think a few hours are going to make a big difference." What is the best course of action for the doctor to take at this time?

- **(A)** Do not treat and determine if the parents are on the way.
- **(B)** Do not treat until a court order is obtained.
- **(C)** Do not treat until obtaining a psychiatric evaluation.
- **(D)** Treat because the patient admits he has a psychiatric disorder.
- **(E)** Treat because the patient has been placed in a psychiatric facility.
- **(F)** Treat because the patient shows signs of paranoia and is thus incompetent.

*(See "Answers and Explanations" at end of chapter.)*

## I. MEDICAL PRACTICE

**A. Seeking medical care**
  1. Patients' behavior when ill and their expectations of physicians are influenced by their **culture** (see Chapter 18), previous experiences with medical care, physical and mental conditions, **personality styles** (not necessarily personality disorders: See Table 14.3) (Table 21.1) and **coping skills**.
  2. Only about **one-third of Americans with symptoms seek medical care**; most people contend with illnesses at home with over-the-counter medications and home management.

**B. Seeking psychiatric care**
  1. In the United States, there is a **stigma** to having a psychiatric illness. Psychiatric symptoms are considered by many Americans to indicate **a moral weakness** or a **lack of self-control**. Because of this stigma, many patients fail to seek help.
  2. It is important for patients to seek help since there is a strong **correlation between psychological illness** and **physical illness**. Morbidity rates and mortality rates are much higher in patients who need psychiatric attention.

**C. The "sick role"**
  1. A person assumes a particular role in society and certain behavioral patterns when he or she is ill (the "sick role," described by T. Parsons). The sick role includes **exemption from**

226 **Behavioral Science**

| table 21.1 | Patient Personality Style and Behavioral Characteristics During Illness |
|---|---|
| **Personality Style** | **Behavioral Characteristics During Illness** |
| Paranoid | Blames the physician for the fact that he or she is ill |
| Schizoid | Becomes even more withdrawn during illness |
| Schizotypal | Bizarre behavior may mask serious illness |
| Histrionic | May be dramatic, emotionally changeable, and approach the physician in an inappropriate sexual fashion during illness |
| Narcissistic | Has a perfect self-image, which is threatened by illness and may refuse needed treatment which can alter his or her appearance |
| Antisocial | May self-write or alter prescriptions and lie to the physician |
| Borderline | Idealizes the physician at first, may make gestures of self-harm when ill |
| Avoidant | Interprets physician health suggestions as criticisms, fears rejection by the doctor, is overly sensitive to a perceived lack of attention or caring |
| Obsessive–compulsive | Fears loss of control and may in turn become more controlling during illness |
| Dependent | Becomes more needy during illness and wants the physician to make all decisions and assume all responsibility |
| Passive–aggressive | Asks for help but then does not adhere to the physician's advice |

**usual responsibilities** and expectation of care by others, as well as working toward becoming healthy and cooperating with health care personnel in getting well.
2. Critics of the sick role theory argue that it **applies only to middle-class** patients with acute physical illness, emphasizes the power of the physician, and undervalues the individual's social support network in getting well.

D. **Telling patients the truth**
1. In the United States, adult patients generally are **told the complete truth** about the diagnosis, the management and its side effects, and the prognosis of their illness. **Falsely reassuring** or **patronizing statements** in response to patient questions (e.g., "Do not worry, we will take good care of you" or "You still have one child" [after a miscarriage]) are not appropriate.
2. Information about the illness must be **given directly to the adult patient** and **not relayed to the patient through relatives. Parents decide** if, how, and when such information will be given to an **ill child**.
    a. With the **patient's permission**, the physician can tell relatives this information in conjunction with, or after, telling the patient.
    b. Relieving the fears of close relatives of a seriously ill patient can bolster the support system, and thus help the patient.

E. **Special situations**
1. Patients may be **afraid to ask questions** about issues that are **embarrassing** (e.g., sexual problems) or **fear-provoking** (e.g., laboratory results). A physician should not try to guess what is troubling a patient; it is the physician's responsibility to ask about such issues in an open-ended fashion (see section III.B.2.b.) and address them truthfully and fully with the patient.
2. Physicians have the primary responsibility for dealing with **adherence issues** (see II below), as well as with **angry, seductive**, or **complaining behavior** by their patients (Table 21.2). Referrals to other physicians should be reserved only for medical and psychiatric problems outside of the treating physician's range of expertise.

# II. ADHERENCE

A. **Patient characteristics associated with adherence**
1. Adherence refers to the extent to which a patient follows the recommendations of the physician, such as taking medications on schedule, having a needed medical test or surgical procedure, and following directions for changes in lifestyle, such as diet or exercise.

table **21.2** Do's and Do Not's for Answering USMLE Questions Involving Common Problems in the Physician–Patient Relationship

| Problem | Do | Do Not |
|---|---|---|
| Angry patient | **Do** acknowledge the patient's anger | **Do not** take the patient's anger personally (the patient is probably fearful about becoming dependent as well as of being ill) |
| Complaining patient: About another doctor | **Do** encourage the patient to speak to the other physician directly if the patient complains about a relationship with another physician | **Do not** intervene in the patient's relationship with another physician unless there is a medical reason to do so |
| Complaining patient: About you or your staff | **Do** speak to your own office staff if the patient has a complaint about one of them | **Do not** blame the patient for problems with you or your office staff |
| Crying patient | **Do** acknowledge the patient's sadness and quietly wait for the patient to speak | **Do not** rush the patient or use patronizing statements such as "do not worry" to comfort the patient<br>**Do not** say "I understand." The patient makes that judgment. |
| Nonadherent patient: Needs to improve health behavior | **Do** examine the patient's willingness to change his or her health-threatening behavior (e.g. smoking); if he or she is not willing, you must address that issue first | **Do not** attempt to scare the patient into adhering (e.g., showing frightening photographs of untreated illness) |
| Nonadherent patient: Needs a test or treatment (e.g., mammogram) | **Do** identify the real reason (e.g., fear) for the patient's refusal to adhere to or to consent to a needed intervention and address it | **Do not** refer the patient to another physician |
| Seductive patient | **Do** call in a chaperone when you are with the patient<br>**Do** gather information using direct rather than open-ended questions<br>**Do** set limits on the behavior that you will tolerate | **Do not** refuse to see the patient<br>**Do not** refer the patient to another physician<br>**Do not** fail to act if the patient crosses a social boundary |
| Suicidal patient | **Do** assess the seriousness of the threat<br>**Do** suggest that the patient remain in the hospital voluntarily if the threat is serious | **Do not** assume that the threat is not serious<br>**Do not** release a hospitalized patient who is a threat to himself or herself (patients who are a threat to self or others can be held involuntarily [see Chapter 23]) |

2. Patients' **unconscious** transference reactions to their physicians, which are based in childhood parent–child relationships, can increase or decrease adherence (see Chapter 6).
3. Only about **one-third of patients adhere fully to management recommendations**, one-third adhere some of the time, and one-third do not adhere to such recommendations.

B. **Factors that increase and decrease adherence**
1. Adherence is **not related to patient intelligence, education**, sex, religion, race, socioeconomic status, or marital status.
2. Adherence is most closely related to **how well the patient likes the doctor**. The strength of the doctor–patient relationship is also the most important factor in whether or not patients sue their doctors when an error or omission is made or when there is a poor outcome (see Chapter 23).
3. Some factors associated with adherence are listed in Table 21.3.

# III. THE CLINICAL INTERVIEW

A. **Communication skills**
1. Patient adherence with medical advice, detection of both physical and psychological problems, and patient satisfaction with the physician are improved by good physician–patient communication.

| table 21.3 | Factors Associated with Adherence to Medical Advice | |
| --- | --- | --- |
| Factors Associated with Increased Adherence | Factors Associated with Decreased Adherence | Comments |
| Good physician–patient relationship | Poor physician–patient relationship | Liking the physician is the most important factor in adherence; it is even more important than the physician's technical skill<br>Physicians perceived as unapproachable have low adherence from patients |
| Patient feels ill and usual activities are disrupted by the illness | Patient experiences few symptoms and little disruption of usual activities | In asymptomatic illnesses, such as hypertension, only about half of the patients initially adhere to management<br>Many asymptomatic patients who initially adhered have stopped adhering within 1 yr of diagnosis |
| Short time spent in the waiting room | Long time spent in the waiting room | Patients kept waiting get angry and then fail to adhere |
| Belief that the benefits of care outweigh its financial and time costs | Belief that financial and time costs of care outweigh its benefits | The "Health Belief Model" of health care |
| Written diagnosis and instructions for management | Verbal diagnosis and instructions for management | Patients often forget what is said during a visit to the physician because they are anxious<br>Asking the patient to repeat your verbal instructions can improve understanding and thus increase adherence |
| Acute illness | Chronic illness | Chronically ill people see physicians more often but are more critical of them than acutely ill people |
| Recommending only one behavioral change at a time | Recommending multiple behavioral changes at once | To increase adherence, instruct the patient to make one change (e.g., stop smoking) this month, and make another change (e.g., start dieting) next month<br>Recommending too many changes at once will reduce the likelihood that the patient will make any changes |
| Simple management schedule | Complex management schedule | Adherence is higher with medications that require once daily dosing, preferably with a meal<br>Patients are more likely to forget to take medications requiring frequent or between-meal dosing |
| Older physician | Younger physician | Usually young physician age is only an issue for patients in the initial stages of management |
| Peer support | Little peer support | Membership in a group of people with a similar problem (e.g., smoking [see Chapter 9]) can increase adherence |

2. One of the most important skills for a physician to have is **how to interview patients**.
   a. The **physical setting** for the interview should be as private as possible. Ideally, there should be **no desk or other obstacle** between the physician and patient, and the participants should interact at **eye level** (e.g., both seated).
   b. During the interview, the physician must first **establish trust in** and **rapport with** the patient and then gather physical, psychological, and social information to identify the patient's problem.
   c. Finally the physician should try to educate the patient about the illness and motivate the patient to adhere to management recommendations.
   d. The physician should obtain backup (e.g., hospital security) if it appears that a patient is **dangerous** or **threatening**.
3. The interview serves to obtain the patient's **psychiatric history**, including information about prior mental problems, drug and alcohol use, sexual activity, current living situation, and sources of stress.
4. When interviewing **young children** the physician should
   a. First establish rapport by interacting with the child in a nonmedical way, for example, drawing pictures.
   b. Use direct rather than open-ended questions, for example, "What is your sister's name?" rather than "Tell me about your family."
   c. Ask questions in the third person, for example, "Why do you think that the little boy in this picture is sad?"

| t a b l e | **21.4** | Aims of the Clinical Interview and Specific Interviewing Techniques | |
|---|---|---|---|
| **Aim** | **Technique** | **Specific Use** | **Example** |
| To establish rapport | Support and empathy | To express the physician's interest, understanding, and concern for the patient | "You must have really been frightened when you realized you were going to fall." |
| | Validation | To give value and credence to the patient's feelings | "Many people would feel the same way if they had been injured as you were." |
| To maximize information gathering | Facilitation | To encourage the patient to elaborate on an answer; can be a verbal question or body language, such as a quizzical expression | "Please tell me more about what happened after that." |
| | Reflection | To encourage elaboration of the answer by repeating part of the patient's previous response | "You said that your pain increased after lifting the package?" |
| | Silence | To increase the patient's responsiveness | Waiting silently for the patient to speak |
| To clarify information | Confrontation | To call the patient's attention to inconsistencies in his or her responses or body language | "You say that you are not worried about tomorrow's surgery, but you seem really nervous to me." |
| | Recapitulation | To sum up all of the information obtained during the interview to ensure that the physician understands the information provided by the patient | "Let's go over what you told me. You fell last night and hurt your side. Your husband called 911. The paramedics came but the pain got worse until they gave you a shot in the emergency room. Have I gotten it right?" |

**B. Specific interviewing techniques**

1. **Direct questions.** Direct questions are used to elicit specific information quickly from a patient in an **emergency** situation (e.g., "Have you been shot?") or when the patient is seductive or overly talkative.

2. **Open-ended questions**

   a. Although direct questions can elicit information quickly, open-ended types of questions are more likely to aid in obtaining information about the patient, and not close off potential areas of pertinent information.

   b. Using open-ended questions (e.g., "What brings you in today?"), the interviewer gives little structure to the patient and **encourages the patient to speak freely**.

3. Table 21.4 lists aims of the clinical interview and gives examples of some specific interviewing techniques.

# Review Test

**Directions:** Each of the numbered items or incomplete statements in this section is followed by answers or by completions of the statement. Select the **one** lettered answer or completion that is **best** in each case.

**1.** After a school bus accident, a 6-year-old boy with an injured leg is brought to the emergency room. The child is awake and alert but is carrying no identifying information. The paramedics report that the child has not spoken since the accident. The most appropriate first step by the physician is to

(A) get crayons and paper and ask the child to draw pictures with her
(B) say to the child "I am very sorry about what happened"
(C) look the child solemnly in the eye and ask him about the accident
(D) say "If you will not talk to me I cannot locate your mother"
(E) leave the child alone so that he can rest

**2.** A woman and her 15-year-old daughter come to a physician's office together. When the physician asks what brings them in, the mother states: "I want you to fit my daughter for a diaphragm." The most appropriate action for the physician to take at this time is to

(A) follow the mother's wishes and fit the girl for a diaphragm
(B) ask the mother why she wants a diaphragm for her daughter
(C) recommend that the girl see a sex-education counselor
(D) ask the mother to leave and speak to the girl alone
(E) ask the girl if there is something she wants to say in private

**3.** A 9-year-old girl who has a terminal illness asks the physician, "Am I going to die?" The child's parents previously told the physician that they do not want the child to know her diagnosis or prognosis. The physician's best response to the child's question is to say

(A) "Do not worry, you will be fine."
(B) "Yes, you will die of this illness."
(C) "Tell me what your parents have told you about your illness."
(D) "Your parents do not want you to know about your illness so I cannot tell you."
(E) "Many children with this kind of illness live a long time."

**4.** A 40-year-old male patient tells his physician that he smokes at least two packs of cigarettes a day but would like to stop. Which of the following is the most effective statement or question the physician can use to encourage the patient to give up smoking?

(A) "You must stop smoking because it causes lung cancer and many other illnesses."
(B) "Why does an intelligent person like you continue to smoke?"
(C) "Do you have any relatives who died of lung cancer?"
(D) "I would like to show you a picture of what lungs look like after a lifetime of smoking."
(E) "Please tell me how I can help you to stop smoking"

**5.** A 50-year-old patient with diabetes tells his physician that he and his wife are having problems in bed. The physician's best response to the patient is to say

(A) "Do not worry; sexual problems are common in diabetes."
(B) "Please tell me what you mean by 'problems in bed.'"
(C) "I think that you and your wife should see a sex therapist."
(D) "I will give you a prescription for Viagra."
(E) "We need to do some laboratory tests to determine what is causing the problem."

**6.** A 50-year-old, poorly groomed woman has monthly appointments with a cardiologist. The patient, who frequently complains about the office and staff during these visits, tells the cardiologist that on this day, the office receptionist (who is well liked by patients and staff) was unfriendly to her. The physician's best response is to

**(A)** not comment and proceed with the examination

**(B)** apologize to the patient and offer to speak to the receptionist

**(C)** refer the patient for psychiatric evaluation

**(D)** ask the receptionist to reschedule the patient's appointment for another day

**(E)** tell the patient that everyone else likes the receptionist

**7.** A 45-year-old man, who was previously a successful businessman and devoted husband and father, now neglects his work and family. At his last visit he confided to the physician that he abuses alcohol. His wife tells the physician that his drinking is ruining the family. Which of the following is the most effective question for initiating a discussion with the patient about the effects of alcohol on his family?

**(A)** "Do you know that most patients who drink as much as you do eventually lose their families?"

**(B)** "Do you feel guilty about what your drinking is doing to your children?"

**(C)** "Do you realize the damage that your drinking is doing to your marriage?"

**(D)** "What do you think is the impact of your drinking on your family?"

**(E)** "Your wife says your drinking is ruining your family. Do you agree?"

**8.** In a hospital emergency room, a 43-year-old male patient shouts "I want a real doctor, not some jerk in training" and then throws his urine sample at the resident who is examining him. The first action the resident should take is to

**(A)** alert hospital security

**(B)** ask an attending physician to take over the case

**(C)** demand that the patient stop shouting and throwing things

**(D)** say to the patient "I see you are upset, what can I do?"

**(E)** ask the patient why he is upset

**(F)** ignore the behavior and continue to examine the patient

**9.** When a physician prescribed fluoxetine (Prozac) for a 35-year-old male patient, she explained the major side effects of the drug. Four months later, the patient asks her whether fluoxetine has any side effects. The physician's best response is to say

**(A)** "The side effects are nervousness, insomnia, and sexual dysfunction."

**(B)** "I will have the nurse go over the side effects with you again."

**(C)** "Please tell me about what you have been experiencing while taking Prozac."

**(D)** "Would you like me to check for possible side effects?"

**(E)** "The side effects are minor; do not worry."

**Questions 10 and 11**

A 38-year-old salesman, who previously had a myocardial infarction, comes to the physician's office for a routine visit. On seeing the physician, he angrily exclaims, "What is the matter with this place? I can never find a parking space around here and everyone is so disorganized!" He then insists on making a phone call while the physician waits to examine him.

**10.** Most appropriately, the physician should now say

**(A)** "I cannot examine you until you calm down."

**(B)** "Are you always this angry?"

**(C)** "You seem upset."

**(D)** "Would you like a referral to another physician?"

**(E)** "I will reschedule your appointment for another day."

**11.** The personality type that best describes this patient is

**(A)** histrionic

**(B)** schizoid

**(C)** obsessive–compulsive

**(D)** passive–aggressive

**(E)** dependent

**Questions 12 and 13**

A 28-year-old woman comes to a physician's office wearing a low-cut blouse. When the physician begins to interview her, the woman puts her hand on his arm and asks him if he is married.

**12.** The physician's most appropriate behavior at this time is to

(A) refuse to examine the patient at this time but give her another appointment

(B) call in a chaperone for the interview and examination

(C) use only open-ended questions in interviewing the patient

(D) refer the patient to a female physician

(E) ask the patient about her personal life

**13.** The personality type that best describes this patient is

(A) histrionic

(B) schizoid

(C) obsessive–compulsive

(D) passive–aggressive

(E) dependent

**14.** A 46-year-old man comes to the emergency department complaining of chest pain. Which of the following statements will elicit the most information from this patient?

(A) "Point to the area of pain in your chest."

(B) "Tell me about the pain in your chest."

(C) "Tell me about the pain."

(D) "Have you been to a physician within the past 6 months?"

(E) "Is there a history of heart disease in your family?"

**15.** A 50-year-old woman presents with a complaint of gastric distress. She seems agitated and says that she is afraid she has cirrhosis of the liver but then stops speaking. Which of the following will best encourage this patient to continue speaking?

(A) "Please go on."

(B) "How much liquor do you drink?"

(C) "Do you drink?"

(D) "Why did you wait so long to come in?"

(E) "There are many ways to treat alcoholism."

**16.** On the day he is to receive the results of a lung biopsy, a patient tells the physician that he feels fine. However, the physician notices that the patient is pale, sweaty, and shaky. Which of the following is the most appropriate statement for the physician to make?

(A) "Tell me again about the pain in your chest."

(B) "How do you feel?"

(C) "You'll be fine."

(D) "You look frightened."

(E) "Are you upset about being in the hospital?"

**17.** Patients are most likely to adhere to medical advice for which of the following reasons?

(A) The illness has few symptoms.

(B) The patient likes the physician.

(C) The physician is young.

(D) The illness is chronic.

(E) The management schedule is complex.

**18.** A 50-year-old African American male patient who is well educated has a herniated disc. The characteristic of this patient most likely to increase his adherence to the management plan is his

(A) race

(B) socioeconomic status

(C) back pain

(D) education

(E) gender

**19.** The "sick role" as described by Parsons

(A) applies mainly to low socioeconomic groups

(B) overvalues people's social support networks

(C) includes lack of cooperation with health care workers

(D) includes exemption from usual responsibilities

(E) applies mainly to chronic illness

**Questions 20 and 21**

A 34-year-old father of four children smokes two packs of cigarettes a day but believes that smoking does not cause him harm. Instead, he believes that smoking prevents him from getting colds.

**20.** To encourage this patient to smoke less, the physician should first

(A) recommend a smoking cessation support group
(B) recommend a nicotine patch
(C) show him photographs of the lungs of patients with lung cancer
(D) determine how willing he is to stop smoking
(E) tell him his children will be fatherless if he continues smoking

**21.** Although the patient has agreed to try to stop smoking, he has not made any progress in 2 months. The most appropriate thing for the physician to say at this time is

(A) "It can be really hard for people to stop smoking."
(B) "How much are you smoking now?"
(C) "Have you been following my instructions?"
(D) "I cannot help you if you do not listen to me."
(E) "I recommend that you start taking bupropion (Zyban)"

**22.** A patient whose father died of prostate cancer says that he cannot take a prostate-specific antigen test because "the needle will leave a mark." The most appropriate next step for the physician to take is to

(A) speak to the patient's wife and ask her to convince him to have the test
(B) reassure the patient that the needle mark will fade with time
(C) show the patient photographs of patients with untreated prostate cancer
(D) reassure the patient that whatever the outcome of the test, he can be cured
(E) ask the patient to describe his feelings about his father's illness

**23.** The parents of a critically ill 6-year-old patient tell the physician that when the child became ill, his 14-year-old brother started to behave badly in school and at home. At this time, the younger child's physician should

(A) refer the teenager to an adolescent psychologist
(B) ask to speak to the teenager alone as soon as possible
(C) ask to speak to the teenager when the younger child is out of danger
(D) tell the parents that the patient is the younger child, not the teenager
(E) tell the parents to concentrate on the younger child

**24.** During a follow-up visit after a mastectomy, a 39-year-old, well-groomed, married woman seems sad and tells her surgeon that she is embarrassed to undress in front of her husband. Most appropriately, the surgeon should now say

(A) "You should not be embarrassed, you still look good."
(B) "There are a number of breast reconstruction procedures that can improve your appearance."
(C) "The most important thing is not how you look, but that we caught the disease in time."
(D) "Please tell me how the surgery has affected your relationship with your husband."
(E) "It is not so bad, you still have one breast."

**25.** A 30-year-old woman visiting a physician for the first time sits silently in the waiting room with her fists clenched. When asked to by a nurse, she refuses to fill out a personal data form. In the examining room she says to the doctor, "Let's get this over with." The most appropriate statement for the physician to make at this time is

(A) "I cannot examine you until you fill out the personal data form."
(B) "Please tell me why you refused to fill out the personal data form."
(C) "You seem to be quite tense."
(D) "Are you frightened?"
(E) "Do not worry, I will take good care of you."

**26.** A lethargic, 19-month-old Mexican American boy with a temperature of 102°F is brought to the emergency room by his mother. The physician finds that the child is dehydrated. When the child refuses to drink water, the doctor offers the child a fruit flavored ice pop. When the child takes it, the mother becomes panicky and takes the ice pop away. She states that in her culture, one never gives food to a child with a fever. What is the physician's next step?

**(A)** Explain that the child needs rehydration and is more likely to eat an ice pop than drink water.

**(B)** Follow the mother's wishes and start an IV to replace fluids.

**(C)** Call in a consultant to convince the mother to allow the child to eat the ice pop.

**(D)** Explain to the mother that you are a licensed physician and know what is best for the child.

**(E)** Explain to the mother that the child can die of dehydration.

**(F)** Elicit a suggestion from the mother about how to best get fluids into the child that fits in with her beliefs.

**27.** A 38-year-old patient asks her primary care doctor, Dr. 1, for a referral because she is moving to a different city. Dr. 1 refers the patient to Dr. 2, an old medical school friend, in the new city. When the patient goes to Dr. 2, he notices that the patient seems depressed and anxious, so he refers her to Dr. 3, who is a psychiatrist. Dr. 3 will be out of town for a while so he refers the patient to Dr. 4. Dr. 4 has no time to see the patient so he refers her to Dr. 5. Ethically, which step in the referral sequence was least appropriate?

**(A)** Dr. 1 to Dr. 2

**(B)** Dr. 2 to Dr. 3

**(C)** Dr. 3 to Dr. 4

**(D)** Dr. 4 to Dr. 5

**28.** A 16-year-old girl has a chronic disorder that occasionally requires an opioid analgesic. She calls the physician when her prescription runs out 2 days prior to her final exams. She lives 2 hours away from the physician. The patient has access to a local medical clinic that renews the prescription when needed but she checked with them and they stated that their wait time for a visit is 3 days. The physician should

**(A)** call the pharmacy to refill the prescription

**(B)** recommend an over-the-counter medication to treat the pain

**(C)** call the medical clinic and request that they see the patient immediately

**(D)** ask a friend who practices near the patient to prescribe the drug

**(E)** drive to the patient's home with a ready prescription

**29.** A 39-year-old woman goes to her physician after discovering a breast mass during self-examination. Two months earlier, at her yearly physical, the same physician had told the patient that all findings were normal. The patient schedules a mammogram and, learning that the mass is suspicious for breast cancer, begins to wonder if the doctor missed finding the lump 2 months ago. This patient is most likely to file a malpractice suit against the physician if

**(A)** the biopsy indicates that she has breast cancer

**(B)** she believes that she can get a significant financial settlement from the doctor's insurance company

**(C)** she has poor communication with the doctor

**(D)** a family member insists that she sue the doctor

**(E)** she learns that the cancer has metastasized

# Answers and Explanations

**The answer is A.** Do not treat and determine if the parents are on the way. This patient apparently understands the risk of waiting but has elected to wait for his parents. Unless a patient is obviously incompetent because of current psychotic or suicidal thinking, or in imminent danger a doctor should follow the patient's wishes. Having a psychiatric illness, being in a psychiatric facility, or having paranoid thoughts does not make this patient incompetent to make health care decisions for himself (and see Chapter 23).

1. **The answer is A.** The physician should first play with the child to build rapport. After the child is more comfortable, the doctor can ask him direct (not open-ended) questions about the accident. Expressing sympathy or coercing the child to talk will be stressful as well as ineffective.

2. **The answer is D.** The physician should first ask to speak to the girl alone. The girl should not be questioned in front of her mother about her (the girl's) need for speaking privately with the physician. The physician does not have to follow the mother's wishes or ask the mother questions. The daughter is the patient. Referring the girl is not appropriate; the physician can deal with this situation.

3. **The answer is C.** While information about an illness is given directly to an adult patient, parents decide if, how, and when such information will be given to an ill child. In this situation, the physician should find out what the child knows about her illness by asking her what her parents have told her. False reassurance is as inappropriate for children as it is for adults.

4. **The answer is E.** The most effective statement or question the physician can use to help the patient stop smoking is, "Please tell me how I can help you to stop smoking." Trying to frighten the patient into adherence (e.g., telling him it will cause lung cancer, showing him pictures of lungs exposed to cigarette smoke, or asking about relatives who died of lung cancer) is less likely to be effective.

5. **The answer is B.** The physician's best response is to identify the specific problem by asking the patient what he means by "problems in bed." The patient's problem must be identified before testing, treatment, or reassurance is given.

6. **The answer is B.** The physician's best response is to apologize to the patient and offer to speak to the receptionist. The physician is responsible for dealing with illness-related emotional needs and problems of patients and should not blame the patient, no matter how unpleasant she is about problems interacting with the office staff. There is no reason to refer this patient for psychiatric evaluation.

7. **The answer is D.** The most effective question is the most open-ended one, for example, "What do you think is the impact of your drinking on your family?" Questions with implied judgment such as "Do you know most patients who drink as much as you do lose their families?", "Do you feel guilty about what you are doing to your children?", "Do you realize the damage that your use of alcohol is doing to your marriage?", or "Your wife says your drinking is ruining your family" can cause the patient to become defensive and/or angry and, as such, are not likely to be helpful.

8. **The answer is A.** Patients who throw things have lost their self-control and are therefore in danger. The most important thing for the resident to do in dealing with this angry patient is to ensure both her own and her patient's safety. Therefore she should immediately alert hospital security. Acknowledging the patient's anger or asking the patient why he is upset are steps that can be taken after everyone's safety, including that of the patient, is ensured. Demanding that an out-of-control patient stop shouting and throwing things is rarely effective.

9. **The answer is C.** The physician's best response is to say, "Please tell me about what you have been experiencing while taking Prozac," an open-ended question meant to encourage the patient to speak freely. It is likely that the patient is having sexual side effects, common with fluoxetine, and is uncomfortable about discussing them. It is not appropriate to just repeat the possible side effects, reassure the patient, or have the nurse do the physician's work by talking to the patient.

10. **The answer is C. 11. The answer is C.** Before examining this patient, the physician should acknowledge his anger by saying, "You seem upset." While directed at the physician via the parking problem, the patient's anger is more likely to be related to his anxiety about having a serious illness. Treating him in a childlike way (e.g., telling him that he cannot be examined until he calms down) will further anger him. The physician is responsible for dealing with illness-related emotional needs and problems of patients. There is no reason to refer this patient to another physician. The personality type that best describes this patient is obsessive–compulsive. Obsessive–compulsive patients fear loss of control and may in turn become controlling (e.g., having the physician wait while he makes a phone call) during illness (Table 21.1).

12. **The answer is B. 13. The answer is A.** The physician's most appropriate behavior is to call in a chaperone when dealing with this seductive patient. Refusing to treat her, asking about her personal life, or referring her to another physician are not appropriate. For seductive patients, closed-ended questions that limit responsiveness are often more appropriate than open-ended questions. The personality type that best describes this patient is histrionic. Histrionic patients are dramatic and, like this patient, may behave in a sexually inappropriate fashion during illness (Table 21.1).

14. **The answer is C.** The most open-ended of these questions, "Tell me about the pain," gives little structure to the patient and can therefore elicit the most information.

15. **The answer is A.** The interview technique known as facilitation is used by the interviewer to encourage the patient to elaborate on an answer. The phrase, "Please go on," is a facilitative statement.

16. **The answer is D.** The physician's statement, "You look frightened," demonstrates the interviewing technique of confrontation, which calls the patient's attention to the inconsistency in his response and his body language and helps him to express his fears.

17. **The answer is B.** Patients are most likely to adhere to medical advice because they like the physician. Adherence is also associated with symptomatic illnesses, older physicians, acute illnesses, and simple management schedules.

18. **The answer is C.** The fact that he is experiencing pain is most likely to increase this patient's adherence to the management plan. There is no clear association between adherence and race, socioeconomic status, education, or gender.

19. **The answer is D.** The "sick role" applies mainly to middle-class patients with acute physical illnesses. It includes the expectation of care by others, lack of responsibility for becoming ill, and exemption from one's usual responsibilities. It undervalues social support networks.

**20. The answer is D. 21. The answer is A.** In order to get this patient to smoke less, the physician should first determine how willing he is to stop smoking. A support group or medication such as bupropion is only useful for motivated patients. This patient is not motivated. In fact, he believes that smoking helps him avoid colds. Scaring patients about the consequences of their behavior is not appropriate or effective in gaining adherence. The best thing for the physician to say after the patient has tried but not succeeded at stopping smoking is a statement that acknowledges the difficulty of the task the patient faces. Thus, the interview technique of validation, for example, "It can be really hard for people to stop smoking," is the most appropriate statement to make at this time. Criticizing the patient's behavior or threatening to abandon the patient is not appropriate. A former smokers' support group can be a useful adjunct to the physician's program, but acknowledging the difficulty of the task is more important at this time.

**22. The answer is E.** The physician's most appropriate behavior with this patient who refuses a needed test is to determine the basis of his refusal—probably his feelings about his father's fatal illness. The reason he refuses to have the test probably has little to do with the mark it will leave. Telling him that he can be cured is patronizing, inappropriate, and possibly untrue. Speaking to his wife also is not appropriate; physicians should deal directly with patients whenever possible. Trying to frighten patients about the consequences of their behavior is not appropriate or effective in gaining adherence (see Table 23.1).

**23. The answer is B.** The younger child's physician should speak to the teenager alone as soon as possible to provide information and relieve his fears. This teenager is likely to be frightened about his sibling's illness and the changed behavior of his parents. Adolescents often "act out" when fearful or depressed (see Chapter 6) It is the physician's role to deal with problems in the 6-year-old patient's support system to reduce stress and thus help in recovery. There is usually no need to refer family members to mental health professionals. Waiting until the younger child is out of danger will needlessly prolong the older child's problem and further stress the family.

**24. The answer is D.** Before offering suggestions (e.g., "There are a number of breast reconstruction procedures that can improve your appearance") the physician should try to address a concern that many patients have after undergoing disfiguring surgery such as this, for example, embarrassment about undressing in front of her husband. The physician should also avoid falsely reassuring or patronizing statements such as, "You still look good," "You still have one breast," or "The most important thing is that we caught the disease in time."

**25. The answer is C.** The most appropriate statement for the physician to make at this time to this woman is to acknowledge what she seems to be feeling by saying, "You seem to be quite tense," since she seems more tense and angry than frightened. Asking her why she refused to fill out a personal data form or insisting that she do so is likely to make her more tense and angry. Falsely reassuring statements (see also question 24) such as "There is nothing to worry about" are patronizing as well as nonproductive.

**26. The answer is F.** If possible, a physician should try to work within a patient's cultural belief system. Thus, this physician's next step in dealing with this case involving a dehydrated toddler is to ask the mother to suggest a means of getting fluid into the child that fits in with her cultural belief system. Starting an IV is not necessary because the child seems ready to take the ice pop by mouth. Calling in a consultant, stating that you know what is best, or warning of the worst possible outcome will not foster adherence or a good physician–patient relationship.

27. **The answer is B.** The step in the referral sequence which was least appropriate is when Dr. 2 referred the patient to Dr. 3 because the patient seemed depressed and anxious. Doctor 2 should have carefully investigated the patient's behavioral symptoms before deciding on a course of action. A primary care physician is expected to address such behavioral symptoms and, because the patient is depressed, evaluate suicide risk. Referrals can be indicated when patients ask for a referral (e.g., if they are moving out of town), or if the physician will not be available (e.g., he or she has a full schedule).

28. **The answer is C.** The most appropriate action for the physician to take is to call the local medical clinic, explain the situation, and ask them to see the patient immediately. While it is not required that the physician drive to the patient's home, the patient must be evaluated by a physician before an opioid prescription is refilled. So, calling the pharmacy is not appropriate. Patients with pain severe enough to require opioids are unlikely to respond to over-the-counter pain medication.

29. **The answer is C.** This patient is most likely to file a malpractice suit if she has poor communication with the doctor. The severity of the illness, the possible financial rewards of a lawsuit, and pressure from family members to sue are unlikely to lead to a lawsuit when a patient likes the doctor.

**Typical Board Question**

Upon returning from a week long vacation in the Caribbean, a 25-year-old African-American woman with no history of psychiatric symptoms, seems agitated and anxious. When she tells her sister that a television newscaster is publically discussing her behavior, the sister brings her to the emergency department. The patient subsequently is admitted to the hospital with fever, fatigue, joint pain, and a butterfly-shaped rash across the bridge of her nose. Hematologic findings include mild anemia and presence of antinuclear antibodies (ANA). Of the following, the most likely explanation of the patient's behavioral symptoms is

**(A)** dissociative fugue
**(B)** generalized anxiety disorder
**(C)** brief psychotic disorder
**(D)** systemic lupus erythematosus (SLE)
**(E)** somatization disorder

*(See "Answers and Explanations" at end of chapter.)*

## I. STRESS AND HEALTH

A. **Psychological factors affecting health.** Psychological factors may initiate or exacerbate symptoms of medical disorders (**psychosomatic symptoms**) involving almost all body systems. These factors include
   1. **Poor health behavior** (e.g., smoking, failure to exercise).
   2. **Maladaptive personality style** (e.g., obsessive–compulsive personality) (see Chapter 21).
   3. **Chronic or acute life stress** caused by emotional (e.g., depression), social (e.g., divorce), or economic (e.g., job loss) difficulties.

B. **Mechanisms of the physiologic effects of stress**
   1. Acute or chronic life stress leads to **activation of the autonomic nervous system**, which in turn affects cardiovascular and respiratory systems.
   2. Stress also leads to **altered levels of neurotransmitters** (e.g., serotonin, norepinephrine), which result in changes in mood and behavior.
   3. Stress can increase the **release of adrenocorticotropic hormone** (ACTH), which leads to the release of cortisol, ultimately resulting in **depression of the immune system** as measured by decreased lymphocyte response to mitogens and antigens and impaired function of natural killer cells.

| table 22.1 | Magnitude of Stress Associated with Selected Life Events According to the Holmes and Rahe Social Readjustment Scale |
|---|---|
| **Relative Stressfulness** | **Life Event (Exact Point Value of Stressor)** |
| Very high | Death of a spouse (100) <br> Divorce (73) <br> Marital separation (65) <br> Death of a close family member (63) |
| High | Major personal loss of health because of illness or injury (53) <br> Marriage (50) <br> Job loss (47) <br> Retirement (45) <br> Major loss of health of a close family member (44) <br> Birth or adoption of a child (39) |
| Moderate | Assuming major debt (e.g., taking out a mortgage) (31) <br> Promotion or demotion at work (29) <br> Child leaving home (29) |
| Low | Changing residence (20) <br> Vacation (15) <br> Major holiday (12) |

C. **Stressful life events.** High levels of stress in a patient's life may be related to an **increased likelihood of medical** and **psychiatric illness**.
  1. The **Social Readjustment Rating Scale** by **Holmes and Rahe** (which also includes "positive" events like holidays) ranks the effects of life events (Table 22.1). Events with the highest scores require people to make the most social readjustment in their lives.
  2. The need for social readjustment is directly correlated with increased risk of medical and psychiatric illness; in studies by Holmes and Rahe, 80% of patients with a **score of 300 points** in a given year became ill during the next year.

D. **Other psychosomatic relationships**
  1. **Medical conditions** not uncommonly present with psychiatric symptoms.
     a. Conditions that present with **depression** or **anxiety** include **neurologic illnesses** (e.g., dementia), **neoplasms** (particularly pancreatic or other gastrointestinal cancers), **endocrine and enzyme disturbances** (e.g., hypothyroidism, diabetes) (see Chapter 5), and **viral illnesses** (e.g., AIDS) (see Table 12.4), blood abnormalities, hypoglycemia, and pheochromocytoma.
     b. Conditions that present with **personality changes** or **psychotic symptoms** include neurological illnesses (e.g., temporal lobe **epilepsy**), tertiary **syphilis**, Wilson disease, **acute intermittent porphyria** (see Chapter 5), connective tissue disorders (e.g., systemic **lupus erythematosus**), **Huntington** disease, AIDS (see later), Cushing disease, and multiple sclerosis.
  2. **Nonpsychotropic medications** can **produce psychiatric symptoms** such as confusion (e.g., antiasthmatics), anxiety and agitation (e.g., antiparkinson's agents), depression (e.g., antihypertensives), sedation (e.g., antihistamines), and psychotic symptoms (e.g., analgesics, antibiotics, antihistamines, steroid hormones).
  3. Medical conditions such as **diabetes** and medications such as antihypertensives also commonly produce **sexual symptoms** such as erectile dysfunction (see Chapter 19). These symptoms in turn can lead to depression or other psychiatric difficulties in patients.
  4. **Vitamin and mineral toxicity.** Although there is **little empirical evidence**, many Americans believe that vitamin and mineral supplements enhance cognitive and emotional functioning. Because of these beliefs, many Americans take excessive amounts of vitamins and minerals which leads to behavioral symptoms related to vitamin and mineral toxicity (Table 22.2) rather than to deficiency.

| table   22.2 | Selected Vitamins and Minerals: Neuropsychological Symptoms of Toxicity and Their Management | |
|---|---|---|
| **Vitamin or Mineral** | **Symptoms of Toxicity** | **Management of Toxicity** |
| Vitamin A | Increased intracranial pressure leading to headache, altered mental status, neurological deficits | Limit further use of supplements and foods containing Vitamin A |
| Vitamin $B_6$ (pyrixidine) | Depression, peripheral neuropathy | Limit further use of supplements and foods containing Vitamin $B_6$ |
| Vitamin $B_{12}$ (cobalamin) | Tingling and burning sensations in the extremities | Limit further use of supplements and foods containing Vitamin $B_{12}$ |
| Vitamin D (pyridoxine) | Confusion, apathy, poor appetite, thirst | IV hydration and corticosteroids or biophosphonate to reduce serum calcium levels |
| Iron (found in prenatal vitamins) | Confusion, seizures, sedation, vomiting "coffee grounds" | Give deferoxamine mesylate |
| Lead (found in some paints) | Depression, cognitive deficits, hyperactivity, aggression | Give ethylenediaminetetraacetic acid (EDTA) |
| Copper | Inappropriate or psychotic behavior | Give d-penicillamine |
| Zinc (found in denture creams) | Nerve damage leading to feelings of burning, numbness, and weakness | Give EDTA |

## II. PSYCHOLOGICAL STRESS IN SPECIFIC PATIENT POPULATIONS

### A. Overview

1. Not uncommonly, medical and surgical patients have concurrent psychological problems. These difficulties cause psychological stress, which can exacerbate the patient's physical disorder.
2. Usually, the treating physician handles these problems by helping to **organize the patient's social support systems** and by using specific psychotropic medications.
3. For severe psychiatric problems (e.g., psychotic symptoms) in hospitalized patients, **consultation–liaison (CL) psychiatrists** may be needed.

### B. Hospitalized patients

1. Common psychological complaints in hospitalized patients include anxiety, sleep disorders, and disorientation, often as a result of **delirium** (see Chapter 14) and **depression**.
2. Patients who are at the **greatest risk** for such problems include those undergoing surgery, or renal dialysis, or those being treated in the intensive care unit (**ICU**) or coronary care unit (**CCU**) (e.g., "ICU psychosis"); in all groups, **elderly patients** are at increased risk.
3. Patients undergoing surgery who are at greatest psychological and medical risk are those who **believe that they will not survive** surgery as well as those who **do not admit that they are worried** before surgery.
4. Psychological and medical risk can be reduced by **enhancing sensory** and **social input** (e.g., placing the patient's bed near a window, encouraging the patient to talk), providing information on what the patient can expect during and after a procedure, and allowing the patient to control the environment (e.g., lighting, pain medication) as much as possible.

### C. Patients undergoing renal dialysis

1. Patients on renal dialysis are at increased risk for psychological problems (e.g., depression, suicide, and sexual dysfunction) in part because their lives **depend on other people** and **on technology**.
2. Psychological and medical risk can be **reduced** through the use of **in-home dialysis units**, which cause less disruption of the patient's life.

**D. Patients with sensory deficits**
   1. Patients with sensory deficits such as **blindness** or **deafness** are also at increased psychological risk in part because they can become more easily disoriented when ill.
   2. Encouraging and accomodating such patients in the use of their support technology or strategy, for example, their seeing-eye dog, can increase a patient's sense of control and thus reduce his or her stress during illness.

## III. PATIENTS WITH CHRONIC PAIN

**A. Psychosocial factors**
   1. Chronic pain (pain lasting at least 6 months) is a **commonly encountered complaint** of patients. It may be associated with physical factors, psychological factors, or a combination of both.
      a. **Decreased tolerance for pain** is associated with depression, anxiety, and life stress in adulthood and physical and sexual abuse in childhood.
      b. **Pain tolerance** can be increased through biofeedback, physical therapy, hypnosis, psychotherapy, meditation, and relaxation training.
   2. Chronic pain often leads to a **loss of independence**, which can lead to depression. Practical suggestions for self-care in addition to pharmacologic management can be helpful for such patients.
   3. Depression may predispose a person to develop chronic pain. More commonly, **chronic pain results in depression**.
   4. People who experience pain after a procedure have a **higher risk of morbidity and mortality** and a **slower recovery** from the procedure.
   5. Religious, cultural, and ethnic factors may influence the patient's expression of pain and the responses of the **patient's support systems** to the pain (see Chapter 18).

**B. Managing pain**
   1. **Pain relief** in pain caused by physical illness is best achieved by **analgesics** (e.g., opioids), using **patient-controlled analgesia (PCA)**, or nerve-blocking surgical procedures.
   2. **Antidepressants**, particularly tricyclics, are useful in the management of pain.
      a. Antidepressants are most useful for patients with **arthritis, facial pain**, and **headache**.
      b. Their analgesic effect may be the result of **stimulation of efferent inhibitory pain pathways**.
      c. Although they have direct analgesic effects, antidepressants may also decrease pain indirectly by **improving mood symptoms**.
   3. According to the **gate control theory**, the perception of pain can be blocked by electric stimulation of large-diameter afferent nerves. Some patients are helped by this treatment.
   4. Patients with pain caused by physical illness also benefit from **behavioral, cognitive**, and **other psychological therapies** (see Chapter 17), by needing less pain medication, becoming more active, and showing increased attempts to return to a normal lifestyle.

**C. Programs of pain management**
   1. **Scheduled administration of an analgesic** before the patient requests it (e.g., every 3 hours) and PCA are more effective than medication administered when the patient requests it (on demand). Scheduled administration separates the experience of pain from the receipt of medication.
   2. Many **patients with chronic pain are undermedicated** because the physician fears that the patient will become addicted to opioids. However, most patients with chronic pain **easily discontinue the use of opioids** as the pain remits.
   3. Pain patients are at **higher risk for depression** than they are for drug addiction.

**D. Pain in children**
   1. Children feel pain and remember pain as much as adults do.
   2. Because children are afraid of injections, the most useful ways of administering pain medications to them are **orally** (e.g., a fentanyl "lollipop"), **transdermally** (e.g., a skin cream to prevent pain from injections or spinal taps), or, in older children and adolescents, via PCA.

## IV. PATIENTS WITH ACQUIRED IMMUNE DEFICIENCY SYNDROME

A. **Psychological stressors.** Acquired immune deficiency syndrome (**AIDS**) and HIV-positive patients must deal with particular psychological stressors not seen together in other disorders.
   1. These stressors include having a **fatal illness**, feeling **guilty** about how they contracted the illness (e.g., sex with multiple partners, intravenous drug use) and about possibly infecting others, and being met with **fear of contagion** from medical personnel, family, and friends.
   2. **HIV-positive** patients who have a **homosexual orientation** may be compelled (because of their illness) to "**come out**" (i.e., reveal their sexual orientation) to others.
   3. Medical and psychological **counseling** can reduce medical and psychological risk for HIV-positive patients.
   4. It is important to note that psychiatric symptoms such as depression or psychosis in AIDS patients may also result from **infection of the brain** with HIV or with an opportunistic infection such as cryptococcal meningitis (see Chapter 14) or cerebral lymphoma.

B. **Contagion**
   1. If they comply with accepted methods of infection control, **HIV-positive physicians do not risk transmitting the virus to their patients**.
   2. **Few health care workers** have contracted HIV from patients. The main risk of transmission is through accidental contamination from needles and other sharps although this risk is very low (see Table 19.6).
   3. Physicians can identify their HIV-positive patients to those they put at imminent risk (e.g., sexual partners) (see Chapter 23).

# Review Test

**Directions:** Each of the numbered items or incomplete statements in this section is followed by answers or by completions of the statement. Select the **one** lettered answer or completion that is **best** in each case.

**1.** A 45-year-old man has a routine yearly physical examination. While taking the history, the doctor determines that during the last year, the patient took out a substantial mortgage and moved to a new house. During the move, he fell and sustained a head injury which required hospitalization. While recuperating, he and his wife of 10 years went on a 2-week vacation. He recovered completely, but after the vacation, the couple separated. According to the Holmes and Rahe scale, which of these social experiences puts this man at the highest risk for physical illness in the next year?

**(A)** Experiencing marital separation
**(B)** Taking out a large mortgage
**(C)** Changing residence
**(D)** Sustaining a serious injury
**(E)** Going on vacation

**Questions 2 and 3**

A 35-year-old woman with a herniated disc has had back pain for the past 2 years. To help control her pain she takes an opioid-based medication daily.

**2.** Which of the following is most likely to be true about this patient?

**(A)** She is at high risk for drug addiction
**(B)** Psychological therapies will not benefit her
**(C)** Her expression of pain is related exclusively to the extent of her pain
**(D)** She is at high risk for depression
**(E)** She is receiving too much pain medication

**3.** Psychological stress engendered by this patient's pain is most likely to result in increased

**(A)** lymphocyte response to mitogens
**(B)** release of adrenocorticotropic hormone (ACTH)
**(C)** function of natural killer cells
**(D)** function of the immune system
**(E)** cortisol suppression

**4.** In the United States, the number of patients confirmed to have contracted HIV from their physicians is

**(A)** fewer than 50
**(B)** between 51 and 100
**(C)** between 101 and 200
**(D)** between 201 and 300
**(E)** more than 300

**Questions 5 and 6**

A 65-year-old male patient is scheduled for cardiac surgery. After the surgery he will be in the intensive care unit (ICU) for about 24 hours and will require a mechanical ventilator.

**5.** To reduce this patient's likelihood of psychological problems in the ICU, the physician should

**(A)** limit visits from his family
**(B)** reduce his exposure to ambient light
**(C)** explain the need for and function of the mechanical ventilator
**(D)** discourage communication between the patient and the staff
**(E)** have the nurses control the patient's lighting level

**6.** During his stay in the ICU after surgery, this patient is most likely to experience which of the following disorders?

**(A)** Panic disorder

**(B)** Obsessive–compulsive disorder

**(C)** Hypochondriasis

**(D)** Somatization disorder

**(E)** Delirium

**7.** A 25-year-old woman with no psychiatric history has a rapid heart rate and feelings of anxiety, which have been present for the past 3 months. The patient has lost 15 pounds and reports that she does not sleep well. Physical examination reveals exophthalmos (bulging eyes) and a neck mass. The most appropriate next step in the management of this patient is

**(A)** an antidepressant

**(B)** an antipsychotic

**(C)** a benzodiazepine

**(D)** psychotherapy

**(E)** a medical evaluation

**8.** A 65-year-old physician with no history of psychiatric problems reports that over the past 3 months he has been having difficulty sleeping through the night and has lost his appetite for food. He states that if he had been a better doctor, some of his patients would not have died, and he expresses guilt about not spending more time with his children when they were young. The patient also reports that he has lost 25 pounds since the previous year. The most appropriate next step in the management of this patient is

**(A)** an antidepressant

**(B)** an antipsychotic

**(C)** a benzodiazepine

**(D)** psychotherapy

**(E)** a medical evaluation

**9.** A 40-year-old woman comes to the doctor with the complaint that she is tired all the time. She also notes that her speaking voice is changing and seems lower than before. Thyroid function tests reveal increased thyroid-stimulating hormone (TSH), and decreased $T_3$ and free $T_4$. Physical examination reveals delayed relaxation phase of the muscle strength reflex and a bone scan reveals early evidence of osteoporosis. This patient is most likely to also show which of the following psychiatric symptoms?

**(A)** Hallucinations and delusions

**(B)** Depression

**(C)** Obsessions and compulsions

**(D)** Panic attacks

**(E)** Unexplained physical complaints

**10.** A 50-year-old patient who was diagnosed with diabetes the previous year tells the physician that he and wife are having problems in bed. The most appropriate next statement for the physician to make is

**(A)** "Sexual problems are common in diabetes."

**(B)** "I can recommend a sex therapist with special expertise in diabetes."

**(C)** "Please tell me about the problems you are having."

**(D)** "Patients with well-controlled diabetes have fewer sexual problems."

**(E)** "I can suggest forms of sexual expression which do not involve sexual intercourse."

**11.** A 30-year-old blind patient with a seeing-eye dog comes to a physician for the first time. When it is time for the patient to go into the examining room the physician should most appropriately

**(A)** allow the patient to be led into the examination room by the dog

**(B)** take the patient by the arm and lead her into the examining room with the dog following

**(C)** ask a member of the office staff to care for the dog during the examination

**(D)** tell the patient that the dog will have to stay in the waiting room during the examination for reasons of sanitation

**(E)** make another appointment for the patient when she can come in without the dog

**12.** A 45-year-old woman with rheumatoid arthritis calls her physician on a Monday morning because she cannot turn on the bathtub faucet because of the pain in her hands and wrists. She is tearful and says, "My husband has already left for work and my hands hurt too much to turn the water on. Now I can't even take a bath." Which of the following is the doctor's most appropriate response?

**(A)** "I sympathize with you. Unfortunately, it looks like your only option is to wait until your husband comes home."

**(B)** "People with rheumatoid arthritis often feel that their independence has been lost because of their pain. Perhaps using a tool like a wrench with a long handle will help."

**(C)** "Come to the office right away and I will give you a cortisone shot."

**(D)** "I know this must be difficult for you, perhaps you can call a plumber."

**(E)** "Many people with rheumatoid arthritis have difficulty turning faucets. Perhaps you would be interested in joining an arthritis support group."

**13.** After a 5-year-old child takes his mother's prenatal vitamins, he throws up material that looks like coffee grounds and then loses consciousness. In the emergency room the physician's next step in pharmacological management is to give this child

**(A)** d-penicillamine
**(B)** ethylenediaminetetraacetic acid (EDTA)
**(C)** biphosphonate
**(D)** deferoxamine mesylate
**(E)** flumazenil

# Answers and Explanations

## Typical Board Question

**The answer is D.** These signs (butterfly rash, fever), symptoms (fatigue, joint pain) and laboratory test results (mild anemia and presence of ANA) suggest that this patient has systemic lupus erythematosus (SLE), a connective tissue disorder. SLE is more common in African-American women of reproductive age and is exacerbated by exposure to the sun (such as this patient experienced on vacation). Personality changes and psychotic symptoms, such as the notion that people on television are referring to her (an idea of reference; see Table 11.1), also occur in connective tissue disorders such as SLE. Dissociative fugue, generalized anxiety disorder, brief psychotic disorder, and somatization disorder are not diagnosed when a medical illness explains the behavioral and physical symptoms.

1. **The answer is A.** According to the Holmes and Rahe scale, marital separation puts this man at the highest risk for physical illness this year. The events in this man's life in decreasing order of stressfulness are marital separation, serious head injury, large mortgage, changing residence, and going on vacation.

2. **The answer is D.** This chronic pain patient is at high risk for depression but at relatively low risk for drug addiction. Pain patients tend to be undermedicated; it is more likely that this patient is receiving too little rather than too much pain medication. Psychological therapies can be of significant benefit to chronic pain patients. This patient's expression of pain is related not only to the extent of her pain, but also to religious, cultural, and ethnic factors.

3. **The answer is B.** Psychological stress engendered by this patient's pain is likely to result in increased release of adrenocorticotropic hormone (ACTH) and cortisol. This, in turn, results in decreased function of the immune system as reflected in decreased lymphocyte response to mitogens and function of natural killer cells.

4. **The answer is A.** In the United States, no physician-to-patient transmission of HIV has been confirmed.

5. **The answer is C. 6. The answer is E.** To reduce this patient's likelihood of psychological problems in the intensive care unit (ICU), the physician should explain the need for and function of the mechanical ventilator and any other mechanical support that he will need. The physician should also encourage visits from family and communication between patient and staff. The patient should also be encouraged to control aspects of his environment
(e.g., lighting level). Outside stimuli (e.g., light) should be increased rather than decreased, for example, placing the patient's bed near a window. Because of the disorienting nature of the ICU, delirium is commonly seen in ICU patients. Panic disorder, obsessive–compulsive disorder, hypochondriasis, and somatization disorder are no more common in ICU patients than in the general population.

7. **The answer is E.** The most appropriate next step in the management of this anxious patient is a medical evaluation, particularly for thyroid function. She has symptoms of an overactive thyroid, including a neck mass (enlarged thyroid gland), exophthalmos (bulging eyes), and weight loss. People with thyroid hyperactivity may also present with anxiety (see Chapter 13) and insomnia. Psychotherapy, antidepressants, and benzodiazepines can manage the associated symptoms but do not address this patient's underlying physical condition.

8. **The answer is E.**  The most appropriate next step in the management of this depressed patient, who has no previous history of psychiatric illness, is a medical evaluation. This patient has symptoms of depression including sleep problems, inappropriate guilt, suicidal ideation, and significant weight loss. Because of his age and because pancreatic cancer and other gastrointestinal cancers not uncommonly present with depression, this patient should be evaluated for such conditions prior to treating his depression. As in question 7, psychotherapy, antidepressants, and benzodiazepines do not address this patient's underlying physical problem.

9. **The answer is B.**  Increased TSH, decreased $T_3$ and free $T_4$ as well as tiredness, coarsening of the voice, and osteoporosis indicate that this patient has hypothyroidism. Patients with hypothyroidism not uncommonly present with behavioral symptoms such as those seen in major depressive disorder. Anxiety symptoms such as those seen in panic disorder and OCD are more closely associated with hyperthyroidism. Somatization disorder is diagnosed when physical findings do not adequately explain the patient's symptoms. In this patient, the physical findings are significant.

10. **The answer is C.**  The most appropriate statement for the physician to make to this patient with diabetes is to first find out what he means by "problems in bed." Anticipating what the problems are and making reassuring statements or specific suggestions can wait until the doctor has all of the information.

11. **The answer is A.**  Patients who use a helper animal should be allowed to take the animal with them in as many situations as possible. Therefore, when it is time for this blind patient to go into the examining room the physician should allow the patient to be led into the examination room by her guide dog. Seeing-eye dogs are trained to take their masters to many places and are commonly allowed where pet animals are not, for example, public buildings and transportation. There is no reason to believe that the dog will increase the risk of infection for the patient.

12. **The answer is B.**  The doctor's most appropriate response to this patient with pain caused by rheumatoid arthritis is to recognize that she is upset because her independence has been lost. A practical suggestion such as using a long-handled tool is helpful. Telling her to wait until her husband comes home or calling a plumber can intensify her feelings of helplessness. Recommending an arthritis support group may be useful in the long term but will not help her with the current problem. A cortisone shot might or might not be helpful but is again not appropriate to deal with the immediate problem.

13. **The answer is D.**  Prenatal vitamins contain iron and this child has taken an iron overdose. The physician's next step in management of an iron overdose is to give deferoxamine mesylate. D-penicillamine, ethylenediaminetetraacetic acid (EDTA), biphosphonate, and flumazenil are used to manage overdoses of copper, lead, Vitamin D, and benzodiazepines, respectively.

# chapter 23

# Legal and Ethical Issues in Medicine

## Typical Board Question

A 30-year-old patient with Down syndrome who lives in an assisted living facility develops pneumonia and is successfully treated. The patient's mother, who rarely comes to visit the patient, leaves a voice message for the doctor asking for information about her daughter's condition. When the patient is informed about her mother's request, she asks that the doctor not give her mother any information. Most appropriately, the doctor should call the mother back and tell her that

  **(A)** he will give her the information that she has requested
  **(B)** he cannot reveal information about his patient to her
  **(C)** the daughter has asked that he not reveal such information to anyone
  **(D)** he will give her the information but requests that she not tell her daughter that he did so
  **(E)** the facility personnel will give her the information that she has requested at a later date

*(See "Answers and Explanations" at end of chapter.)*

## I. LEGAL COMPETENCE

**A. Definition**
  **1.** To be **legally competent** to make health care decisions, a patient must understand the **risks, benefits**, and likely outcome of such decisions.
  **2. All adults** (persons 18 years of age and older) are assumed to be legally competent to make health care decisions for themselves.

**B. Minors**
  **1. Minors** (persons younger than 18 years of age) usually are **not** considered legally competent.
  **2. Emancipated minors** are people under 18 years of age who are considered legally competent adults and can give consent for their own medical care.
  **3.** To be considered an emancipated minor an individual must meet at least one of the following criteria.
    **a.** Be **self-supporting**.
    **b.** Be in the **military**.
    **c.** Be **married**.
    **d.** Have **a child** for whom he or she cares.

**C. Questions of decision-making capacity and competence**
  **1.** If an adult's competence is in question (e.g., a person with mental retardation or dementia), physicians involved in the case can evaluate and testify to the **capacity** of the patient to make health care decisions. However, only **a judge** (with input from the patient's family or physicians) can make **the legal determination** of competence.

2. If a person is found to be **incompetent**, a **legal guardian** will be appointed by the court to make decisions for that person. The legal guardian may or may not be a family member.
3. A person **may meet the legal standard** for competence to accept or refuse medical management **even if she is mentally ill**, has mental retardation or is incompetent in other areas of her life (e.g., with finances).
4. **The Folstein Mini-Mental State Examination** (MMSE) (see Table 5.3) correlates to some extent with clinicians' evaluation of **capacity**. While a total score of 23 or higher suggests competence and a total score of 18 or lower suggests incompetence, the MMSE score alone cannot be used to make a determination of legal competence.

# II. INFORMED CONSENT

A. **Overview.** With the exception of life-threatening emergencies (e.g., when the time taken to obtain consent would further endanger the patient), a physician must inform and obtain consent (verbal or nonverbal) from a competent adult patient before proceeding with **any medical or surgical treatment**.
   1. Although a signature may not be required for minor medical procedures, patients usually sign a **document of consent** for major medical procedures or for surgery.
   2. **Other hospital personnel** (e.g., nurses) usually **cannot** obtain informed consent.

B. **Components of informed consent**
   1. Before patients can give consent to be treated by a physician, they must be informed of and understand the **health implications** of their diagnosis.
   2. Patients must also be informed of the **health risks and benefits** of treatment **and the alternatives** to treatment.
   3. Patients must know the likely **outcome if they do not consent** to the treatment.
   4. They must also be informed that they can **withdraw consent for treatment at any time** before the procedure.
   5. Physicians must also obtain informed consent before entering a patient in a **research study**. However, if a patient's condition worsens during the study as a result of lack of treatment, placebo treatment, or exposure to experimental treatment, the patient must be taken out of the study and given the standard treatment for his or her condition.

C. **Special situations**
   1. **Competent patients** have the **right to refuse to consent** to a needed test or procedure for religious or other reasons, even if their health will suffer or death will result from such refusal.
   2. Although medical or surgical intervention may be necessary to protect the health or life of the fetus, a **competent pregnant woman has the right to refuse** such intervention (e.g., cesarean section) even if the fetus will die or be seriously injured without the intervention.
   3. While all of the medical findings are generally provided to a patient, a physician can **delay** telling the patient the diagnosis if the physician believes that such knowledge will **adversely affect the patient's health** (e.g., a coronary patient), or until the patient indicates that he or she is ready to receive the news.
   4. The **opinions of family members**, while helpful for information about the patient's state of mind, cannot dictate what information the physician tells the patient. **At the patient's request**, family members may be present when the physician provides the diagnosis.

D. **Unexpected findings**
   1. If an **unexpected finding** during surgery necessitates a **nonemergency** procedure for which the patient has not given consent (e.g., biopsy of an unsuspected ovarian malignancy found during a tubal ligation), the patient must be given the opportunity to provide informed consent before the additional procedure can be performed.
   2. In an **emergency** in which it is impossible to obtain consent without further endangering the patient (e.g., a "hot" appendix is found during a tubal ligation), the procedure can be done without obtaining consent.

E. **Treatment of minors**
1. Only the **parent** or **legal guardian** can give consent for surgical or medical treatment of a minor.
2. Parental consent is **not required** in the treatment of minors in the following instances.
   a. **Emergency** situations (e.g., when the parent or guardian cannot be located and a delay in treatment can potentially harm the child).
   b. Treatment of sexually transmitted diseases (**STDs**).
   c. Prescription of **contraceptives**.
   d. Medical care during **pregnancy**.
   e. Treatment of **drug or alcohol dependence**.
3. Most states require parental notification or consent when a minor seeks an **abortion**.
4. **A court order** can be obtained from a judge (within hours if necessary) if a child has a life-threatening illness or accident and the **parent or guardian refuses to consent** to an established (but not an experimental) medical procedure for religious or other reasons.
5. Because the likelihood of a poor outcome is extremely high, **non-initiation of resuscitation after delivery** is usually appropriate for infants born **before the 23rd gestational** week, at birth weight **less than 400 g**, or with **anencephaly**, or **trisomy 13 or 18**.
6. Testing for **genetic disorders**
   a. If the disorder has a pediatric onset and preventive therapy or treatment is available (e.g., cystic fibrosis), genetic testing should be offered or even required.
   b. If there are **no preventive therapies** or treatments for the disorder and it has a **pediatric onset** (e.g., Tay–Sachs disease), **parents should have the discretion** as to whether or not to test the child.
   c. Because the child can make the decision to be tested or not when he or she is an adult, genetic testing should generally **not be done**
      (1) If the disorder has an **adult onset** and there are no preventative therapies (e.g., Huntington disease) or
      (2) To determine whether a prepubescent child is a **carrier of a genetic** disorder that will affect his or her offspring (e.g., fragile X syndrome).
   d. If genetic testing reveals information (e.g., **issues of paternity**) unrelated to the presence or absence of the genetic disorder, it is not necessary for the physician to divulge such information to anyone.

# III. CONFIDENTIALITY

A. Although physicians are **expected ethically to maintain patient confidentiality**, they are not required to do so if:
1. Their patient is suspected of **child or elder abuse**.
2. Their patient has a significant **risk of suicide**.
3. Their patient poses a serious **threat to another person**.
4. Their patient poses a **risk to public safety** (e.g., an impaired driver).

B. Intervention by the physician if the **patient poses a threat**.
1. The physician must first ascertain the **credibility** of the threat or danger.
2. If the threat or danger is credible, the physician must **notify** the appropriate law enforcement officials or social service agency and **warn** the intended victim (the Tarasoff decision).

# IV. REPORTABLE ILLNESSES

A. Most states require physicians to **report** certain infectious illnesses to their **state health departments** (reportable illnesses). State health departments report these illnesses to the federal Centers for Disease Control and Prevention (**CDC**) for statistical purposes.

B. Specific illnesses
   1. **"B A SSSMMART Clam or Chicken or you're Gone."** In most states hepatitis **B** and **A**, **S**almonellosis, **S**higellosis, **S**yphilis, **M**easles, **M**umps, **A**IDS, **R**ubella, **T**uberculosis, **C**hlamydia, **C**hickenpox, and **G**onorrhea are reportable.
   2. **STDs** that are reportable in most states include **AIDS**, HIV-positive status is not reportable in all states; genital herpes is not reportable in most states.
   3. Infection with **hepatitis A** is related to exposure to **infected feces** as a result of:
      a. **Poor access to clean drinking water.** Hepatitis A is less common in the United States, Canada, Western Europe, Australia, and Japan than in countries with poorer public sanitation such as Mexico and India.
      b. **Anal sexual contact.** Hepatitis A is more common in men who have unprotected anal sex with men.

# V. ETHICAL ISSUES INVOLVING HIV INFECTION

A. **HIV-positive doctors.** Physicians are **not required to inform** either patients or the medical establishment about another physician's HIV-positive status since, if the physician follows procedures for infection control, he or she does not pose a risk to patients (see Chapter 22).

B. **HIV-positive patients**
   1. Ethically and legally, a physician **cannot refuse** to treat HIV-positive patients because of fear of infection.
   2. **A pregnant patient** at high risk for HIV infection **cannot be tested or treated** for the virus (e.g., with zidovudine [AZT] and/or nevirapine [Viramune]) **against her will**, even if the fetus could be adversely affected by such refusal. After the child is born, however, the mother cannot refuse to allow the child to be tested and treated for the virus.
   3. If a **health care provider** is exposed to the body fluids of a patient who may potentially be infected with HIV (e.g., a nurse is stuck with a needle while obtaining blood from a patient whose HIV status is unknown), it is acceptable to **test the patient for HIV infection** even if the patient refuses to consent to the test.
   4. Physicians are **not required to maintain confidentiality** when an HIV-positive patient habitually puts an identified person at risk by engaging in unprotected sex (see section III.B above).

# VI. INVOLUNTARY AND VOLUNTARY PSYCHIATRIC HOSPITALIZATION

A. Under certain circumstances, patients in psychiatric **emergency situations** who will not or cannot agree to be hospitalized may be hospitalized against their will or without consent (involuntary hospitalization) with certification by **one or two physicians.** Such patients may be hospitalized for up to 90 days (depending on state law) before a court hearing.

B. Even if a psychiatric patient **chooses voluntarily to be hospitalized**, he or she may be required to wait 24–48 hours before being permitted to sign out against medical advice.

C. **Patients,** who are confined to mental health facilities, whether voluntarily or involuntarily, have the **right to receive treatment** and **to refuse treatment** (e.g., medication, electroconvulsive therapy). Patients who are actively psychotic or suicidal, however, generally cannot refuse treatment aimed at stabilizing their condition.

## VII. ADVANCE DIRECTIVES

A. **Overview**
   1. Advance directives are instructions given by patients **in anticipation of the need for a medical decision**. A durable power of attorney and a living will are examples of advance directives.
      a. A **durable power of attorney** is a directive in which a competent person **designates another person** (e.g., spouse, friend) as his or her legal representative (i.e., health care proxy) to make decisions about his or her health care when he or she can no longer do so.
      b. A **living will** is a written **document or oral statement** in which a competent person gives directions for his or her future health care if he or she becomes incompetent to make decisions when he or she needs care.
      c. The **most recent information** about the patient's wishes is the most relevant advance directive.
   2. Health care facilities that receive Medicare payments (most hospitals and nursing homes) **are required to ask patients** whether they have advance directives and, if necessary, help patients to write them. They must also inform patients of their **right to refuse** treatment or resuscitation.

B. **Persistent vegetative state (PVS)**. A person in a PVS may **appear to be awake with eyes open** but is not aware of others or of the environment and is not expected to ever recover brain function. Whether to maintain a PVS patient on life support is dependent upon his or her advance directives or on the decisions of surrogates.

C. **Surrogates**
   1. If an incompetent patient does not have an **advance directive**, people who know the patient, for example, family members (**surrogates**), must determine **what the patient would have done if he or she were competent** (the substituted judgment standard). The **personal wishes of surrogates are irrelevant** to the medical decision.
   2. The **priority order** in which family members make this determination is the **(1) spouse, (2) adult children, (3) parents, (4) siblings**, and, finally, **(5) other relatives**. If there is a conflict among family members at the same priority level and discussion among family members does not settle the issue, the ethics committee of the hospital may make the decision. For intractable disagreement, legal intervention (e.g., by a judge) may be necessary.
   3. Even if a health care proxy or surrogate has been making decisions for an incompetent patient, if the patient **regains function** (competence) even briefly or intermittently, he or she regains the right during those periods to make decisions about his or her health care.

## VIII. DEATH AND EUTHANASIA

A. **Legal standard of death**
   1. In the United States, the legal standard of death (when a person's heart is beating) is **irreversible cessation of all functions of the entire brain**, including the brain stem. This standard differs among states but commonly involves **absence of:**
      a. Response to external events or painful stimuli.
      b. Spontaneous respiration.
      c. Cephalic reflexes (e.g., pupillary, corneal, pharyngeal).
      d. Electrical potentials of cerebral origin over 2 mV from symmetrically placed electrodes more than 10 cm apart.
      e. Cerebral blood flow for more than 30 minutes.
   2. **Physicians certify** the **cause of death** (e.g., natural, suicide, accident) and sign the death certificate.
   3. If the patient is dead according to the legal standard, the physician is authorized to **remove life support**. A court order or relative's permission is not necessary.

**B. Organ donation**
1. A patient's **organs cannot be harvested after death** unless the patient (or parent if the patient is a minor) has signed a document (e.g., an organ donor card) or informed surrogates of his or her wish to donate.
2. A **minor** (but not an adult) **can be compelled to donate** tissue (e.g., bone marrow, skin) to a close relative if he or she
   a. Is the only appropriate source and
   b. Will not be harmed seriously by the donation.

**C. Euthanasia.** According to medical codes of ethics (e.g., those of the American Medical Association and medical specialty organizations), **euthanasia** (directly killing a patient for compassionate reasons) **is a criminal act** and is **never appropriate**.
1. **Physician-assisted suicide** (providing a means for a patient to commit suicide for compassionate reasons) is legal in only a few states, but is not generally an indictable offense in other states as long as the physician does not actually perform the killing (e.g., the patient injects himself).
2. There is **no ethical distinction** between **withholding** and **withdrawing** life-sustaining treatment.
   a. If requested by a competent patient, food, water, and medical care can be withheld from a patient who has **no reasonable prospect of recovery**.
   b. If a competent patient **requests removal of artificial life support** (e.g., ventilator support), it is **both legal and ethical** for a physician to comply with this request. Such an action by the physician is not considered euthanasia or assisted suicide.

## IX. MEDICAL MALPRACTICE

**A. Overview**
1. Medical malpractice occurs when harm comes to a patient as a result of the action or inaction of a physician. The elements of malpractice (**the 4 Ds**) are
   a. **Dereliction**, or negligence (i.e., deviation from normal standards of care), of a
   b. **Duty** (i.e., there is an established physician–patient relationship) that causes
   c. **Damages** (i.e., injury)
   d. **Directly** to the patient (i.e., the damages were caused by the negligence, not by another factor).
2. **Surgeons** (including obstetricians) and **anesthesiologists** are the specialists most likely to be sued for malpractice. Psychiatrists and family practitioners are the least likely to be sued.
3. Malpractice is a **tort**, or **civil wrong**, not a crime. A finding for the plaintiff (the patient) results in a financial award to the patient from the defendant physician or his or her insurance carrier, not a jail term or loss of license.
4. Recently, there has been an increase in the number of malpractice claims. This increase is mainly a result of a **breakdown** of the traditional **physician–patient relationship** because of:
   a. **Technological advances** in medicine, which reduce personal contact with the physician.
   b. **Limits on time for personal interaction** and physician autonomy, partly as a result of the growth of managed care.

**B. Damages.** The patient may be awarded compensatory damages only, or both compensatory and punitive damages.
1. **Compensatory damages** are given to **reimburse** the patient for medical bills or lost salary and to compensate the patient for pain and suffering.
2. **Punitive damages** are awarded to the patient to **punish the physician** and set an example for the medical community. Punitive damages are rare and are awarded only in cases of wanton carelessness or gross negligence (e.g., a drunk surgeon who cuts a vital nerve).

**C. Relationships with patients**
1. Sexual relationships with current or former patients are **inappropriate** and are **prohibited** by the ethical standards of most specialty boards.
2. Patients who claim that they had a sexual relationship with a physician may **file an ethics complaint or a medical malpractice complaint**, or both.

3. Physicians should **avoid treating family members, close friends, or employees** since personal feelings can interfere with professional objectivity, and familiarity may limit questions or physical examinations of a sensitive nature.
4. Physicians should **avoid accepting valuable gifts** (e.g., things that can be sold) from patients.

# X. IMPAIRED PHYSICIANS

A. **Causes** of impairment in physicians include:
   1. Drug or alcohol abuse.
   2. Physical or mental illness.
   3. Impairment in functioning associated with old age.

B. **Removing** an impaired colleague, medical student, or resident from contact with patients is an ethical requirement because patients must be protected and the impaired colleague must be helped. The legal requirement for reporting impaired colleagues varies among states.
   1. An **impaired medical student** should be reported to the **Dean** of the medical school or the Dean of students.
   2. An **impaired resident** or **attending physician** should be reported to the person directly in charge of him or her (e.g., the residency training director or the chief of the medical staff, respectively).
   3. **Impaired physicians** in private practice should be reported to the state licensing board or the impaired physicians program, usually run by physicians who are associated with the state medical society.
      Table 23.1 provides "**Do's**" and "**Do Not's**" for answering questions on the USMLE involving legal and ethical issues.

| table 23.1 Do's and Do Not's for Answering USMLE Ethical and Legal Questions | |
| --- | --- |
| **Do** | **Do Not** |
| **Do** tell patients the complete truth about their illness and prognosis in language they can understand | **Do not** cover up the truth about a patient's condition or explain the diagnosis and prognosis using medical terms that the patient does not understand |
| **Do** tell patients the truth about your qualifications (e.g., "I am a third-year medical student") | **Do not** cover up the true status of medical students or residents (e.g., "I am a member of the doctor's team") |
| **Do** speak to competent adult patients directly | **Do not** discuss issues concerning patients with their relatives (e.g., spouse, adult children) or anyone else (e.g., insurance companies) without the patients' permission |
| **Do** ask competent patients to consent to their own treatment | **Do not** ask a relative for consent to treat a patient unless the relative has durable power of attorney or is the legal guardian |
| **Do** encourage competent patients to make their own health care choices (i.e., be autonomous) | **Do not** make decisions about health care choices for patients; supply them with the information they need to make such decisions |
| **Do** take care of your patient yourself | **Do not** refer your patient (no matter how difficult or offensive) to another student, resident, or physician |
| **Do** spend time with your patient | **Do not** delegate your responsibilities (e.g., giving lengthy medical instructions to patients) to office staff (e.g., nurses) |
| **Do** make health care decisions based on what is best for the health of the patient | **Do not** limit health care based on expense in time or money |
| **Do** discuss all treatment options with patients, even if their insurance companies do not cover such options | **Do not** restrict information about uncovered treatment options (such insurance company-generated "gag clauses" are ethically unacceptable) |
| **Do** discuss with a pregnant patient the practical issues of having and caring for the child | **Do not** advise a patient to have an abortion (unless she is at medical risk) no matter what the age of the mother (e.g., teenage) or the condition of the fetus (e.g., Down syndrome) |
| **Do** encourage a pregnant minor to make her own decision about whether or not to have an abortion. At the same time, encourage discussion between the woman and her parents about the best course of action | **Do not** accede to the demand of the pregnant woman's parents to perform an abortion (even if the woman or her unborn child is mentally impaired) |
| **Do** provide medically needed analgesia to a terminally ill patient even if it coincidentally may shorten the patient's life | **Do not** administer an analgesic overdose with the purpose of shortening a terminally ill patient's life |

**Directions:** Each of the numbered items or incomplete statements in this section is followed by answers or by completions of the statement. Select the **one** lettered answer or completion that is **best** in each case.

**1.** A 73-year-old patient has been in the intensive care unit for 2 weeks after a stroke. The patient has had a flat line EEG for 24 hours, shows no corneal reflexes, and is on ventilator support. Hospital records note that at age 53 the patient stated that he wanted all measures taken to continue his life as long as possible. His son, with whom he lives, says his father would want life support only if he could live a normal life. His daughter, who lives in another state, wants everything done to continue life support. The physician tests the patient's brain stem reflexes, and after 48 hours life support is discontinued. This action by the doctor is justified because

(A) the son lived with the patient
(B) the son had expressed his father's wishes
(C) the son, daughter, and ethics committee of the hospital decided to stop life support
(D) the daughter did not live with the patient
(E) the physician declared the patient brain dead

**2.** A 19-year-old man who is HIV positive tells his physician that he is regularly having unprotected sex with his 18-year-old girlfriend. The girlfriend does not know the patient's HIV status and the patient refuses to tell her. The physician has notified state health authorities about the situation, but cannot confirm that the state has contacted the girlfriend. At this time the physician should

(A) inform the police about the patient's HIV status
(B) keep the information about the patient's HIV status confidential
(C) inform the girlfriend of the patient's HIV status
(D) inform the girlfriend's parents of the patient's HIV status
(E) advise the girlfriend not to have unprotected sex with the patient but do not tell her why

**3.** A 15-year-old patient who has contracted genital herpes consults her family physician. In addition to treating her infection, the physician should

(A) notify her parents
(B) notify her sexual partner
(C) get written permission from her parents
(D) counsel her on safe sex practices
(E) report the case to state health authorities

**4.** A clearly competent 50-year-old woman who has religious beliefs that preclude blood transfusion is scheduled for major surgery. Prior to the surgery, she states that the physician is not to give her a blood transfusion, although she may need it during surgery. If a transfusion becomes necessary during surgery, the physician should

(A) replace lost body fluids but not give the woman the transfusion
(B) get a court order to do the transfusion
(C) get permission from the woman's family to do the transfusion
(D) give the woman the transfusion but not tell her about it
(E) give the woman the transfusion and inform her of it when she recovers from the anesthetic

**5.** A 30-year-old man and his 10-year-old son are injured in a commuter train accident. Both of them need surgery within the next 12 hours. The father is clearly mentally competent but refuses the surgery, for religious reasons, for both himself and his son. The physician should

(A) get a court order for the surgery on the child but do not operate on the father
(B) get a court order for the surgery for both the father and child
(C) get permission for the surgery for both the father and child from the mother
(D) have the father moved to another hospital
(E) follow the father's wishes and do not operate on either the father or the child

**6.** A 60-year-old man has a suspicious mass biopsied. He is clearly mentally competent but has been very depressed over his wife's recent death. His daughter asks the physician not to tell the patient the diagnosis if the results show a malignancy because she fears that he will kill himself. If the mass proves to be malignant, the physician should

**(A)** follow the daughter's wishes and not tell the patient the diagnosis
**(B)** tell the patient the diagnosis immediately
**(C)** tell the patient not to worry and that he will be well cared for
**(D)** ask the patient when he would like to receive the diagnosis
**(E)** have the daughter tell the patient the diagnosis

**7.** A 10-year-old boy who was injured during gym class is brought to the emergency department. He has a severe laceration that requires immediate suturing. His parents are on vacation and cannot be located and an aunt is babysitting for the child. The most appropriate action for the physician to take at this time is to

**(A)** obtain consent from the aunt
**(B)** obtain consent from the gym teacher
**(C)** suture the laceration without obtaining consent
**(D)** keep the patient comfortable until the physician reaches the parents
**(E)** obtain consent from the child himself

**8.** On his surgery rotation, medical student X frequently smells alcohol on the breath of medical student Y. Medical student Y denies that he has been drinking. The most appropriate action for medical student X to take at this time is to

**(A)** ask medical student Y why he is drinking on the floor
**(B)** warn medical student Y that he will be reported if he continues to drink on the floor
**(C)** report medical student Y to the dean of students
**(D)** report medical student Y to the police
**(E)** ask that medical student Y be transferred to another rotation site

**9.** A surgeon to whom an internist has regularly referred patients tells the internist in confidence that he (the surgeon) is HIV positive. At the same time, the surgeon assures the internist that he always complies with accepted procedures for infection control. The most appropriate action for the internist to take at this time is to

**(A)** stop referring patients to the surgeon
**(B)** report the surgeon to the state health authorities
**(C)** report the surgeon to the hospital administration
**(D)** continue to refer patients to the surgeon
**(E)** continue to refer patients to the surgeon but first tell them about his HIV status

**10.** A 25-year-old man who is HIV positive comes to a physician's office for treatment of a skin lesion. Because she is afraid of infection, the physician refuses to treat him. This physician's refusal to treat the patient is best described as

**(A)** unethical and illegal
**(B)** ethical and legal
**(C)** unethical but legal
**(D)** ethical but illegal

**11.** A legally competent, terminally ill 70-year-old patient on life support asks her physician to turn off the machines and let her die. The physician follows the patient's wishes and discontinues life support. The physician's action is best described as

**(A)** unethical and illegal
**(B)** ethical and legal
**(C)** unethical but legal
**(D)** ethical but illegal

**12.** A legally competent 65-year-old man signs a document that states that he does not want any measures taken to prolong his life if he becomes mentally impaired. Five days later he has a stroke and requires life support. Extensive evaluation reveals that he will never fully recover consciousness but will instead remain in a vegetative state. The patient's wife urges the physician to keep her husband alive. The physician should

**(A)** get a court order to start life support
**(B)** follow the wishes of the wife and start life support
**(C)** carry out the patient's prior request and not start life support
**(D)** ask the patient's adult children for permission to start life support
**(E)** turn the case over to the ethics committee of the hospital

**13.** A married 17-year-old woman sustains brain damage after an unsuccessful suicide attempt. She is in a coma, shows no spontaneous respiration, and requires life support. Clinical examination and electroencephalogram reveal lack of response to external events or painful stimuli; absence of pupillary, corneal, or pharyngeal reflexes; and absence of electrical potentials of cerebral origin. The patient's father insists that the physician not withdraw life support. The most appropriate action for the physician to take at this time is to

**(A)** explain to the family that the patient is legally dead and withdraw life support
**(B)** continue life support until a family member authorizes its withdrawal
**(C)** get a court order to withdraw life support
**(D)** get the patient's husband to authorize withdrawal of life support
**(E)** get the patient's mother to authorize withdrawal of life support

**14.** A 55-year-old woman undergoes surgery to repair a torn knee ligament. After the surgery, she has partial paralysis of the affected leg and sues the surgeon for malpractice. The lawsuit will be successful if the patient can prove that

**(A)** the physician did not follow the usual standards of professional care
**(B)** the paralysis is permanent
**(C)** the physician was not board certified in orthopedic surgery
**(D)** her marriage is negatively affected by the paralysis
**(E)** she will lose a significant amount of time from work because of the paralysis

**15.** A 35-year-old man who has paranoid-type schizophrenia and lives in a subway station is brought to the emergency department. The best reason to hospitalize this patient against his will is if he

**(A)** is dirty and disheveled
**(B)** is malnourished
**(C)** has attempted to push a passenger onto the train tracks
**(D)** is hearing voices
**(E)** believes the FBI is listening to his conversations

**16.** Although she previously agreed to allow a medical student to attend the delivery, a 27-year-old woman, who is about to give birth, states that she does not want the medical student in the delivery room. The most appropriate action for the medical student to take at this time is to

**(A)** stay, but keep to a part of the room where the patient cannot see him
**(B)** tell the patient that she must let him stay because she is in a teaching hospital
**(C)** ask the attending physician for permission to stay
**(D)** inform the attending physician and then leave the delivery room
**(E)** remind the patient that she already gave permission for him to stay

**17.** A 58-year-old man is scheduled for open-heart surgery. The night before the surgery, the patient seems anxious and worried. When the surgeon obtains informed consent from the patient she should include

(A) the risks of the anesthesia only
(B) the risks of the surgery only
(C) the risks of both the surgery and anesthesia, omitting the risk of death
(D) the risks of both the surgery and anesthesia, including the risk of death
(E) none of the risks of the surgery or anesthesia

**18.** A 90-year-old patient who was recently transferred to a nursing home from the hospital experiences cardiac arrest and a physician is called. Although they believe that the patient signed a do not resuscitate (DNR) order, the staff cannot locate the patient's chart containing the advance directive. Most appropriately, the physician should now

(A) resuscitate the patient
(B) not resuscitate the patient
(C) ask the family if she should resuscitate the patient
(D) ask the nursing home staff if she should resuscitate the patient
(E) provide supportive management only

**19.** A clearly competent 25-year-old woman, who is 5-months pregnant, tells her obstetrician that over the past year she has been using illegal intravenous drugs and has had at least five different sexual partners. The physician explains the risk to her fetus if she is HIV positive and how prenatal treatment with an antiretroviral agent can reduce the risk. He then suggests that she be tested for the virus. The woman refuses to be tested. The most appropriate action for the physician to take at this time is to

(A) perform the HIV test on a blood sample obtained for another purpose
(B) give the patient a prescription for an antiretroviral agent
(C) refer the patient to another obstetrician
(D) note in the patient's chart that she has refused to be tested and continue caring for her
(E) get a court order to do the HIV test

**20.** A nurse, who works in a physician's office, asks her employer to become her primary care physician. The physician's best response is

(A) "I can be your primary care physician and I will start a chart for you."
(B) "I can be your primary care physician but only if I am not paid."
(C) "I cannot be your primary care physician because I am your employer."
(D) "I cannot be your primary care physician but I can treat you without starting a chart."
(E) "I cannot be your primary care physician but I can write prescriptions for you occasionally."

**21.** A competent 30-year-old patient who is 38 weeks pregnant refuses to have a cesarean delivery despite the fact that without the surgery the fetus will probably die. Both her physician and a consultation-liaison psychiatrist have failed to convince her to have the surgery. The most appropriate action for her physician to take at this time is to

(A) get permission from the patient's husband to do the surgery
(B) ask a judge to issue a court order to do the surgery
(C) tell the patient that she can be criminally prosecuted if the child dies
(D) deliver the child vaginally
(E) refer the patient to another physician

**22.** Which of the following patients is most likely to be infected with hepatitis A?

(A) A heterosexual Mexican man
(B) A homosexual Mexican man
(C) A heterosexual French man
(D) A homosexual French man
(E) A heterosexual Canadian man
(F) A homosexual Canadian man

**23.** A 62-year-old man who has been in a serious automobile accident is brought to the hospital. After the patient is stabilized, medical evaluation reveals that he will never recover consciousness but will instead remain in a vegetative state. A decision must be made about whether or not to continue life support. Prior to the accident, the patient was declared the legal guardian for his wife who has Alzheimer disease and lives in a nursing home. The patient's sister, with whom the patient lives, urges the physician to keep her brother alive at any cost. The patient's adult son tells the physician that his father would not want to be kept alive in a vegetative state. Most correctly, which of the following will make the decision regarding continuing life support for this patient?

**(A)** The hospital ethics committee
**(B)** The wife
**(C)** The son
**(D)** The physician
**(E)** The sister

**24.** At an evening going-away party a 40-year-old physician drinks 10 glasses of beer. The physician then gets a page to go to the hospital. Despite the fact that a colleague tells him not to go, the physician says, "I am fine," and leaves for the hospital. What is the most appropriate action for the colleague to take?

**(A)** Chase the physician and physically restrain him
**(B)** Immediately notify those in charge at the hospital that the physician is likely to be impaired
**(C)** Report the physician to the hospital ethics committee the next day
**(D)** Report the physician to the State Board of Medical Examiners as soon as possible
**(E)** Ask to speak to the physician alone as soon as possible

**25.** A physician determines that a 40-year-old patient with Down syndrome needs hepatic surgery within 72 hours. When the physician explains this to her, the patient points to her stomach and says, "Tummy hurt." At this time the physician should

**(A)** declare an emergency and operate immediately
**(B)** ask the patient's parents for permission to operate
**(C)** consider the patient competent and then operate
**(D)** get substituted judgment from the patient's parents and then operate
**(E)** determine whether the patient has the capacity to give consent

**26.** A surgeon is about to perform a cholecystectomy on an obese patient. After the anesthesia takes effect, the anesthesiologist laughs and says, "If she wasn't so fat she would not have gall bladder problems." At this time the surgeon should

**(A)** ask the anesthesiologist to leave and find a replacement
**(B)** leave and ask another surgeon to do the procedure
**(C)** scold the anesthesiologist for his lack of empathy
**(D)** carry out the operation and then report the incident to the ethics committee
**(E)** carry out the operation and then speak to the anesthesiologist alone

**27.** A pregnant woman and her husband ask their physician to do genetic testing to determine if the fetus she is carrying is at risk for cystic fibrosis. The test shows that the husband is not the child's biological father. With respect to the paternity finding the physician should

**(A)** tell only the mother
**(B)** tell only the husband
**(C)** tell both the mother and the husband
**(D)** write it in the chart but do not tell the couple
**(E)** neither write it in the chart nor tell the couple

**28.** Parents of a 10-year-old girl want to find out if she is a carrier of the fragile X gene. With respect to genetic testing of her carrier status, most appropriately the physician should advise the parents to have her tested

(A) when she reaches reproductive maturity and requests the test
(B) when she decides to get married
(C) when she decides to have children
(D) as soon as possible
(E) when she reaches reproductive maturity

**29.** Parents of a 9-year-old child with leukemia are offered a chance to enroll the child in a randomized study of a new experimental treatment developed by a respected pediatric oncologist. When the parents hear that the study is randomized, they refuse to have the child participate. At this time the child's physician should

(A) randomize the patient without the parents' permission
(B) offer the standard treatment only
(C) offer the experimental treatment only
(D) offer a combination of the standard and the experimental treatment
(E) refer the child to a different physician

**30.** An attending surgeon asks a first-year surgery resident to obtain informed consent from a patient for a surgical procedure. The resident knows little about the surgery or its risks and complications. At this time, the resident should

(A) obtain consent and answer any questions that he feels able to answer at this time
(B) obtain consent and tell the patient to talk to the attending surgeon later if she has any questions
(C) obtain consent and then research and answer the patient's questions at a later time
(D) ask the attending surgeon to get consent from the patient himself
(E) ask the nurse to get consent from the patient

**31.** A physician has just told a couple that their 3-year-old son has fragile X syndrome. The woman tells the doctor that her sister-in-law is currently pregnant but that she and her husband do not want to tell anyone in their family about their own child's diagnosis. Which of the following actions by the physician is most appropriate concerning informing the sister-in-law?

(A) Ask for a third party to mediate the communication between the couple and the sister-in-law
(B) Insist that the couple tell the pregnant woman
(C) Keep the diagnosis confidential
(D) Offer to contact the pregnant woman directly
(E) Recommend family counseling

**32.** A physician is treating a17-year-old patient with kidney failure. The doctor tells the patient's parents that, without a kidney transplant, she will die within 3–4 weeks. The only person whose kidney matches for a transplant is the patient's 18-year-old brother. However, when asked to donate his kidney, the brother gets very upset, crying and shouting and refuses to donate to his sister. The doctor's best course of action at this time is to

(A) tell the parents to put more pressure on the brother to donate
(B) prescribe an antianxiety agent for the brother and reapproach him the following week about donating his kidney
(C) apply for a court order to do the transplant
(D) accept the brother's decision and do not do the transplant
(E) reapproach the brother the following week and ask him if he has reconsidered

**33.** An 84-year-old man with cancer who is receiving chemotherapy and pain medication tells the doctor that he was told that death from cancer is very painful. He then asks the doctor if he can have extra pain medication if he needs it in the future. At this time the physician should

(A) tell the patient that it is unethical to prescribe high doses of pain medication
(B) ask the patient what else he was told
(C) assure the patient that his death will not be painful
(D) reassure the patient that he can have as much pain medication as he needs
(E) tell the patient that not all cancer patients experience extreme pain

**34.** A mildly mentally retarded 16-year-old girl, who is 16-weeks pregnant with a child who has Down syndrome, wants to keep the baby. She is healthy and the pregnancy is uncomplicated. Her parents want her to have an abortion. The most appropriate action for the physician to take at this time is to

(A) refer the family to an adoption agency
(B) facilitate discussion between the girl and her parents
(C) follow the parents' wishes and do the abortion
(D) refuse to do the abortion
(E) convince the parents to let the girl keep the child

# Answers and Explanations

**The answer is B.** Most appropriately, the doctor should tell the mother that he cannot reveal information about his patient to her. It is not appropriate to reveal information about an adult patient (even a mentally retarded person) to anyone without the patient's consent. The doctor should also not tell the mother that the patient has requested such confidentiality.

1. **The answer is E.** Discontinuing life support is justified in this case because the physician declared the patient brain dead. A court order, ethics committee decision, or relatives' permission is not necessary in the decision to remove life support when a patient is brain dead.

2. **The answer is C.** If the patient refuses to tell his girlfriend, the physician herself must notify public health authorities and, if they do not act on this information, in some jurisdictions, also inform the endangered partner. If the patient had agreed to tell his girlfriend about his HIV status, the physician should set up an appointment to see the patient and partner together to ensure that the patient discloses his HIV status to the partner. The usual standards of physician–patient confidentiality do not apply here since the patient's failure to use condoms poses a significant threat to his girlfriend's life (Tarasoff decision). If the patient is using condoms, the physician does not have to inform his partner of his HIV-positive status. However, even if he is using condoms, the physician should encourage the patient to disclose his medical condition to his sexual partner. Not all states require reporting of HIV-positive patients.

3. **The answer is D.** In addition to treating the patient the physician should counsel her on safe sexual practices. There is no need to break physician–patient confidentiality by telling the sexual partner, since genital herpes is not life threatening. Parental consent is not required for treating minors in cases of sexually transmitted disease, pregnancy, and substance abuse. Genital herpes is not generally reportable to state health authorities.

4. **The answer is A.** The physician can use means to replace lost body fluids but should not give the patient a blood transfusion. Legally competent patients may refuse treatment even if death will result. Getting a court order or obtaining permission from the woman's family to do the transfusion is not appropriate or ethical. Failing to tell a patient the truth (e.g., giving the woman the transfusion but not telling her about it), or going against a competent patient's expressed wishes (e.g., informing her of the transfusion when she recovers from the anesthetic), is never appropriate.

5. **The answer is A.** As noted above, a patient (e.g., the father) who is legally competent can refuse lifesaving treatment for himself for religious or other reasons, even if death will be the outcome. However, a parent (or guardian) cannot refuse lifesaving treatment for his child for any reason. When there is time (here, 12 hr), a court order should be obtained before treatment is started. In an emergency, the physician can proceed without a court order.

6. **The answer is D.** Since there is some question here about the patient's emotional state, asking him when he would like to receive the diagnosis is the best choice. Only the physician (not a family member) should tell the patient the results of a medical test. If the physician believes that the patient's health will be adversely affected by the news of a malignancy, he or she can delay telling the patient the diagnosis until he or she is ready to receive the biopsy report. The opinions of family members may be helpful to inform the physician about the patient's state of mind, but the determination of whether and when to inform the patient must be made by the physician.

7. **The answer is C.** Only the parent or legal guardian can give consent for surgical or medical treatment of a minor. In an emergency such as this, if the parent or guardian cannot be located, treatment may proceed without consent. The babysitting aunt and gym teacher have no legal standing to make health care decisions for this child. Waiting to act until the parents are reached could be harmful to the child.

8. **The answer is C.** The most appropriate action for medical student X to take is to report medical student Y to the Dean of students. Reporting of an impaired colleague is required ethically because patients must be protected and the impaired colleague must be helped. Even if medical student X asks Y why he is drinking or warns Y about his drinking, there is no guarantee that Y will listen and that the patients will be protected. Reporting Y to the police is not appropriate.

9. **The answer is D.** The most appropriate action for the internist to take is to continue to refer patients to the surgeon without mentioning his HIV status, provided that the surgeon is physically and mentally competent to treat patients and that he complies with standard precautions for infection control. Physician-to-patient transmission of HIV has never been confirmed in the United States. Physicians are not required to inform either patients or the medical establishment about a colleague's HIV-positive status.

10. **The answer is A.** It is legal for a physician to refuse to treat a patient for a number of reasons (e.g., the physician has no room in his or her practice). However, a federal appeals court has ruled recently that it is illegal under the Americans with Disabilities Act for a health care worker to refuse to treat a patient with HIV due to fear of transmission. It is also unethical for a physician to refuse to manage a patient with a communicable disease.

11. **The answer is B.** If a competent patient requests cessation of artificial life support, it is both legal and ethical for a physician to comply with this request.

12. **The answer is C.** In this case, the physician should carry out the patient's request and not provide life support. This decision is based on the patient's prior instructions as put forth in his living will. The wife's or adult children's wishes are not relevant to this decision. Under these circumstances, the patient's wishes are clear, and there is no need to approach the court or the ethics committee of the hospital.

13. **The answer is A.** The most appropriate action for the physician to take is to withdraw life support. If a patient is legally dead (brain dead), the physician is authorized to remove life support without a court order or consent from family (and see question 1).

14. **The answer is A.** The lawsuit will be successful if the patient can prove that the physician did not follow the usual standards of professional care. An unfavorable outcome alone (e.g., paralysis of the leg as an unavoidable complication of the surgical procedure) or negative effects on functioning because of the injury do not constitute malpractice. Licensed physicians are legally permitted to perform any medical or surgical procedure; they do not have to be boarded in a specialty.

15. **The answer is C.** The best reason that this patient can be hospitalized involuntarily is if he poses a significant danger to himself or to others. Trying to push a passenger onto the tracks is such a danger. Self-neglect (e.g., poor grooming, malnutrition) or psychotic symptoms (e.g., hearing voices or having delusions—see Chapter 11) can also be grounds for

involuntary hospitalization when they constitute a significant, imminent danger to this patient's life or to others.

16. **The answer is D.** The most appropriate action for the medical student to take when a patient asks him to leave the delivery room is to follow the patient's wishes. Thus, the student should inform the attending physician and then leave. Asking the resident for permission or arguing with the patient (e.g., telling her that she must let him stay because it is a teaching hospital or because she already agreed) are not appropriate. Patients can refuse to have trainees of any kind present at any time and for any reason.

17. **The answer is D.** The surgeon should explain the risks of complications from both the surgery and anesthesia, including the risk of death. Although patients scheduled for major surgery are often worried, they have the right to be informed of all risks before giving consent for a procedure.

18. **The answer is A.** In the absence of other instructions (e.g., a DNR), the physician must resuscitate the patient. Asking the family or nursing home staff what action to take is not appropriate.

19. **The answer is D.** The most appropriate action for the physician to take is to note in the patient's chart that she has refused to be tested and continue to care for her. Although providing zidovudine (AZT) and/or nevirapine (Viramune) to an HIV-positive woman during pregnancy can significantly reduce the danger of HIV transmission to the unborn child (see Table 19.6), a pregnant woman has the right to refuse medical tests or treatment even if the fetus will die or be seriously injured as a result. After the child is born, the mother cannot refuse to have it tested or treated for HIV.

20. **The answer is C.** The physician's best response is, "I cannot be your primary physician because I am your employer." Except in emergency situations, physicians should not manage the care of family members, close friends, or employees since personal feelings can interfere with medical decision making. Also, such patients are likely to be uncomfortable answering questions concerning sensitive information, or having intimate physical examinations when needed. Physicians should not treat patients without keeping appropriate records nor should they write prescriptions for individuals other than patients.

21. **The answer is D.** The most appropriate action for the physician to take is to deliver the child vaginally. Competent pregnant women, like all competent adults, can refuse medical treatment, even if the fetus will die as a result. Neither the patient's husband (even if he is the father) nor the court has the right to alter this decision. Trying to frighten the patient by telling her that she can be criminally prosecuted if the child dies or referring her to another physician are not appropriate actions (see also answer to Question 19).

22. **The answer is B.** Hepatitis A is related both to poor water quality and to oral–anal contact. Thus, a Mexican man with a homosexual orientation (who engages in oral–anal sex) is most likely to be infected with this virus.

23. **The answer is C.** The priority order in which family members make this determination is the (1) spouse, (2) adult children, (3) parents, (4) siblings, and (5) other relatives. The fact that the spouse has a legal guardian indicates that she has been declared incompetent. Therefore, the son makes the decision. The hospital ethics committee may be called in if there is a difference between family members at the same priority level (not necessary in this case).

24. **The answer is B.** This impaired physician is a potential danger to patients. Thus, the colleague should immediately notify those in charge at the hospital that the physician is likely to be impaired. Reporting him or speaking to him the next day will not protect patients he is likely to see that evening. Also, it may not be possible for the colleague to physically stop the physician from seeing patients.

25. **The answer is E.** It is not clear whether or not this patient with Down syndrome understands enough about her condition to give informed consent. However, since there is time to make this determination the situation is not emergent. Therefore, the physician should evaluate the patient's capacity with input from consultants.

26. **The answer is E.** Most appropriately, the surgeon should carry out the operation and then speak to the anesthesiologist alone about his insensitive behavior. The ethics committee does not have to be notified if the patient is not endangered and if the anesthesiologist's behavior improves in the future. Asking the anesthesiologist to leave or another surgeon to take over can prolong the procedure and endanger the anesthetized patient. It would not be helpful or professional to scold the other doctor in a public venue.

27. **The answer is E.** With respect to the paternity finding the physician should neither write it in the chart nor tell the couple. According to the American Medical Association Code of Medical Ethics, it is not appropriate for physicians to divulge information obtained serendipitously in the course of genetic testing and unrelated to the purpose of the testing.

28. **The answer is A.** Most appropriately, this girl's parents should be advised not to test the girl for the fragile X gene until she is reproductively mature and requests the test for herself. According to the American Medical Association Code of Medical Ethics, "Genetic testing for carrier status should be deferred until either the child reaches maturity, or the child needs to make reproductive decisions."

29. **The answer is B.** The child's physician should offer the standard treatment only. Parents can refuse experimental treatment of their child for any reason.

30. **The answer is D.** The first-year resident should ask the attending surgeon to get consent from the patient himself. Consent cannot be obtained until the patient has been informed and understands the health implications of her diagnoses, health risks and benefits of treatment, the alternatives to treatment, likely outcome if she does not consent to the treatment, and that she can withdraw consent for treatment at any time. It is not appropriate for the resident (or the nurse) to get consent since he cannot provide the patient with this information at the time that consent is obtained.

31. **The answer is C.** Keep the diagnosis confidential as the parents have requested. This information does not pose a threat to the sister-in-law so the physician is not compelled to reveal the diagnosis.

32. **The answer is E.** The doctor's best course of action at this time is to reapproach the brother the following week and ask him if he has reconsidered. People may be frightened at first by the prospect of organ donation, but may come around in time. The antianxiety agent will not increase the chance that he will comply. Ultimately however, it may be necessary to accept the brother's decision not to donate. Since he is an adult, the brother cannot be compelled to donate by either his parents or the court. Putting more pressure on him is unlikely to change his mind at this time.

33. **The answer is B.** The physician should first ask the patient what else he was told. The doctor can then address all of the patient's concerns about his illness and its management.

34. **The answer is B.** The most appropriate action for the physician to take at this time is to facilitate discussion between the girl and her parents concerning their disagreement. Because the pregnancy is not threatening her life or health, the parents cannot force the girl to have an abortion. However, helping the family to come to an agreement on this issue is a better choice than simply refusing to do the abortion, or recommending adoption.

# chapter 24

# Health Care in the United States

**Typical Board Question**

Parents bring their 8-year-old son in for a school physical. The parents relate that the child is doing well in school. They also tell the doctor that after school they drive their son to soccer practice, and on weekends they all go swimming in the county pool. The child also likes to ride his bicycle around the neighborhood. The parents also reveal that, while they are trying to cut back, both of them smoke cigarettes in the home. In order to protect the child's life and health, what is the most important suggestion the physician can give the parents?

(A) Stop smoking to reduce the child's exposure to secondhand smoke
(B) Put smoke alarms in the home
(C) Have the child wear a helmet while bicycling
(D) Learn cardiopulmonary resuscitation
(E) Ensure that the child wears a seat belt in the car

*(See "Answers and Explanations" at end of chapter.)*

## I. HEALTH CARE DELIVERY SYSTEMS

A. **Hospitals**
   1. According to the American Hospital Association, the United States has close to 6,000 hospitals with about 1,000,000 beds. Currently, at least one-third of hospital beds (especially in city hospitals) are unoccupied.
   2. The average length of a **hospital stay is 4.8 days**, and has been steadily decreasing. Types of hospitals and their ownership are listed in Table 24.1.

B. **Nursing homes** and other health care facilities
   1. In 2011, there were about 15,500 **nursing homes** with a capacity of 1.6 million beds in the United States. In the **elderly, falls leading to broken bones** (e.g., hip fracture) commonly lead to the need for nursing home care (see Chapter 3).
   2. Rehabilitation centers, visiting nurses associations, and hospices provide alternatives to hospital and nursing home care (Table 24.2).

C. **Physicians**
   1. Currently, there are about **130 accredited allopathic medical schools** and **26 accredited schools of osteopathic medicine** in the United States, annually graduating over 16,000 medical doctors (**MDs**) and 3,600 doctors of osteopathy (**DOs**).
      a. Due to the increasing need for physicians, the number of schools and the number of students enrolled in these schools are increasing. At least 15 institutions have notified

| table **24.1** | Types of Hospitals in the United States | |
|---|---|---|
| Type | Number | Category Includes |
| Community hospitals<br>• Nongovernment not-for-profit<br>• Investor-owned (for-profit)<br>• State and local government | Total = 5,008<br>2,919<br>998<br>1,092 | Nonfederal and short-term general and other special hospitals (e.g., obstetrics and gynecology; rehabilitation, orthopedic), and academic medical centers or other teaching hospitals accessible to the general public |
| Federal government hospitals | 211 | Veterans administration (VA) and military hospitals that are federally owned and reserved for individuals who have served (veterans) or are currently serving in the military |
| Nonfederal psychiatric hospitals (often owned and operated by state governments) | 444 | Hospitals for chronically mentally ill patients |
| Nonfederal long-term care hospitals | 117 | Hospitals for chronically physically ill patients |

From American Hospital Association. *Hospital Statistics.* Chicago, IL: American Hospital Association; 2011.

the Liaison Committee on Medical Education (**LCME**) of their intention to start new medical schools.

   **b.** Both MDs and DOs are correctly called "physicians." There are currently about **950,000 physicians** in the United States.

   **c.** Training and practice are essentially the same for DOs as for MDs; however, the philosophy of osteopathic medicine stresses the **interrelatedness of body systems** and the use of **musculoskeletal manipulation** in the diagnosis and treatment of physical illness.

   **d.** Overall, physicians earn an average income of **$200,000 annually**. Psychiatrists, pediatricians, and family practitioners typically earn less than this average figure and surgeons typically earn more.

**2. Primary care** physicians, including family practitioners, internists, and pediatricians, provide initial care to patients and account for at least one-third of all physicians. This number is increasing and soon is expected to make up one-half of all physicians.

**3.** The **ratio of physicians to patients** is higher in the northeastern states and in California than in the southern and mountain states.

**4.** People in the United States average **fewer yearly visits** to physicians than people in developed countries with systems of government-funded medical care.

**5.** Seventy-five percent of people visit physicians in a given year. In all age groups, the two **most common medical conditions** for which treatment is sought are **upper respiratory ailments** and **injuries**.

| table **24.2** | Other Health Care Facilities | |
|---|---|---|
| Type of Care or Facility | Services Provided | Comments |
| Residential assisted living facility, intermediate care facility and nursing home (i.e., skilled care) facility | Long-term care<br>Room and board<br>Assistance with self-care<br>Nursing care | Average costs range from about $36,000/yr (residential assisted living facility) to at least $75,000/yr (skilled care facility), depending on geographical area |
| Rehabilitation centers and halfway house | Short-term care<br>Room and board | Goal is to help hospitalized patients reenter society |
| Visiting nurse association | Nursing care, physical and occupational therapy, and social work services<br>Care given in a patient's own home | Funded by Medicare<br>Serves as a less expensive alternative to hospitalization or nursing home placement |
| Hospice organization | Supportive care to terminally ill patients (i.e., those expected to live, <6 mos)<br>Care usually given in a patient's own home | Funded by Medicare<br>Goal is to allow patients to die at home to be with their families and preserve their dignity<br>Pain medication is used liberally |

| table **24.3** Health Care Expenses and Payment | |
| --- | --- |
| **Origin of Health Care Expenses (in Decreasing Order of Magnitude)** | **Sources of Payment for Health Care Expenses (in Decreasing Order of Magnitude)** |
| Hospitals | Private health insurance (36%) |
| Physicians' fees | Federal government (34%) |
| Nursing homes | State and local governments (11%) |
| Medications and medical supplies | Individuals (15%) |
| Mental health services | |
| Dental and other care | |

## II. COSTS OF HEALTH CARE

**A. Health care expenditures**

1. Health care expenditures in the United States make up **more than 14% of the total economy, more than in any other industrialized society**.
2. Health care expenditures have increased because of the **increasing age** of the population, advances in medical technology, and the availability of health care to the poor and elderly through Medicaid and Medicare, respectively (see section III.E.).

**B. Allocation of health care funds.** The origins of health care expenses and the sources of payment for health care are listed in Table 24.3.

## III. PAYMENT FOR HEALTH CARE: HEALTH INSURANCE

**A. Overview**

1. The United States is one of the few industrialized countries that do not have publicly mandated health care insurance coverage funded by the government for all citizens. This is one reason that the **United States** has **higher infant mortality** rates (see Figure 1.1) and **lower life expectancies** than most other developed countries.
2. Most Americans must obtain **health insurance** through their employers or on their own.
   **a.** Typically, the employer and the employee share the cost of health insurance.
   **b.** In 2007, health insurance costs averaged $12,100 per year for a family of four and have been increasing.
   **c.** About 15% of Americans have **no health insurance**, while many others are "**underinsured.**" Such people must pay all or part of the costs of health care themselves. Fifty percent of **bankruptcy** filings are related to the inability to pay medical expenses.
3. More than 40 million Americans **cannot afford adequate health care** and go without prescription drugs, eyeglasses, or dental treatment.
4. Certain citizens have government-funded health care insurance through **Medicaid** and **Medicare** (see section III.E.).
5. No matter what the insurance, the **privacy of health information** (e.g., insurance claims, referral authorization requests) that is held or transmitted in any form (e.g., paper, electronic) is legally protected by the **Health Insurance Portability and Accountability Act (HIPAA)** implemented by The Standards for Privacy of Individually Identifiable Health Information (i.e., Privacy Rule).

**B. Private health insurers**

1. **Blue Cross/Blue Shield (BC/BS)**, a nonprofit private insurance carrier, is regulated by insurance agencies in each state.

    **a.** BC/BS pays for hospital costs (Blue Cross) and physician fees and diagnostic tests (Blue Shield) for up to half of the working people in the United States.

    **b.** Almost half of BC/BS subscribers are enrolled in some type of managed care plan.

  **2.** Individuals can also contract with one of at least 1,000 other private insurance carriers, such as **Aetna** or **Prudential**.

**C.  Fee-for-service care versus managed care**

  **1.** Whichever the insurance carrier, patients usually can choose between a traditional fee-for-service indemnity plan and at least one type of managed care plan.

    **a.** A traditional **fee-for-service** indemnity plan has no restrictions on provider choice or referrals. It also commonly has higher premiums.

    **b.** A **managed care** plan has restrictions on provider choice and referrals and lower premiums.

  **2.** Many insurance plans have a **deductible** (i.e., the amount the patient must pay out of pocket before the insurance company begins to cover expenses), a **co-payment** (i.e., a percentage, typically 20%, of the total bill that the patient must pay), or both.

**D.  Managed care**

  **1. Managed care** describes a health care delivery system in which all aspects of an individual's health care are coordinated or managed by a group of providers to enhance cost effectiveness.

  **2.** Although cost is controlled in managed care, **patients are restricted** in their choice of a physician. Thus, while the number of managed care plans is increasing, **managed care is more popular with the government** than with the public.

  **3.** Because fewer patient visits result in lower costs, the philosophy of managed care stresses **primary, secondary**, and **tertiary prevention** (Table 24.4) rather than acute treatment.

  **4.** Types of managed care plans including health maintenance organizations (**HMOs**), preferred provider organizations (**PPOs**), and point of service (**POS**) plans are described in Table 24.5.

**E.  Federal- and state-funded insurance coverage**

  **1. Medicare and Medicaid** are government-funded programs that provide medical insurance to certain groups of people. Medicare Part D (added in 2006) covers some, but not all, prescription drug costs. Eligibility requirements and coverage provided by these programs are outlined in Table 24.6.

  **2. Diagnosis-related groups (DRGs)** are used by Medicare and Medicaid to pay hospital bills. The amount paid is based on an estimate of the cost of hospitalization for each diagnosis rather than the actual charges incurred.

**t a b l e    24.4**    Primary, Secondary, and Tertiary Prevention in Health Care

| Type of Prevention | Goal | Examples |
|---|---|---|
| Primary | To reduce the incidence of a disorder by reducing its associated risk factors | Immunization of infants to prevent infectious illnesses<br>Improved obstetrical care to avoid premature birth and its associated problems |
| Secondary | To reduce the prevalence of an existing disorder by decreasing its severity | Early identification and management of otitis media in children to prevent hearing loss<br>Mammography for the early identification and management of breast cancer |
| Tertiary | To reduce the prevalence of problems caused by an existing disorder | Physical therapy for stroke patients so that they can care for themselves<br>Occupational training for mentally retarded persons so that they can gain the skills needed to join the work force |

| table **24.5** Managed Care Plans | | |
|---|---|---|
| **Type of Plan** | **Definition** | **Comments** |
| HMO (staff model or closed panel) | Physicians and other health care personnel are paid a salary to provide medical services to a group of people who are enrolled voluntarily and who pay an annual premium<br>HMOs may operate their own hospitals and clinics<br>Services include hospitalization, physician services; preventive medicine services; and often dental, eye, and podiatric care | These plans are the most restrictive for the patient in terms of choice of doctor<br>Patient is assigned a "gatekeeper" (a primary care doctor from within the network who decides if and when a patient needs to see a specialist) |
| HMO (independent practice association [IPA] model) | Physicians in private practice are hired by an HMO to provide services to HMO patients<br>About 65% of HMOs have IPA Components | Private practice physicians receive a fee, or capitation, for each HMO patient they are responsible for |
| Preferred provider organization (PPO) | A third-party payer (e.g.. a union trust fund, insurance company, or corporation) contracts with physicians in private practice and with hospitals to provide medical care to its subscribers<br>Participants choose physicians from a list of member practitioners (the network)<br>Physicians in the network receive capitation for each patient | These plans guarantee doctors in private practice a certain volume of patients<br>By paying a larger share of the cost, patients can choose a doctor who is not in the network<br>There is no "gatekeeper" physician |
| Point of service plan (POS) | Variant of a PPO in which a third-party payer contracts with physicians in private practice to provide medical care to its subscribers<br>Physicians in the network receive capitation for each patient | As with a PPO, patients can choose a doctor who is not in the network by paying an extra fee<br>As with an HMO, there is a "gatekeeper" physician |

# IV. DEMOGRAPHICS OF HEALTH IN THE UNITED STATES

## A. Lifestyle, habits, and attitudes

1. Lifestyle and poor dietary and other habits, particularly smoking and drinking alcohol, are responsible for much **physical and mental illness**.

2. **Social attitudes** involving health care issues also affect health care delivery. For example, although organ transplants can save many lives, fewer transplant procedures are done than are needed. This is due largely to the fact that not enough people are willing to donate their organs at death.

| table **24.6** Medicare and Medicaid | | |
|---|---|---|
| **Source of Funding** | **Eligibility** | **Coverage** |
| ***Medicare*** | | |
| The federal government (through the Social Security system) | People eligible for Social Security benefits (e.g., those older than 65 yrs of age regardless of income)<br>People of any age with chronic disabilities or debilitating illnesses<br>Covers about 35 million people | Part A: Inpatient hospital care, home health care, medically necessary nursing home care (for up to 90 days after hospitalization), hospice care<br>Part B: Physician fees, dialysis, physical therapy, laboratory tests, ambulance service, medical equipment (Part B is optional and has a 20% co-payment and a $100 deductible)<br>Part D: Is optional and covers a share of prescription drug costs<br>Medicare does not cover long-term nursing home care |
| ***Medicaid (MediCal in California)*** | | |
| Both federal and state governments (the state contribution is determined by average per capita income of the state) | Indigent (very low income) people<br>One-third of all funds is allocated for nursing home care for indigent elderly people<br>Covers about 25 million people | Inpatient and outpatient hospital care<br>Physician services<br>Home health care, e.g., hospice care, laboratory tests, dialysis, ambulance service, medical equipment<br>Prescription drugs<br>Long-term nursing home care<br>Dental care, eyeglasses, hearing aids<br>No co-payment or deductible |

B. **Socioeconomic status (SES) and health**
   1. SES, which is determined by **occupation and educational level** as well as place of residence and income, is directly associated with mental and physical health.
   2. Approximately 85% of people with low SES are African American or Latino (see Chapter 18).
      a. **High-income patients** are more likely to seek treatment and to visit private doctor's offices than are low-income patients.
      b. **Low-income patients** are more likely to seek treatment in hospital emergency departments and to **delay** seeking treatment, in part because of the cost. Illnesses often become more severe when patients delay seeking treatment.
   3. Hospitals are legally required to provide care to anyone needing emergency management whether they have the means to pay or not via the Emergency Medical Treatment and Active Labor Act (**EMTALA**).

C. **Gender and health**
   1. **Women are more likely to seek medical treatment** than men.
   2. **Men** have shorter life expectancies and are more likely to have heart disease than women.
   3. While they have less heart disease overall, **women** are more likely than men to **die during their first heart attack** or to die during the year after a heart attack.
   4. Women are also at higher risk than men for developing:
      a. Autoimmune diseases (e.g., rheumatoid arthritis)
      b. Multiple sclerosis
      c. Alcohol- and smoking-related illnesses
      d. AIDS (when they are already HIV positive and have the same viral load as a man)
      e. Cataracts
      f. Thyroid disease

D. **Age and health**
   1. Children and the elderly are more likely to require medical care than people of other ages.
   2. The **elderly** comprise about 12% of the population, but currently incur over **30% of all health care costs**; this figure is expected to rise to 50% by the year 2020.
   3. The leading causes of death differ by age group (Table 24.7).

**table 24.7** Leading Causes of Death by Age Group (Across Sex and Ethnic Group)

| Age Group | Causes of Death (in Decreasing Order of Frequency) |
|---|---|
| Infants (<1 yr of age) | Congenital anomalies<br>Sudden infant death syndrome (SIDS)<br>Prematurity/low birth weight |
| Children (1–4 yrs of age) | Accidents (in motor vehicles and in the home)<br>Congenital anomalies<br>Cancer (primarily leukemia and central nervous system [CNS] malignancies) |
| Children (5–14 yrs of age) | Accidents (most in motor vehicles)<br>Cancer (primarily leukemia and CNS malignancies)<br>Homicide and legal intervention |
| Adolescents and young adults (15–24 yrs of age) | Accidents (most in motor vehicles)<br>Homicide and legal intervention<br>Suicide |
| Adults (25–44 yrs of age) | Accidents (most in motor vehicles)<br>AIDS<br>Cancer |
| Adults (45–64 yrs of age) | Cancer<br>Heart disease<br>Stroke and other cerebrovascular diseases |
| Elderly (65 yrs of age and over) | Heart disease<br>Cancer<br>Stroke and other cerebrovascular diseases |
| All ages combined | Heart disease<br>Cancer (lung, breast/prostate, and colorectal, in decreasing order)<br>Stroke and other cerebrovascular diseases |

# Review Test

**Directions:** Each of the numbered items or incomplete statements in this section is followed by answers or by completions of the statement. Select the **one** lettered answer or completion that is **best** in each case.

**1.** A 79-year-old woman who lives in her own home and is in good health has just been diagnosed with osteoporosis. To help prevent fractures, the physician should first recommend that this patient

(A) initiate safety measures in (i.e., safe-proof) the home
(B) take calcium supplements
(C) take alendronate sodium (Fosamax)
(D) begin a regular exercise program
(E) increase dairy products in the diet
(F) apply for admission to an assisted living facility

## Questions 2 and 3

A 45-year-old stockbroker with three children must choose a health insurance plan at work.

**2.** In which of the following plans will she have the most choice in choosing a physician?

(A) A health maintenance organization (HMO)
(B) A preferred provider organization (PPO)
(C) A point of service (POS) plan
(D) A fee-for-service plan

**3.** In which of the following plans will she have the least choice in choosing a physician?

(A) A health maintenance organization (HMO)
(B) A preferred provider organization (PPO)
(C) A point of service (POS) plan
(D) A fee-for-service plan

**4.** Of the following patients, the one likely to use the least Medicare services and funds during his or her lifetime is a(n)

(A) African-American man
(B) African-American woman
(C) white man
(D) white woman
(E) Latino man

## Questions 5 and 6

A first-year resident who has recently started working in a hospital emergency department sees four patients during his first hour on the service.

**5.** Which of these patients is likely to be healthiest when first seen by the resident?

(A) A 45-year-old man from a low socioeconomic group
(B) A 45-year-old woman from a low socioeconomic group
(C) A 45-year-old man from a high socioeconomic group
(D) A 45-year-old woman from a high socioeconomic group

**6.** Which of these patients is likely to be the most ill when first seen by the resident?

(A) A 45-year-old man from a low socioeconomic group
(B) A 45-year-old woman from a low socioeconomic group
(C) A 45-year-old man from a high socioeconomic group
(D) A 45-year-old woman from a high socioeconomic group

**7.** In the United States, the percentage of the gross domestic product spent on health care is currently about

(A) 1%
(B) 8%
(C) 14%
(D) 30%
(E) 50%

**8.** In the United States, the largest percentage of personal health care expenses is paid by which of the following sources?

**(A)** The federal government
**(B)** State governments
**(C)** Municipal governments
**(D)** Private health insurance
**(E)** Personal funds

**9.** In the United States, the largest percentage of health care expenditures is for

**(A)** physician fees
**(B)** nursing home care
**(C)** medications
**(D)** hospital care
**(E)** mental health services

**10.** A mother brings her 2-month-old daughter to the physician for a checkup. In the United States, the most common cause of death in infants between birth and 1 year of age is

**(A)** leukemia
**(B)** sudden infant death syndrome (SIDS)
**(C)** congenital anomalies
**(D)** accidents
**(E)** respiratory distress syndrome

**Questions 11 and 12**

A 70-year-old female patient is hospitalized for a fractured hip. The patient, who has $100,000 in savings, was brought to the hospital by ambulance. She stayed in the hospital for 5 days and, when released, required physical therapy and a walker for help with mobility for the next 6 weeks.

**11.** This patient can expect that Medicare Part A will cover which of the following costs related to this injury?

**(A)** Inpatient hospital care
**(B)** The walker
**(C)** Ambulance service
**(D)** Physician bills
**(E)** Physical therapy

**12.** After 6 months at home, it is determined that this patient is unable to care for herself and requires care in a residential nursing home facility, probably for the rest of her life. Which of the following will pay for the first few years of this care?

**(A)** Medicare Part A
**(B)** Medicare Part B
**(C)** Blue Cross
**(D)** Blue Shield
**(E)** The patient's savings

**13.** Which of the following are the three leading causes of death in the United States in order of magnitude (higher to lower)?

**(A)** AIDS, heart disease, cancer
**(B)** Heart disease, cancer, stroke
**(C)** Cancer, heart disease, AIDS
**(D)** Heart disease, cancer, AIDS
**(E)** Stroke, heart disease, cancer

**14.** In women in the United States, which is the most common cause of cancer death?

**(A)** Cervical cancer
**(B)** Colorectal cancer
**(C)** Breast cancer
**(D)** Lung cancer
**(E)** Uterine cancer

**15.** Most patients in the United States can expect to receive care in which of the following types of hospital?

**(A)** Federal government
**(B)** Nongovernment not-for-profit
**(C)** Investor-owned
**(D)** Local government
**(E)** State government

**16.** An educational program is developed to teach mentally ill adults skills necessary to help them get and keep paying jobs. This program is an example of

**(A)** primary prevention
**(B)** secondary prevention
**(C)** tertiary prevention
**(D)** managed care

**17.** Parents bring their 2-year-old child to a well-child clinic. In order to protect the child's life and health, the most important suggestion the physician can make is to tell the parents to

**(A)** keep ipecac in the medicine cabinet
**(B)** put smoke alarms in the home
**(C)** initiate safety measures in (i.e., safeproof) the home
**(D)** learn cardiopulmonary resuscitation
**(E)** have the child immunized against measles, mumps, and rubella

# Answers and Explanations

## Typical Board Question

**The answer is E.** While house fires, bicycling accidents and drowning cause accidental death in children, failure to wear seat belts is the major cause of accidental death in children 4–14 years of age. While it has been associated with increased childhood upper respiratory symptoms, secondhand smoke has not been shown to significantly affect survival in children.

1. **The answer is A.** The most important recommendation for the physician to make at this time to prevent fractures in this woman with osteoporosis is to safe-proof the home environment to reduce the likelihood of falls (e.g., remove scatter rugs, install shower grab bars) (see Chapter 3). Calcium supplements, medications such as alendronate sodium (Fosamax), exercise, and increasing dairy products in the diet are all important for prophylaxis in osteoporosis; none will help prevent fractures in the short term. Since this patient does well living on her own, there is no reason for her to move to an assisted living facility.

2. **The answer is D. 3. The answer is A.** Patients have the most choice in choosing a physician in a traditional fee-for-service indemnity plan. In this type of plan there are no restrictions on provider choice or referrals. Managed care plans (e.g., health maintenance organizations [HMOs], preferred provider organizations [PPOs], and point of service [POS] plans) have restrictions on physician choice. Patients have the least choice in choosing a physician in an HMO. HMOs are the most restrictive of managed care plans for the patient in terms of choice of physician. Rather than choosing a physician from the network as in a PPO or POS, in an HMO the patient is assigned a physician.

4. **The answer is A.** Medicare pays for health care services for persons 65 years of age and older and others who are eligible to receive Social Security benefits. These benefits continue for the life of the individual. Because statistically he is likely to have a shorter life than a white or Latino man, an African-American woman, or a white woman, an African-American man is likely to use the least Medicare services over the course of his lifetime (see Table 3.1).

5. **The answer is D. 6. The answer is A.** A woman from a high socioeconomic group is likely to be healthiest when the resident first sees her. Women and people from higher socioeconomic groups are more likely to seek treatment and therefore to be less ill when first seen by a physician than men and people from low socioeconomic groups. A man from a low socioeconomic group is likely to be most ill when the resident first sees him. Low-income patients and male patients are more likely to delay seeking treatment. Delay in seeking treatment commonly results in more severe illness.

7. **The answer is C.** The percentage of the gross domestic product (GDP) spent on health care is about 14%, a percentage that is larger than that of any other developed country.

8. **The answer is D.** The largest percentage of personal health care expenses is paid by private health insurance. In decreasing order, other sources of payment for health care expenses are the federal government, state governments, and personal funds. Municipal governments pay a relatively small percentage of these expenses.

9. **The answer is D.** In the United States, most health care expenditures are for hospital care. In decreasing order, other sources of health care expenses are physician fees, nursing home care, medications, mental health services, and dental services.

10. **The answer is C.** The most common cause of death in infants up to 1 year of age is congenital anomalies. Sudden infant death syndrome (SIDS) and prematurity/low birth weight are the second and third leading causes of death in this age group.

11. **The answer is A. 12. The answer is E.** Medicare Part A will cover inpatient hospital costs. Part B covers ambulance services, physician fees, medical equipment (the walker), and therapy. The patient herself is responsible for long-term residential nursing home facility costs since neither Part A or Part B of Medicare nor Blue Cross/Blue Shield will cover such costs. After the patient's $100,000 is exhausted (probably within 1.5 years at about $75,000 per year), she will be indigent and therefore eligible for Medicaid. Medicaid pays for residential nursing home care and all other health care for indigent people.

13. **The answer is B.** The leading cause of death in the United States is heart disease, followed by cancer and stroke.

14. **The answer is D.** In women, as in men, the most common cause of cancer death in the United States is cancer of the lung. In women, this is followed by breast cancer and colorectal cancer. The number of women getting lung cancer is increasing with increased smoking rates in women.

15. **The answer is B.** More patients in the United States receive care in nongovernment, not-for-profit hospitals than in federal, state, local-government, or investor-owned hospitals.

16. **The answer is C.** This educational program for adults with mental illness is an example of tertiary prevention. Tertiary prevention is aimed at reducing the prevalence of problems caused by an existing disorder, mental illness in this case. Primary prevention is aimed at reducing the occurrence or incidence of a disorder by reducing its associated risk factors (e.g., immunization against measles). Secondary prevention is aimed at reducing the prevalence of an existing disorder by reducing its severity (e.g., early identification and management of breast cancer using mammography). Managed care is a system of health care in which all aspects of health care are coordinated by providers to control costs.

17. **The answer is C.** While accidental poisoning, house fires, and drowning are causes of death in children, in children 1–4 years of age, accidents in the home are a more important cause of accidental death. Infectious illness due to lack of immunization is not a common cause of death in American children (see also the TBQ).

### Typical Board Question

A new laboratory test to detect osteoporosis in women >80 years of age has a sensitivity of 90% and a specificity of 75%. Autopsy studies suggest that osteoporosis has a prevalence of 30% for women in this age group. Using this information, the likelihood that a woman with a positive test actually has osteoporosis is best estimated as

    **(A)** 12.5%
    **(B)** 30%
    **(C)** 60%
    **(D)** 70%
    **(E)** 85%

*(See "Answers and Explanations" at end of chapter.)*

## I.  MEDICAL EPIDEMIOLOGY: INCIDENCE AND PREVALENCE

Medical epidemiology is the study of the factors affecting the occurrence and distribution of diseases in human populations.

**A.** **Incidence. Incidence rate** is a ratio of the number of individuals in the population who **develop an illness** in a given time period (commonly 1 year) divided by the total number of individuals at risk for the illness during that time period (e.g., the number of IV drug abusers newly diagnosed with AIDS in 2013 divided by the number of IV drug abusers in the population during 2013).

**B.** **Prevalence. Prevalence rate** is a ratio of the number of individuals in the population who **have an illness** (e.g., AIDS) divided by the total number of individuals at risk for the illness.
    **1.** **Point prevalence** is a ratio of the number of individuals who have an illness at a specific **point in time** (e.g., the number of people who have AIDS on August 31, 2013, divided by the total population who could have the illness on that date).
    **2.** **Period prevalence** is a ratio of the number of individuals who have an illness during a specific **time period** (e.g., the number of people who have AIDS in 2013 divided by the total population who could have the illness mid-year in 2013).

**C.** **Relationship between incidence and prevalence**
    **1.** Prevalence rate is equal to incidence rate multiplied by the average **duration** of the disease process (if incidence and duration are stable).

2. Prevalence rate is greater than incidence rate if the disease is long term. For example, because diabetes lasts a lifetime, its prevalence is much higher than its incidence. In contrast, the prevalence of influenza, an acute illness, is approximately equal to the incidence.
3. Health interventions that prevent disease (i.e., **primary prevention**, see Chapter 24) decrease the incidence rate of an illness and ultimately its prevalence rate as well.
4. People with a specific illness can leave the population of prevalent cases either **by recovering or by dying**.

## II. RESEARCH STUDY DESIGN

Research studies identify relationships between factors or variables. Types of research studies include cohort, case-control, and cross-sectional studies.

A. **Cohort studies**
 1. Cohort studies begin with the identification of specific populations (cohorts), who are **free of the illness** under investigation at the start of the study.
 2. Following assessment of exposure to a **risk factor** (a variable linked to the cause of an illness [e.g., smoking]), incidence rates of illness between exposed and unexposed members of a cohort are compared. An example of a cohort study would be one that followed healthy adults from early adulthood through middle age to compare the health of those who smoke versus those who do not smoke.
 3. Cohort studies can be **prospective** (taking place in the present time) or **historical** (some activities have taken place in the past).
 4. **A clinical treatment trial** is a special type of cohort study in which members of a cohort with a specific illness are given one treatment and other members of the cohort are given another treatment or a placebo. The results of the two treatments are then compared. An example of a clinical treatment trial would be one in which the differences in survival rates between men with prostate cancer who receive a new drug and men with prostate cancer who receive a standard drug are compared.

B. **Case-control studies**
 1. Case-control studies begin with the identification of subjects who have a specific disorder (cases) and subjects who do not have that disorder (controls).
 2. Information on the **prior exposure of cases and controls to risk factors** is then obtained. An example of a case-control study would be one in which the smoking histories of women with and without breast cancer are compared.

C. **Cross-sectional studies**
 1. Cross-sectional studies begin when information is collected from a group of individuals who provide a **snapshot in time** of disease activity.
 2. Such studies can provide information on the relationship between risk factors and health status of a group of individuals at one specific point in time (e.g., a random telephone sample conducted to determine if male smokers are more likely to have an upper respiratory infection than male non-smokers). They can also be used to calculate the prevalence of a disease in a population.

## III. QUANTIFYING RISK

A. **Risk factors are variables that are linked to the cause of a disease.**
 1. **Measures.** Absolute risk, relative risk, attributable risk, and the odds (or odds risk) ratio are measures used to quantify risk in population studies.
  a. **Absolute, relative, and attributable risks** are calculated for **cohort** studies.
  b. **The odds ratio** is calculated for **case-control** studies.

2. **Absolute risk** is equal to the incidence rate.
3. **Absolute risk reduction** (ARR) is the difference in absolute risks. For example, if the incidence rate of lung cancer among the people in Newark and in Trenton, New Jersey, in 2013 is 20/1,000 and 15/1,000 respectively, the absolute risk is 20/1,000 or 2.0% in Newark and 1.5% in Trenton, and the ARR is 2.0% minus 1.5% or 0.5%.
4. **Relative risk.** Relative risk compares the incidence rate of a disorder among individuals exposed to a risk factor (e.g., smoking) with the incidence rate of the disorder in unexposed individuals.
   a. For example, the incidence rate of lung cancer among smokers in a city in New Jersey is 20/1,000, while the incidence rate of lung cancer among nonsmokers in this city is 2/1,000. Therefore, **the fold increase** in risk of lung cancer (the relative risk) for smokers vs. nonsmokers in this New Jersey population is 20/1,000 divided by 2/1,000, or 10.
   b. A relative risk of 10 means that in this city, if an individual smokes, his or her risk of getting lung cancer is 10 times that of a nonsmoker.
5. **Attributable risk**
   a. Attributable risk is useful for determining what would happen in a study population if the risk factor were removed (e.g., determining how common lung cancer would be in a study if people did not smoke).
   b. To calculate attributable risk, the incidence rate of the illness in unexposed individuals is subtracted from the incidence rate of the illness in those who have been exposed to a risk factor.
   c. For the example above, the risk of lung cancer attributable to smoking (the attributable risk) in this New Jersey city's population is 20/1,000 minus 2/1,000, or 18/1,000.
6. **Odds ratio.** Since incidence data are not available in a case-control study, the odds ratio (i.e., odds risk ratio) can be used as an estimate of relative risk (Example 25.1) in such studies.

---

**Example 25.1 Calculating the Odds Ratio**

Of 200 patients in the hospital, 50 have lung cancer. Of these 50 patients, 45 are smokers. Of the remaining 150 hospitalized patients who do not have lung cancer, 60 are smokers. Use this information to calculate the odds ratio for smoking and lung cancer in this hospitalized patient population.

| | Smokers | Nonsmokers |
|---|---|---|
| People with lung cancer | A = 45 | B = 5 |
| People without lung cancer | C = 60 | D = 90 |

$$\frac{(AD) = (45)(90)}{(BC) = (5)(60)} = 13.5 = \textbf{Odds ratio}$$

An odds ratio of 13.5 means that in this population, a person with lung cancer was 13.5 times more likely to have smoked than a person without lung cancer.

---

B. **Number needed to treat and number needed to harm**
   1. Number needed to treat (**NNT**)
      a. NNT is the number of persons who need to take a treatment for one person to benefit from the treatment.
      b. NNT is 1 divided by the ARR.
      c. NNT allows comparison of the effectiveness of different treatments or of treatment versus no treatment or placebo (Example 25.2).
   2. Number needed to harm (**NNH**)
      a. NNH is the number of persons who need to be exposed to a risk factor for one person to be harmed who would otherwise not be harmed.
      b. NNH is 1 divided by the attributable risk.

**Example 25.2  Number Needed to Treat**

A research study is done to determine if a new drug (Drug S) will prevent stroke in men aged 55–65 with hypertension.

Four thousand hypertensive men in this age group are randomly assigned to a group taking Drug S ($n = 2,000$) or a placebo ($n = 2,000$).

Over 10 years there were 1,200 strokes in the placebo group and 200 strokes in the Drug S group.

Based on these data, how many men would have to be treated with Drug S to prevent one case of stroke?

The absolute risk of stroke in the placebo group is $1,200/2,000 = 60\%$.

The absolute risk of stroke in the Drug S group is $200/2,000 = 10\%$.

The absolute risk reduction is therefore $60\% - 10\% = 50\%$.

Since 50% of the hypertensive men were saved from stroke by the drug, the NNT is $1/0.5 = 2.0$.

Therefore, two men would have to be treated with the Drug S to prevent one case of stroke.

# IV.  BIAS, RELIABILITY, AND VALIDITY

To be useful, testing instruments must be bias-free, reliable, and valid.

**A. Bias**
   1. A biased test or research study is one constructed so that **one outcome is more likely to occur than another**.
   2. Some ways that a research study or clinical treatment trial can be biased can be found in Table 25.1.

table  **25.1**  Types of Bias

**Example: Six research studies were conducted on the effectiveness of a new (fictitious) drug, "Flashless" vs. placebo for relieving menopausal symptoms. One hundred women aged 50–70 were recruited for each study and each subject was paid $1,000. Although Flashless ultimately proved to be a useful drug which significantly reduced menopausal symptoms, because all 6 studies were biased in different ways (see Table below) all failed to show the usefulness of Flashless.**

| Study # | Type of Bias | Explanation | Reason for Flashless Study Failure is that When Compared to the General Population, the Subjects |
|---|---|---|---|
| 1 | Selection | Rather than making random assignments, the subjects or the investigators are permitted to choose whether an individual will go into the drug group or the placebo group | Who had more severe symptoms to start with chose or were chosen to take Flashless rather than placebo and so also had more severe symptoms at the end of the study |
| 2 | Sampling | Subjects who volunteer to be in a study are not representative of the population being studied because factors unrelated to the subject of the study (e.g., money) have led them to volunteer | Only joined the study because they needed the money and as such did not represent the typical population of women using drugs such as Flashless |
| 3 | Recall | Knowledge of the presence of a disorder alters the way the subject remembers his or her history | Seemed to have more severe menopausal symptoms because they were asked about their symptoms to be in the study |
| 4 | Lead-time | Early detection of disease is confused with increased survival or length of time that the symptoms have been present | Seemed to have had menopausal symptoms for a longer period of time because they were identified early to be in the study |
| 5 | Surveillance | People who are aware that they are being followed for the development of a disease are more likely to seek testing for and thus to be identified with the disease | Went to the doctor more often because they were in the study which increased the likelihood of being diagnosed with menopausal symptoms |
| 6 | Late-look | People who are most ill are not included in the sample | Who had severe menopausal symptoms chose not to participate in the study, so those who did participate had few symptoms |

B. **Reducing bias in clinical treatment trials.** Blind studies, placebos, crossover studies, and randomized studies are used to reduce bias.
   1. **Blind studies.** The expectations of subjects can influence the effectiveness of treatment. Blind studies attempt to reduce this influence.
      a. In a **single-blind study**, the subject does not know what treatment he or she is receiving.
      b. In a **double-blind study**, neither the subject nor the clinician-evaluator knows what treatment the subject is receiving.
   2. **Placebo responses**
      a. In a blind drug study, a subject may receive a placebo (an inactive substance) rather than the active drug.
      b. People receiving the **placebo** are the **control group**; those receiving the **active drug** are the **experimental group**.
      c. A number of subjects in research studies respond to the treatment with placebos alone (the placebo effect – and see Chapter 4).
   3. **Crossover studies**
      a. In a crossover study, subjects are randomly assigned to one of the two groups. Subjects in Group 1 first receive the drug and subjects in Group 2 first receive the placebo.
      b. Later in the crossover study, the groups switch—those in Group 1 receive the placebo, and those in Group 2 receive the drug.
      c. Because all of the subjects receive both drug and placebo, **each subject acts as his or her own control**.
   4. **Randomization.** In order to ensure that the proportion of sicker and healthier people is the same in the treatment and control (placebo) groups, subjects are randomly assigned to the groups. The number of subjects in each group does not have to be equal.

C. **Reliability and validity**
   1. **Reliability** refers to the reproducibility or dependability of results.
      a. **Interrater reliability** is a measure of whether the results of the test are similar when the test is administered by a different rater or examiner.
      b. **Test-retest reliability** is a measure of whether the results of the test are similar when the person is tested a second or third time.
   2. **Validity** is a measure of the appropriateness of a test, that is, whether the test assesses what it was designed to assess (e.g., Does a new IQ test really measure IQ or does it instead measure educational level?) (see Chapter 8). Sensitivity and specificity are components of validity.

D. **Sensitivity and specificity** (Example 25.3)
   1. **Sensitivity** measures how well a test identifies truly ill people.
      a. **True positives** (TP) are ill people whom a test has correctly identified as being ill.
      b. **False negatives** (FN) are ill people whom a test has incorrectly identified as being well (i.e., healthy).
      c. **Sensitivity** is calculated using only people who are, in fact, ill (TP and FN) by dividing TP by the sum of TP and FN.
         (1) Tests with high sensitivity identify most or all possible cases.
         (2) They are most useful when identifying an ill person as healthy can lead to severe consequences (e.g., cancer which can metastasize if not identified early).
   2. **Specificity** measures how well a test identifies truly well people.
      a. **True negatives** (TN) are well people whom a test has correctly identified as being well.
      b. **False positives** (FP) are well people whom a test has incorrectly identified as being ill.
      c. **Specificity** is calculated by dividing TN by the sum of TN and FP.
         (1) Tests with high specificity identify most or all well people.
         (2) They are most useful when identifying a healthy person as ill can lead to dangerous, painful, or unnecessary treatment (e.g., a healthy man who tests positive for prostate cancer has a prostate biopsy requiring general anesthesia).

---

**Example 25.3  Sensitivity, Specificity, Predictive Value, and Prevalence**

A new blood test to detect the presence of HIV was given to 1,000 patients. Although 200 of the patients were actually infected with the virus, the test was positive in only 160 patients (TP); the other 40 infected patients had negative tests (FN) and thus were not identified by this new test. Of the 800 patients who were not infected, the test was negative in 720 patients (TN) and positive in 80 patients (FP).

Use this information to calculate sensitivity, specificity, positive predictive value, and negative predictive value of this new blood test and the prevalence of HIV in this population.

|  | Patients Infected with HIV | Patients Not Infected with HIV | Total Patients |
|---|---|---|---|
| Positive HIV blood test | 160 (TP) | 80 (FP) | 240 (those with a + test) |
| Negative HIV blood test | 40 (FN) | 720 (TN) | 760 (those with a − test) |
| Total patients | 200 | 800 | 1,000 |

$$\text{Sensitivity} = \frac{160\,(\text{TP})}{160\,(\text{TP}) + 40\,(\text{FN})} = \frac{160}{200} = 80.0\%$$

$$\text{Specificity} = \frac{720\,(\text{TN})}{720\,(\text{TN}) + 80\,(\text{FP})} = \frac{720}{800} = 90.0\%$$

$$\text{Positive predictive value} = \frac{160\,(\text{TP})}{160\,(\text{TP}) + 80\,(\text{FP})} = \frac{160}{240} = 66.67\%$$

$$\text{Negative predictive value} = \frac{720\,(\text{TN})}{720\,(\text{TN}) + 40\,(\text{FN})} = \frac{720}{760} = 94.7\%$$

$$\text{Prevalence} = \frac{200\,(\text{total of those infected})}{1,000\,(\text{total patients})} = 20.0\%$$

---

E.  **Predictive value** (Example 25.3)
   1.  **The predictive value** of a test is a measure of the percentage of test results that match the actual diagnosis. Predictive values (but not sensitivity or specificity) vary according to the prevalence of the disorder in the population.
       a.  **Positive predictive value** (PPV) is the probability that someone with a positive test is actually ill. PPV is calculated by dividing TP by the sum of TP and FP.
       b.  **Negative predictive value** (NPV) is the probability that a person with a negative test is actually well. NPV is calculated by dividing TN by the sum of TN and FN.
   2.  The **higher the prevalence** of a disorder in the population, the **higher the PPV** and the **lower the NPV** of a test used to detect it. If the prevalence of a disorder in the population is low, even tests with very high specificity may have a low PPV because there are likely to be a high number of FP relative to TP.

F.  **Receiver operating characteristic (ROC) curves**
   1.  ROC curves are graphic representations of the **relationship of sensitivity to specificity.**
   2.  The true positive rate (sensitivity) is plotted as a function of the false positive rate (100 minus specificity) for different cutoff points (Figure 25.1).
   3.  A screening test with perfect discrimination (100% sensitivity and 100% specificity) has an ROC curve that passes through the upper left corner of the curve.

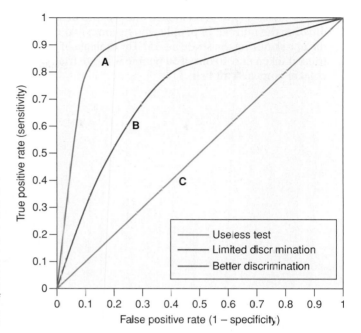

FIGURE 25.1. ROC curve. Graphic representation of the relationship between sensitivity and 1 − specificity for a screening test. The closer the curve to the diagonal (C), the less the discriminating ability; the closer the curve "hugs" the y axis (A), the better the discriminating ability of the screening test (Reprinted with permission from Goroll AH, Muley AG. *Primary Care Medicine: Office Evaluation and Management of the Adult Patient.* 6th ed. Philadelphia, PA: Lippincott Williams & Wilkins; 2009.)

# V. CLINICAL PROBABILITY AND ATTACK RATE

A. Clinical probability is the number of times an **event actually occurs** divided by the number of times the **event can occur** (Example 25.4).

---

**Example 25.4  Clinical Probability**

After 3 years of clinical trials of a new medication to treat migraine headache, it is determined that 20% of patients taking the new medication develop hypertension. If two patients (patients A and B) take the drug, calculate the following probabilities.

1. **The probability that both patient A and patient B will develop hypertension:**

   This is calculated by multiplying the probability of A developing hypertension by the probability of B developing hypertension (the multiplication rule for independent events).

   The probability of A developing hypertension = 0.20 = 20%.

   The probability of B developing hypertension = 0.20 = 20%.

   The probability of both A and B developing hypertension = 0.20 × 0.20 = 0.04 = 4%.

2. **The probability that at least one of the two patients (either A or B or both A and B) will develop hypertension:**
   This is calculated by adding the probability of A developing hypertension to the probability of B developing hypertension and then subtracting the probability of both A and B developing hypertension (the addition rule).

   0.20 + 0.20 − 0.04 = 0.36 = 36%.

3. **The probability that neither patient A nor patient B will develop hypertension:**

   This is calculated by multiplying the probability of patient A being normotensive by the probability of patient B being normotensive: Probability of both being normotensive = (1 − probability of A being hypertensive) × (1 − probability of B being hypertensive) = 0.80 − 0.80 = 0.64 = 64%.

B. **Attack rate** is a type of incidence rate used to describe disease outbreaks. It is calculated by dividing the number of people who become ill during a study period by the number of people at risk during the study period. **For example**, if, after a picnic, 20 out of 40 people who ate fried chicken and 10 out of 50 people who ate fried fish become ill, the attack rate is 50% for chicken and 20% for fish.

# Review Test

**Directions:** Each of the numbered items or incomplete statements in this section is followed by answers or by completions of the statement. Select the **one** lettered answer or completion that is **best** in each case.

**1.** Using the data in the table below, the chance of surviving for 2 years after being diagnosed with ovarian cancer is $360/500 = 72\%$ and the chance of surviving for 4 years is $135/500 = 27\%$. What is the chance of surviving for 4 years after the original diagnosis, given that the patient is alive at the end of the second year?

| Year | Number of Women in the Beginning of the Year | Number of Women Who Died During the Year | Percent of Women Who Survived Each Year (%) |
|------|------|------|------|
| 0–1 | 500 | 100 | 80 |
| 1–2 | 400 | 40 | 90 |
| 2–3 | 360 | 90 | 75 |
| 3–4 | 270 | 135 | 50 |

**(A)** $40/400 = 10\%$
**(B)** $135/500 = 27\%$
**(C)** $40/135 = 29.6\%$
**(D)** $135/360 = 37.5\%$
**(E)** $135/270 = 50\%$

**2.** A type of gynecological cancer has the same incidence rate in white women and African-American women in the United States, but the prevalence rate of this type of cancer is lower in African American than in white women. The most likely explanation for this difference in prevalence rates is that when compared to white women, African-American women are more likely to

**(A)** recover from this type of cancer
**(B)** have natural immunity to this type of cancer
**(C)** have increased access to treatment for this type of cancer
**(D)** be resistant to this type of cancer
**(E)** die from this type of cancer

## Questions 3 and 4

A town in the western United States has a population of 1,200. In 2012, 200 residents of the town are diagnosed with a disease. In 2013, 100 more residents of the town are discovered to have the same disease. The disease is lifelong and chronic but not fatal.

**3.** The incidence rate of this disease in 2013 among this town's population is

**(A)** $100/1,200$
**(B)** $200/1,200$
**(C)** $300/1,200$
**(D)** $100/1,000$
**(E)** $300/1,000$

**4.** The prevalence rate of this disease in 2013 among the town's population is

**(A)** $100/1,200$
**(B)** $200/1,200$
**(C)** $300/1,200$
**(D)** $100/1,000$
**(E)** $300/1,000$

**5.** A study is designed to determine the relationship between emotional stress and peptic ulcer. To do this, the researchers use hospital records of patients diagnosed with peptic ulcer disease and patients diagnosed with other disorders over the period from July 2002–July 2012. The emotional stress each patient was exposed to was determined from these records and was then quantified with a score of 1 (least stress) to 100 (most stress). This study is best described as a

**(A)** cohort study
**(B)** cross-sectional study
**(C)** case-control study
**(D)** historical cohort study
**(E)** clinical treatment trial

**6.** A study is done to determine the effectiveness of a new antihistamine. To do this, 25 allergic patients are assigned to one of the two groups, the new drug (13 patients) or a placebo (12 patients). The patients are then followed over a 6-month period. This study is best described as a

(A) cohort study
(B) cross-sectional study
(C) case-control study
(D) historical cohort study
(E) clinical treatment trial

**7.** An intelligence quotient (IQ) test has high interrater reliability. This means that

(A) the test involves structured interviews
(B) a new assessment strategy is being used
(C) the test actually measures IQ and not educational level
(D) the results are very similar when the test is administered a second time
(E) the results are very similar when the test is administered by a different examiner

**8.** There are 100,000 people in Hobart, Tasmania. On January 1, 2013, 50 of these people have Disease Y. Fifty divided by 100,000 on that date gives which of the following measures for Disease Y?

(A) Point prevalence
(B) Period prevalence
(C) Incidence rate
(D) Odds ratio
(E) Relative risk

**9.** In which of the following infectious illnesses is prevalence most likely to exceed incidence?

(A) Measles
(B) Influenza
(C) Leprosy
(D) Rubella
(E) Rabies

**Questions 10–13**

A patient is given a new screening test for tuberculosis. Although the patient is infected, the test indicates that the patient is well.

**10.** This test result is known as

(A) false positive
(B) false negative
(C) true positive
(D) true negative
(E) predictive

**11.** To identify all patients infected with tuberculosis, the cutoff point for this test should be set at the point of highest

(A) sensitivity
(B) specificity
(C) positive predictive value
(D) negative predictive value
(E) accuracy

**12.** If this new screening test has a sensitivity of 90% and a specificity of 70% in a group of young Russian prisoners in which the prevalence of tuberculosis is 50%, the positive predictive value of this test is best estimated as

(A) 12.5%
(B) 25%
(C) 30%
(D) 75%
(E) 90%

**13.** If the test is given only to old prisoners in whom the incidence and prevalence of tuberculosis is higher than in young prisoners, the positive predictive value and sensitivity of this screening test will respectively change in which of the following ways?

| Positive Predictive Value | Sensitivity |
| --- | --- |
| (A) Increase | Increase |
| (B) Decrease | Decrease |
| (C) Increase | Not change |
| (D) Not change | Not change |
| (E) Increase | Decrease |

**14.** A case-control study is done to determine if elderly demented patients are more likely to be injured at home than elderly patients who are not demented. The results of the study show an odds ratio of 3. This figure means that if an elderly patient was injured at home, that patient

(A) should be placed in an extended-care facility
(B) was one-third more likely to be demented than a patient who was not injured at home
(C) was no more likely to be demented than a patient who was not injured at home
(D) was three times more likely to be demented than a patient who was not injured at home
(E) should be kept at home

## Questions 15–17

A study is undertaken to determine if pre-natal exposure to marijuana is associated with low birth weight in infants. Mothers of 50 infants weighing less than 5 lbs (low birth weight) and 50 infants weighing more than 7 lbs (normal birth weight) are questioned about their use of marijuana during pregnancy. The study finds that 20 mothers of low-birth-weight infants and 2 mothers of normal-birth-weight infants used the drug during pregnancy.

**15.** In this study, the odds ratio associated with smoking marijuana during pregnancy is

(A) 10
(B) 16
(C) 20
(D) 30
(E) 48

**16.** An odds ratio of X, calculated in the preceding question, means that

(A) the incidence of low birth weight in infants whose mothers smoke marijuana is X
(B) an infant of low birth weight was X times as likely as an infant of normal birth weight to have had a mother who used marijuana during pregnancy
(C) a child has a 1/X chance of being born of low birth weight if its mother uses mari-juana
(D) the risk of low birth weight in infants whose mothers use marijuana is no dif-ferent from that of infants whose moth-ers do not use the drug
(E) the prevalence of low birth weight in infants whose mothers smoke marijuana is X

**17.** This study is best described as a

(A) cohort study
(B) cross-sectional study
(C) case-control study
(D) historical cohort study
(E) clinical treatment trial

## Questions 18–21

A new blood test to detect prostate cancer by measuring prostate specific antigen (PSA) was given to 1,000 male members of a large HMO. Although 50 of the men actually had prostate cancer, the test was positive (PSA> 4 ng/mL) in only 15; the other 35 patients with prostate cancer had negative tests. Of the 950 men without prostate cancer, the test was positive in 200 men and negative in 750.

**18.** The specificity of this test is approximately

(A) 15%
(B) 30%
(C) 48%
(D) 79%
(E) 86%

**19.** The positive predictive value of this blood test is

(A) 7%
(B) 14%
(C) 21%
(D) 35%
(E) 93%

**20.** If the cutoff value indicating a positive test is lowered from PSA 4 ng/mL to PSA 3 ng/mL, this change would

(A) increase negative predictive value
(B) decrease sensitivity
(C) increase false negative rate
(D) increase positive predictive value
(E) increase specificity

**21.** With this change in the cutoff value, the incidence and prevalence of prostate cancer would

| Incidence | Prevalence |
| --- | --- |
| (A) Increase | Increase |
| (B) Decrease | Decrease |
| (C) Increase | Not Change |
| (D) Not Change | Not Change |
| (E) Increase | Decrease |

**22.** A study is designed to compare a new medication for Crohn disease with a standard medication. To do this, each of 50 Crohn disease patients is allowed to decide which of these two treatment groups to join. The major reason that the results of this study may not be valid is because of

**(A)** selection bias
**(B)** recall bias
**(C)** sampling bias
**(D)** differences in the sizes of the two groups
**(E)** the small number of patients in the study

**23.** After a new antidepressant has been on the market for 5 years, it is determined that of 2,400 people who have taken the drug, 360 complained of persistent nausea. If a physician has two patients on this antidepressant, the probability that both of them will experience persistent nausea is approximately

**(A)** 2%
**(B)** 9%
**(C)** 24%
**(D)** 30%
**(E)** 64%

**24.** A blood test reveals that a 35-year-old woman at 18 weeks gestation has increased serum alpha-fetoprotein (AFP). Of the following measures, which has the greatest influence in determining the predictive value of this test for neural tube defects in the fetus?

**(A)** Absolute concentration of AFP in the maternal serum
**(B)** Family history of dizygotic twin pregnancy
**(C)** Prevalence of neural tube defects in the population in question
**(D)** Specificity of the blood test
**(E)** Sensitivity of the blood test

**25.** In people with no known risks for tuberculosis, a positive reaction to the purified protein derivative (PPD) tuberculin skin test requires 15 mm or more of hard swelling at the site. A group of physicians decide that they are going to change the criterion for a positive test in a group of people with no known risk for tuberculosis to a hard swelling of 10 mm or more at the site. With respect to the PPD test, this change in the cutoff point is most likely to

**(A)** increase sensitivity
**(B)** decrease sensitivity
**(C)** decrease negative predictive value
**(D)** increase positive predictive value
**(E)** increase specificity

**26.** A research study is done to determine if intravenous (IV) ibandronate sodium (Boniva) will decrease the incidence rate of hip fractures in perimenopausal women. There are 2,600 women in the ibandronate sodium group, of whom 130 develop hip fractures. Of the 2,600 women in the placebo group, 260 develop hip fractures. Based on these data, how many women need to be treated with ibandronate sodium to prevent one hip fracture?

**(A)** 1
**(B)** 5
**(C)** 10
**(D)** 15
**(E)** 20

# Answers and Explanations

## Typical Board Question

**The answer is C.** Assuming a total of 1,000 women over age 80 years and a prevalence rate of 30% in this age group, 300 women have osteoporosis and 700 are well. Of the 300 who have osteoporosis, a screening test with a sensitivity of 90% would identify 270 TP and 30 FN. Of the 700 who are well, a screening test with a specificity of 75% would identify 525 TN and 175 FP. Using these data (see table below), the likelihood that a woman with a positive test actually has osteoporosis [positive predictive value (TP/TP + FP)] is 270/270 + 175 = 60%.

|  | Disease Present | Disease Absent | Total |
|---|---|---|---|
| Positive test | 270 (TP) | 175 (FP) | 445 |
| Negative test | 30 (FN) | 525 (TN) | 555 |
| Total | 300 | 700 | 1,000 |

1. **The answer is D.** The table shows that of the 360 ovarian cancer patients who survived the second year, 135 survived the fourth year. Therefore, the chance of surviving for 4 years given that the patient is alive at the end of the second year is 135/360 = 37.5%.

2. **The answer is E.** Prevalence rate of an illness is decreased either when patients recover or when they die. Because when compared to white patients, African-American patients tend to have lower incomes and decreased access to health care (see Chapter 18), they are less likely to receive early treatment for disorders such as cancer, and thus more likely to die. Decreased prevalence in African-American women is thus more likely to be due to early death than to recovery from this type of cancer. Resistance to an illness or immunity to an illness affects incidence rate, which is equal in both groups of women in this example.

3. **The answer is D. 4. The answer is C.** The incidence rate of the disease in 2013 is 100/1,000, the number diagnosed with the illness divided by the number of people at risk for the illness. Because the 200 people who got the disease in 2012 are no longer at risk for getting the illness in 2013, the denominator in the equation (number of people at risk) is 1,000 (rather than 1,200). The prevalence rate of this disease in 2013 is 300/1,200. This figure represented the people who were diagnosed in 2013 and still have the disease (100) plus the people who were diagnosed in 2012 and still have the disease (200) divided by the total population at risk (1,200).

5. **The answer is C.** Case-control studies begin with the identification of subjects who have a specific disorder (cases, i.e., ulcer patients) and subjects who do not have that disorder (controls i.e., those diagnosed with other disorders). Information on the prior exposure of cases and controls to risk factors is then obtained. In this case-control study, the investigators used cases (ulcer patients) and controls (patients with other disorders), and looked into their histories (hospital records) to determine the occurrence of and quantify the level of the risk factor (i.e., emotional stress) in each group. Cohort studies begin with the identification of specific populations (cohorts), who are free of illness at the start of the study and can be prospective (taking place in the present time) or historical (some activities have taken place in the past). Clinical treatment trials are cohort studies in which members of a cohort with a specific illness are given one treatment and other members of the cohort are given another treatment or a placebo. The results of the two treatments are then compared. Cross-sectional

studies involve the collection of information on a disease and risk factors in a population at one point in time.

6. **The answer is E.** This study is best described as a clinical treatment trial, a study in which a cohort receiving a new antihistamine is compared with a cohort receiving a placebo (see also answer to Question 5).

7. **The answer is E.** Interrater reliability is a measure of how similar test findings are when used by two different examiners.

8. **The answer is A.** Point prevalence is the number of people who have an illness at a specific point in time (e.g., January 1, 2013) divided by the total population at that time. Incidence rate is the number of individuals who develop an illness in a given time period (commonly 1 year) divided by the total number of individuals at risk for the illness during that time period. Period prevalence is the number of individuals who have an illness during a specific time period. Relative risk compares the incidence rate of a disorder among individuals exposed to a risk factor (e.g., smoking) with the incidence rate of the disorder in unexposed individuals. The odds ratio is an estimate of the relative risk in case-control studies.

9. **The answer is C.** In leprosy, a long-lasting, infectious illness, the number of people in the population who have the illness (prevalence) is likely to exceed the number newly developing the illness in a given year (incidence). Measles, influenza, rubella, and rabies are shorter-lasting illnesses than leprosy.

10. **The answer is B. 11. The answer is A. 12. The answer is D. 13. The answer is C.** A false negative result occurs if a test does not detect tuberculosis in someone who truly is infected. True positives are ill people whom a test has correctly identified as being ill. True negatives are well people whom a test has correctly identified as being well. False positives are well people whom a test has incorrectly identified as being ill. In order to identify all truly infected people (TP and FN), the cutoff point for the test should be set at the point of highest sensitivity, that is, the point at which there are the fewest number of FN. Using the data provided and assuming there are a total of 200 young prisoners, the positive predictive value (TP/TP + FP) of this test is 90/90 + 30 = 75%.

|  | Disease Present | Disease Absent | Total |
|---|---|---|---|
| Positive test | 90 (TP) | 30 (FP) | 120 |
| Negative test | 10 (FN) | 70 (TN) | 80 |
| Total | 100 | 100 | 200 |

Positive predictive value: 90 TP/(90 TP + 30 FN) = 90/120 = 75%.

Calculations shown below indicate that if prevalence of the disease is increased in a population (e.g., 200 old men), positive predictive value increases, but sensitivity does not change.

|  | Disease Present | Disease Absent | Total |
|---|---|---|---|
| Positive test | 172 (TP) | 6 (FP) | 178 |
| Negative test | 18 (FN) | 14 (TN) | 32 |
| Total | 180 | 20 | 200 |

If the prevalence of the disease is increased, both TP and FN will increase to the same extent, and sensitivity will not change. However, with increased prevalence, TP will increase and FP will decrease, so positive predictive value will increase. Also, because with increased prevalence, FN increases but TN decreases, negative predictive value will decrease (see also TBQ).

**14. The answer is D.** An odds ratio of 3 means that an elderly patient who was injured at home was three times more likely to be demented than a patient who was not injured at home. This number does not indicate whether or not certain people should remain at home or be cared for by others.

**15. The answer is B. 16. The answer is B. 17. The answer is C.** The odds ratio is 16 and is calculated as follows:

|  | Mother Smoked Marijuana | Mother Did Not Smoke Marijuana |
| --- | --- | --- |
| Low-birth-weight babies | A = 20 | B = 30 |
| Normal-birth-weight babies | C = 2 | D = 48 |

**Odds ratio** = (AD)/(BC) or (20)(48)/(30)(2) = 960/60 = 16.

The odds ratio of 16 means that an infant of low birth weight was 16 times as likely as an infant of normal birth weight to have had a mother who used marijuana during pregnancy. This study is best described as a case-control study; the risk factor here is fetal exposure to marijuana (see also the explanation for Question 5).

**18. The answer is D. 19. The answer is A. 20. The answer is A. 21. The answer is D.** Calculations shown below indicate that the specificity of this blood test is 79% and the positive predictive value is 7%.

|  | Those Who Have Prostate Cancer | Those Who Do Not Have Prostate Cancer | Total |
| --- | --- | --- | --- |
| Positive blood test | 15 (TP) | 200 (FP) | 215 |
| Negative blood test | 35 (FN) | 750 (TN) | 785 |
| Total patients | 50 | 950 | 1,000 |

**Specificity:** 750 (TN)/[750 (TN) + 200 (FP)] = 0.789 or 78.9%.

**Positive predictive value:** 15 (TP)/[15 (TP) + 200 (FP), i.e., all those with a + test) = 0.07 or 7.0%.

Decreasing the lower limit of this reference test value (i.e., the cutoff value) can be expected to both decrease the number of false negatives and increase the number of false positives. Such alterations will both increase sensitivity (TP/TP + FN) and negative predictive value (TN/TN + FN) and decrease specificity (TN/TN + FP) and positive predictive value (TP/TP + FP) of the test. A change in the reference interval would not affect the incidence or prevalence of prostate cancer in the population.

**22. The answer is A.** The major reason that the results of this study are not valid is because of selection bias (i.e., the subjects were able to choose which group to go into). If very ill people were more likely to choose the standard treatment, people in the experimental treatment group (who were healthier to begin with) would have had a better outcome. In recall bias, knowledge of the presence of a disorder alters the way subjects remember their histories. In sampling bias, subjects are chosen to be in a study because of the factors that may be unrelated to the subject of the study but distinguish them from the rest of the population. A study can be valid even though two groups may be of different sizes or there are a small number of patients in a study.

**23. The answer is A.** The probability of both patients (A and B) taking this antidepressant experiencing nausea equals the probability of A experiencing nausea (360/2,400 = 0.15) times the probability of B experiencing nausea (360/2,400 = 0.15) = 0.15 × 0.15 = 0.0225, that is, about 2%.

24. **The answer is C.** The prevalence of neural tube defects in the population in question has the greatest influence in determining the predictive value of this test for this patient since prevalence is directly related to predictive value. The higher the prevalence, the higher the positive predictive value (PPV) and the lower the negative predictive value (NPV). Sensitivity and specificity relate to whether the test indicates that there is a neural tube defect in an affected fetus (sensitivity) or the absence of a neural tube defect in a healthy fetus (specificity). While AFP in the maternal serum or family history of dizygotic twin pregnancy may or may not be related to whether or not the fetus has a neural tube defect, they are not related to the predictive value of a screening test.

25. **The answer is A.** With respect to the PPD test, this change in the cutoff point is most likely to increase sensitivity and negative predictive value. This is because there will be fewer false negatives, that is, fewer people who are actually at risk for TB will be identified as not at risk. This change in the cutoff point will also decrease specificity and positive predictive value (see also answer to Question 20).

26. **The answer is E.** Twenty women need to be treated with IV ibandronate sodium to prevent one hip fracture. The number needed to treat is calculated as 1/absolute risk reduction. Of the 2,600 women in the placebo group, 260 develop hip fractures. Of the 2,600 women in the ibandronate sodium group, 130 develop hip fractures. The incidence rate of hip fractures in the placebo group is therefore 260/2,600 (0.1 or 10%) and the incidence rate of hip fractures in the ibandronate sodium group is 130/2,600 (0.05 or 5%). Therefore, absolute risk reduction (ARR) is 10% − 5% = 5%. If 5% of women were prevented from having a hip fracture by the drug, the NNT is 1.0 divided by .05, or 20.

# chapter 26  Statistical Analyses

## Typical Board Question

At an American medical school, a study is done to evaluate the relationship between parental income (in thousands of dollars per year) and USMLE Step 1 scores. Which of the following is most likely to be the correlation coefficient ($r$) for this relationship as shown by these data?

**(A)** 1.40
**(B)** 0.50
**(C)** 0
**(D)** −0.25
**(E)** −0.75

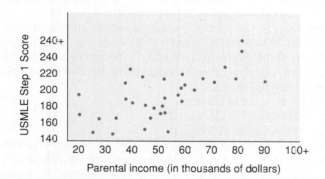

*(See "Answers and Explanations" at end of chapter.)*

## I. ELEMENTS OF STATISTICAL ANALYSES

### A. Overview

1. **Descriptive statistics** summarize the data obtained from research studies.
2. **Inferential statistics** provide a way to generalize results to an entire population by observing a sample of that population.
3. **A variable** is a quantity that can change under different experimental situations; variables may be independent or dependent.
   a. An **independent variable** is a predictive factor that has an impact on a dependent variable (e.g., the amount of fat in the diet).
   b. A **dependent variable** is the outcome that reflects the effects of changing the independent variable (e.g., body weight under different dietary fat regimens).

| table 26.1 | Calculating Standard Deviation, Standard Error of the Mean, $z$ Score, and Confidence Interval | |
|---|---|---|
| **Measure** | **Comment** | **Formula** |
| Standard deviation ($S$) | Average distance of observations from their mean | $S = \sqrt{\dfrac{\Sigma(X - \bar{X})^2}{n-1}}$ |
| Standard error of the mean ($SE$) | Estimate of the quality of the sample | $SE = \dfrac{S}{\sqrt{n}}$ |
| $z$ score ($z$) | Difference between one score in the distribution and the population mean in units of standard deviation | $z = \dfrac{(X - \bar{X})}{S}$ |
| Confidence interval ($CI$) | Specifies the high and low limits of the interval in which the true population mean lies | $CI = \bar{X} \pm z(SE)$ |

$n$, number of subjects; $X$, observed value; $\bar{X}$, mean.
From Fadem B. *Behavioral Science in Medicine*. 2nd ed. Philadelphia, PA: Lippincott Williams & Wilkins; 2012:318.

B. **Measures of dispersion** (Table 26.1)
   1. **Standard deviation** ($S$) is the average distance of observations from their mean ($\bar{X}$). Standard deviation is calculated by squaring each deviation from the mean in a group of scores, then adding the squared deviations; this sum is then divided by the number of scores in the group ($n$) minus 1, and the square root of the result is determined.
   2. A standard normal value, or $z$ **score**, is the difference between an individual variable and the population mean in units of standard deviation.
   3. **Standard error of the mean** or standard error ($SE$) is the standard deviation divided by the square root of the number of scores in a sample ($n$).
   4. **Confidence interval** ($CI$). The mean of a sample is only an estimate. The $CI$ specifies the high and low limits between which a given percentage (e.g., 95% is conventionally used in medical research) of the population would be expected to fall (i.e., the interval in which the true population mean lies). The $CI$ is equal to the mean of the sample ($\bar{X}$) plus or minus the $z$ score multiplied by the $SE$.
      a. For the 95% $CI$, a $z$ score of 2 is used.
      b. For the 99% $CI$, a $z$ score of 2.5 is used.
      c. For the 99.7% $CI$, a $z$ score of 3 is used.
   5. In estimating the mean, **precision** reflects how reliable the estimate is and **accuracy** reflects how close the estimate is to the true mean. The wider the $CI$, the less precise the estimate. However, wider CIs are also more accurate as they have a greater likelihood of containing the true mean.

C. **Measures of central tendency**
   1. The **mean**, or average, is obtained by adding a group of numbers and dividing the sum by the quantity of numbers in the group.
   2. The **median**, 50th percentile value, is the middle value in a **sequentially ordered** group of numbers (i.e., the value that divides the data set into two equal groups).
   3. The **mode** is the value that appears most often in a group of numbers.

D. **Normal distribution.** A **normal** distribution, also referred to as a **gaussian** or **bell-shaped** distribution, is a theoretical distribution of scores in which the mean, median, and mode are equal.
   1. The highest point in the distribution of scores is the **modal peak**. In a **bimodal distribution**, there are two modal peaks (e.g., two distinct populations).
   2. In a normal distribution, approximately 68% of the population scores fall within one, 95% fall within two, and 99.7% fall within three standard deviations of the mean, respectively (Figure 26.1).

E. **Skewed distributions.** In a skewed distribution, the modal peak shifts to one side (Figure 26.2).
   1. In a **positively skewed** distribution (skewed to the right), the tail is toward the right and the modal peak is toward the left (i.e., scores cluster toward the low end).
   2. In a **negatively skewed** distribution (skewed to the left), the tail is toward the left and the modal peak is toward the right (i.e., scores cluster toward the high end).

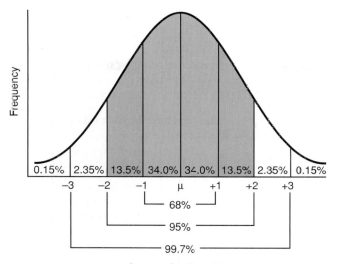

**Area under the curve**

**FIGURE 26.1.** The normal (gaussian) distribution. The number of standard deviations (S) (−3 to +3) from the mean is shown on the x-axis. The percentage of the population that falls under the curve within each S is shown. (From Facem B. *High-Yield Behavioral Science.* 4th ed. Baltimore, MD: Lippincott Williams & Wilkins; 2013:126.)

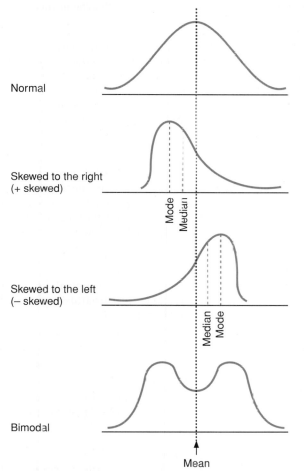

**FIGURE 26.2.** Frequency distributions. (From Fadem B. *High-Yield Behavioral Science.* 4th ed. Baltimore, MD: Lippincott Williams & Wilkins; 2013:126.)

## II. HYPOTHESIS TESTING

A. A **hypothesis** is a statement based on inference, existing literature, or preliminary studies that postulates that a difference exists between groups. The possibility that this difference occurred by chance is tested using statistical procedures.

B. The **null hypothesis**, which postulates that **no difference** exists between groups, can either be rejected or not rejected following statistical analysis.

**Example of the null hypothesis**:
1. A group of 20 patients who have similar systolic blood pressures at the beginning of a study (Time 1) is divided into two groups of 10 patients each. One group is given daily doses of an experimental drug meant to lower blood pressure (experimental group); the other group is given daily doses of a placebo (placebo group). Blood pressure in all 20 patients is measured 2 weeks later (Time 2).
2. The null hypothesis assumes that there are no significant differences in blood pressure between the two groups at Time 2.
3. If, at Time 2, patients in the experimental group show systolic blood pressures similar to those in the placebo group, **the null hypothesis** (i.e., there is no significant difference between the groups) **is not rejected**.
4. If, at Time 2, patients in the experimental group have significantly lower or higher blood pressures than those in the placebo group, **the null hypothesis is rejected**.

C. Type I ($\alpha$) and type II ($\beta$) error
1. **Power** (1 minus $\beta$) is the ability to detect a difference between groups if it is truly there. The larger the sample size, the more power a researcher has to detect this difference.
2. A **type I error** occurs when the null hypothesis is rejected, although it is true (e.g., the drug really does not lower blood pressure).
3. A **type II error** occurs when the null hypothesis is not rejected, although it is false (e.g., the drug really does lower blood pressure), but there may not have been enough power to detect this difference.

D. Statistical probability
1. $\alpha$ is a preset level of **significance**, usually set at **0.05** by convention.
2. The **$P$ (probability) value** is the chance of a type I error occurring.
3. If a $P$ value is equal to or less than 0.05, the preset $\alpha$ level, it is unlikely that a type I error has been made (i.e., a type I error is made 5 or fewer times out of 100 attempts).
4. Therefore, a $P$ value equal to or less than 0.05 is generally considered to be **statistically significant**.

E. Statistical versus clinical significance
1. Statistical significance itself does not translate into clinical importance or significance.
2. Therefore, the question about whether a new treatment should be used in practice requires evaluating its **importance in the real world**.

## III. STATISTICAL TESTS

Statistical tests are used to analyze data from medical studies. The results of statistical tests indicate whether to reject or not reject the null hypothesis. Statistical tests can be parametric or nonparametric.

A. Parametric statistical tests for continuous data
1. Parametric tests use population parameters (e.g., mean scores) and are usually used to identify the presence of statistically significant differences between groups when the distribution of scores in a population is normal and when the sample size is large.

2. Commonly used parametric statistical tests include **$t$-tests, analysis of variance (ANOVA)**, and **linear correlation** (Example 26-1).
3. **Linear correlation** refers to the degree of relationship between two continuous variables that can be assessed using linear correlation coefficients ($r$) that range between **−1 and +1** (see Typical Board Question).
   a. If the two variables move in the same direction, $r$ is **positive** (e.g., as height increases, body weight increases, or as calorie intake decreases, body weight decreases).
   b. If the two variables move in opposite directions, $r$ is **negative** (e.g., as time spent exercising increases, body weight decreases).
   **Meta-analysis** is a statistical method of combining the statistical results of a number of studies to form an overarching conclusion.

B. **Nonparametric statistical tests**
   1. If the distribution of scores in a population is not normal or if the sample size is small, nonparametric statistical tests are used to evaluate the presence of statistically significant differences between groups.
   2. Commonly used nonparametric statistical tests include Wilcoxon's (rank sum and signed rank), Mann–Whitney, and Kruskal–Wallis.

C. **Categorical tests.** To analyze categorical data or compare proportions, the **chi-square test** or **Fisher's Exact test** (when the sample size is small) (Example 26-1) is used.

---

**EXAMPLE 26-1. Commonly Used Statistical Tests**

A consumer group would like to evaluate the success of three different commercial weight loss programs. To do this, male and female subjects are assigned to one of three programs (group A, group B, and group C). The mean weight of the subjects is not significantly different among the three groups at the start of the study (Time 1). Each group follows a different diet regimen. At the end of the 6-week study (Time 2), the subjects are weighed and their high density lipoprotein (HDL) levels are obtained. Examples of how statistical tests can be used to analyze the results of this study are given below.

*The t-test: Difference between the means of two samples*

**Independent (nonpaired) test:** Tests the mean difference in body weights of the subjects in group A and the subjects in group B at Time 1 (i.e., two groups of subjects are sampled on one occasion).

**Dependent (paired) test:** Tests the mean difference in body weights of the subjects in group A at Time 1 and Time 2 (i.e., the same people are sampled on two occasions).

*Analysis of variance (ANOVA): Differences among the means of more than two samples*

**One-way ANOVA:** Tests the mean differences in body weights of the subjects in group A, group B, and group C at Time 2 (i.e., one variable: Group).

**Two-way ANOVA:** It tests the mean differences in body weights of men and women and in body weights of group A, group B, and group C at Time 2 (i.e., two variables: Sex and group).

*Correlation: Mutual relation between two continuous variables*

Tests the relation between HDL and body weight in all subjects at Time 2. Correlation coefficients (r) are negative (0 to −1) if the variables move in opposite directions (e.g., as body weight decreases, HDL increases) and positive (0 to +1) if the variables move in the same direction (e.g., as body weight decreases, HDL decreases).

*Chi-square test: Differences between frequencies in a sample; and Fisher's exact probability: Differences between frequencies in a small sample.*

Tests the difference among the percentage of subjects with body weight of 140 lbs or less in groups A, B, and C at Time 2.

From Fadem B. *Behavioral Science in Medicine.* 2nd ed. Baltimore, MD: Lippincott Williams & Wilkins; 2012:319.

# Review Test

**Directions:** Each of the numbered items or incomplete statements in this section is followed by answers or by completions of the statement. Select the **one** lettered answer or completion that is **best** in each case.

**Questions 1 and 2**

A research study is designed to identify the mean body weight of women between the ages of 30 and 39 in Los Angeles. To do this, a researcher obtains the body weights of an unbiased sample of 81 women in Los Angeles in this age group. The mean body weight of the women in the sample is 135 pounds with a standard deviation of 18.

**1.** What is the estimated standard error of the mean for this population?

(A) 0.05
(B) 0.10
(C) 1.0
(D) 2.0
(E) 3.0

**2.** What are, respectively, the 95% and 99% confidence intervals for this sample?

(A) 131–139 and 130–140 pounds
(B) 130–140 and 131–139 pounds
(C) 129–141 and 130–135 pounds
(D) 130–135 and 129–141 pounds
(E) 131–139 and 129–141 pounds

**3.** When compared to the 99% confidence interval, the 95% confidence interval is

(A) less precise and less accurate
(B) more precise but less accurate
(C) more precise and more accurate
(D) less precise and more accurate

**Questions 4–6**

Systolic blood pressure is normally distributed with a mean of 120 mm Hg and a standard deviation of 10.

**4.** What percentage of people in a population selected at random would be expected to have systolic blood pressure at or above 140 mm Hg?

(A) 1.9%
(B) 2.5%
(C) 13.5%
(D) 34.0%
(E) 64.2%

**5.** In a population of 500 people selected at random, how many people would be expected to have systolic blood pressure between 110 mm Hg and 120 mm Hg?

(A) 80
(B) 100
(C) 125
(D) 170
(E) 250

**6.** What percentage of the population can be expected to have blood pressure that falls within one standard deviation of the mean?

(A) 0.15%
(B) 2.35%
(C) 34%
(D) 68%
(E) 95%

**7.** Which of the following statistical tests is most appropriately used to evaluate the difference in the percentage of women who lose weight on a protein-sparing diet versus the percentage who lose weight on a high-protein diet?

(A) Paired $t$-test
(B) Analysis of variance
(C) Chi-square test
(D) Correlation
(E) Independent $t$-test

**8.** Which of the following statistical tests is most appropriately used to evaluate differences between initial body weight and final body weight for each woman on a protein-sparing diet?

**(A)** Paired *t*-test
**(B)** Analysis of variance
**(C)** Chi-square test
**(D)** Correlation
**(E)** Independent *t*-test

**9.** Which of the following statistical tests is most appropriately used to evaluate the relationship between body weight and systolic blood pressure in a group of 25-year-old women?

**(A)** Paired *t*-test
**(B)** Analysis of variance
**(C)** Chi-square test
**(D)** Correlation
**(E)** Independent *t*-test

**10.** In a study to determine the usefulness of a new antihypertensive medication, 12 hypertensive patients are given the new drug and 10 hypertensive patients are given a placebo. The dependent variable in this study is

**(A)** the experimenter's bias
**(B)** giving the patients the drug
**(C)** giving the patients a placebo
**(D)** the patients' blood pressure following treatment with the drug or placebo
**(E)** the daily variability in the patients' blood pressure before the drug treatment

**11.** Analysis of the data from a large research study reveals a *P* value of 0.001. These results indicate that the researcher

**(A)** has committed a type I error
**(B)** has committed a type II error
**(C)** can reject the null hypothesis
**(D)** cannot reject the null hypothesis
**(E)** has biased the study

**Questions 12–14**

On a gross anatomy quiz, test scores of 10, 10, 10, 70, 40, 20, and 90 are obtained by seven students in a laboratory group.

**12.** Which of the following correctly describes these quiz scores?

**(A)** Positively skewed
**(B)** A normal distribution
**(C)** Negatively skewed
**(D)** The mode is higher than the mean
**(E)** The mode is equal to the mean

**13.** The median of these quiz scores is

**(A)** 10
**(B)** 20
**(C)** 40
**(D)** 70
**(E)** 90

**14.** If the class teaching assistant erred and recorded the grade of one student who got a 10 as 100, the mean, median, and mode would, respectively

**(A)** increase, increase, increase
**(B)** increase, not change, not change
**(C)** increase, increase, not change
**(D)** increase, not change, not change
**(E)** not change, increase, not change

**15.** A pharmaceutical company claims that their new drug for genital herpes decreases the persistence of an outbreak from 5.5 days to 5.3 days. This difference is significant at the 95% confidence interval. This result

**(A)** is clinically significant but not statistically significant
**(B)** is not clinically significant but is statistically significant
**(C)** is neither clinically nor statistically significant
**(D)** is both clinically and statistically significant

**16.** For a group of 20 elderly patients aged 85 to 90, blood pressure measurements are taken and recorded three times per day over a 2-week period. At the end of the 2 weeks, the patients' blood pressures are taken and recorded four times per day for the next 2 weeks. If the patients' blood pressures fall within a normal distribution, what will be the effect of taking the blood pressures four times per day rather than three times per day on the standard deviation and shape of the resulting curve?

**(A)** Standard deviation decreases; shape of the curve does not change
**(B)** Standard deviation increases; shape of the curve does not change
**(C)** Standard deviation decreases; shape of the curve is positively skewed
**(D)** Standard deviation increases; shape of the curve is negatively skewed
**(E)** Standard deviation does not change; shape of the curve does not change

# Answers and Explanations

## Typical Board Question

**The answer is B.** The correlation between parental income and USMLE Step 1 scores as shown by these data is positive (i.e., as parental income increases, scores increase). Since a correlation coefficient ($r$) cannot be more than 1, the only possible answer is 0.50 (for information on a similar study see Fadem, Schuchman, and Simring, *Academic Medicine*, 1995).

1. **The answer is D.** The estimated standard error of the mean (*SE*) equals the sample standard deviation (18) divided by the square root of $81 = 9$. The *SE* is therefore $18/9 = 2$.

2. **The answer is A.** Confidence interval (*CI*) specifies the interval in which the true population mean lies. The *CI* is equal to the mean of the sample ($\bar{X}$) plus or minus the $z$ score. The 95% *CI* and 99% *CI* equal the mean plus or minus 2.0 (*SE*) and 2.5 (*SE*) respectively, i.e., $135 \pm 4$ (95% confidence interval), and $135 \pm 5$ (99% confidence interval).

3. **The answer is B.** With respect to estimating the mean, precision reflects how reliable the estimate is and accuracy reflects how close the estimate is to the true mean. The wider the *CI*, the less precise and the more accurate the estimate of the mean. When compared to a 99% confidence interval, a 95% confidence interval will be more precise (smaller *SE* and width of the confidence interval) but less accurate (the sample is less likely to be representative).

4. **The answer is B. 5. The answer is D. 6. The answer is D.** Systolic blood pressure of 140 mm Hg is two standard deviations above the mean (120 mm Hg). The area under the curve between two and three standard deviations above the mean is about 2.35% plus about 0.15% (everything above three standard deviations). Thus, a total of about 2.5% of the people will have blood pressures of 140 mm Hg and above. Systolic blood pressure between 110 and 120 mm Hg is one standard deviation below the mean. The percentage of people in this area on a normal curve is 34%. Thus, 34% of 500 people, or 170 people, will have systolic blood pressure in the range of 110–120 mm Hg. "Within" includes one standard deviation below (34%) plus one standard deviation above (34%) the mean for a total of 68%. Thus, a total of 68% of the population can be expected to have blood pressure that falls within one standard deviation of the mean.

7. **The answer is C.** The chi-square test is used to examine differences between frequencies in a sample, in this case, the percentage of women who lose weight on a protein-sparing diet versus the percentage of women who lose weight on a high-protein diet.

8. **The answer is A.** The *t*-test is used to examine differences between means of two samples. This is an example of a paired *t*-test because the same women are examined on two different occasions.

9. **The answer is D.** Correlation is used to examine the relationship between two continuous variables—in this case, systolic blood pressure and body weight.

10. **The answer is D.** The dependent variable is a measure of the outcome of an experiment. In this case, blood pressure following treatment with the drug or placebo is the dependent variable. The independent variable is a characteristic that an experimenter examines to see if it changes the outcome. In this case, giving the patient a drug or placebo is the independent variable.

11. **The answer is C.** With a $P$ value of 0.001 (which is smaller than the preset $\alpha$ level of 0.05), the findings are statistically significant and the researcher can reject the null hypothesis. A type I error occurs when the null hypothesis is rejected, although it is true. A type II error occurs when the null hypothesis is not rejected, although it is false. There is no evidence of a type I or type II error or that the study is biased (see Chapter 25).

12. **The answer is A. 13. The answer is B. 14. The answer is C.** Because of all the low scores, the distribution of these test scores is skewed to the right (positively skewed). Also, the mode (10) of these scores is lower than the mean (35.7), a characteristic of a positively skewed distribution. In a negatively skewed distribution (skewed to the left), the tail is toward the left (i.e., scores cluster toward the high end). In a normal distribution, the mean, median, and mode are equal. When they are sequentially ordered, the median (middle value) of these scores is 20. If the class teaching assistant erred and recorded the grade of one student who got a 10 as 100, the mean would increase to 48.6 and the median would increase to 40; the mode would stay the same at 10.

15. **The answer is B.** It is unlikely that patients will take the new drug (and deal with its side effects) to secure this small reduction (i.e., 0.2 days) in length of outbreaks. Therefore, although these results are statistically significant they are unlikely to be of clinical significance.

16. **The answer is A.** When patients' blood pressures are measured four rather than three times per day, because there is a higher $n$ (i.e., more data points are used to calculate the mean), the standard deviation decreases. However, the increased number of data points does not affect the shape of the curve.

# Comprehensive Examination

**Directions:** Each of the numbered items or incomplete statements in this section is followed by answers or by completions of the statement. Select the **one** lettered answer or completion that is **best** in each case.

**1.** A 34-year-old female police officer comes to the physician for a yearly physical. The officer tells the doctor that she smokes one-half package of cigarettes a day, eats hamburger and steak at least twice a week, and drinks one glass of red wine daily with dinner. She also notes that while she wears a seat belt in the patrol car, she rarely wears a seat belt in her own car. The most important recommendation the doctor can make to modify this patient's long-term mortality risk is to recommend that she

**(A)** stop smoking
**(B)** start using a seat belt regularly
**(C)** reduce red meat in her diet
**(D)** get a different job
**(E)** stop drinking alcohol

**2.** A physician working at a large state college sees a 19-year-old student in the student health service. The student, who started college 1 month ago, tells the doctor that since school started she has been calling home every night. She also notes that she starts crying as soon as her mother answers the phone. She says that while she still enjoys going out occasionally with friends, she misses her family so much that she has not been going to class and is in danger of failing her mid-term exams. There is no previous history of emotional problems and the student denies having suicidal feelings. Physical examination is unremarkable. The most likely explanation for this clinical picture is

**(A)** major depressive disorder
**(B)** adjustment disorder
**(C)** generalized anxiety disorder
**(D)** normal "homesickness"
**(E)** acute stress disorder

**3.** A 48-year-old man who has been employed by a company for the past 2 years believes that, although they deny it, his fellow employees are conspiring to get him fired. He believes that they have wires on his phone and that they follow him home. He frequently checks his home for cameras that he believes his fellow employees have hidden there and insists that his wife also check when he is at work. He denies having auditory hallucinations and, aside from the conspiracy idea, has no evidence of a thought disorder. Which of the following is the most appropriate diagnosis for this man?

**(A)** Paranoid schizophrenia
**(B)** Catatonic schizophrenia
**(C)** Delusional disorder (paranoid type)
**(D)** Paranoid personality disorder
**(E)** Schizoid personality disorder

**4.** A 45-year-old man presents in the emergency room with sinus tachycardia (112/bpm), flattening of T waves, and prolonged QT interval. The patient tells the physician that the previous week he began taking "nerve pills." Which of the following medications is this patient most likely to be taking?

**(A)** Bupropion
**(B)** Fluoxetine
**(C)** Lorazepam
**(D)** Sertraline
**(E)** Imipramine

**5.** A 50-year-old patient, who has had diabetes for the past 3 years, tells his physician that he and his wife are having problems in bed. The physician's most appropriate response to the patient is

**(A)** "Tell me about the problems."
**(B)** "Sexual problems are normal in diabetes."
**(C)** "Sexual problems are common in diabetes."
**(D)** "A sex therapist can be helpful with these problems."
**(E)** "Are the sexual problems affecting your relationship with your wife?"

**6.** Just prior to a serious operation, a 75-year-old patient asks the physician not to put him on life support if he requires it during or after the surgery. The physician agrees to follow the patient's wishes and documents the conversation in the patient's chart. After the surgery, the patient requires life support. The patient's son produces a written will by the patient drafted 2 years previously stating, "Do whatever you can to keep me alive." What should the physician do at this time?

**(A)** Have the hospital chaplain counsel the son
**(B)** Put the patient on life support as the will states
**(C)** Do not put the patient on life support
**(D)** Contact the hospital ethics committee
**(E)** Get a court order to put the patient on life support

**7.** A 76-year-old man whose wife died 1 month ago tells his physician that sometimes he feels that life is not worth living since she died. The patient shows no evidence of psychotic thinking or suicidal plans. He also reports that he sleeps well most nights and that his appetite is normal. Of the following, the most appropriate description of the patient's behavior at this time is

**(A)** adjustment disorder with depression
**(B)** adjustment disorder with anxiety
**(C)** major depressive disorder
**(D)** normal bereavement
**(E)** dysthymic disorder

**8.** A 29-year-old woman who has been brought to the emergency room by a friend tells the physician that she has not slept in 3 days. She says she is staying awake because Jesus and Allah asked her to do a project to bring physics and science into one entity. Her history reveals that she had an episode of depression at the age of 19 but, until last week, showed no other mood episodes or abnormal behavior. The most appropriate diagnosis for this patient at this time is

**(A)** major depressive disorder
**(B)** bipolar I disorder
**(C)** bipolar II disorder
**(D)** brief psychotic disorder
**(E)** schizophrenia

**9.** A 6-year-old child shows seizures, cognitive deficits, and behavior suggestive of autism. The child also shows raised discolored areas on her forehead (forehead plaques). Which of the following chromosomes is most likely to be involved in the etiology of this child's symptoms?

**(A)** 4
**(B)** 11
**(C)** 12
**(D)** 16
**(E)** 21

**10.** The parents of a 10-year-old boy report that he often fights with his brother and sister and has tried to strangle the family cat. His teachers report that he shows problematic behavior at school and was recently found setting a fire in the coat closet. The most likely cause of this picture is

**(A)** oppositional defiant disorder
**(B)** attention deficit hyperactivity disorder
**(C)** problems with his parents
**(D)** conduct disorder
**(E)** adjustment disorder

**11.** An obese 14-year-old boy is brought to the doctor by his mother and his 18-year-old brother. The mother, who cooks all of the family's meals, would like information on how best to prepare food for the boy. His brother, who exercises regularly and is of normal body weight, wants to coach the boy on physical fitness. Most appropriately, the doctor should first talk to

**(A)** the patient alone
**(B)** the mother alone
**(C)** the mother and patient together
**(D)** the patient, mother, and brother together
**(E)** the brother and patient together

**12.** An 18-year-old male patient who has a mental age of 2 years is enrolled in a day care program with other teens who have disabilities. The most likely reason that this patient would not hit the other patients in the day care center is that he would

**(A)** feel badly afterward
**(B)** invoke anger in the teacher
**(C)** not want to hurt them
**(D)** be afraid that they would not like him
**(E)** not want them to hit him back

**13.** While in her teens, a 22-year-old woman had anorexia nervosa for a 5-year period. She has recovered but is now at highest risk for which of the following conditions?

**(A)** Dermatitis
**(B)** Osteoarthritis
**(C)** Amenorrhea
**(D)** Osteoporosis
**(E)** Biliary atresia

**14.** Which of the following agents used to treat patients with Alzheimer disease is not an acetylcholinesterase inhibitor?

**(A)** Galantamine
**(B)** Rivastigmine
**(C)** Memantine
**(D)** Tacrine
**(E)** Donepezil

**15.** An overweight middle-aged woman has just been diagnosed with sleep apnea. Medical examination and laboratory test results are unremarkable. Which of the following is the most appropriate medication to manage sleep apnea in this patient?

**(A)** Diazepam
**(B)** Protriptyline
**(C)** Medroxyprogesterone acetate
**(D)** Imipramine
**(E)** Alprazolam

**16.** During a routine physical examination, a physician discovers that an alert 88-year-old man in a nursing home has bruises on his right leg and right arm but no other medical findings. When the doctor asks the patient about the bruises, the patient says, "At my age what are you going to do about it?" The doctor notes that while speaking with him the patient avoids making eye contact. What is the physician's next step in management?

**(A)** Ask the patient about his relationship with his caretakers
**(B)** Suggest that the staff restrain the patient for his safety
**(C)** Assess the patient to rule out dementia
**(D)** Assess the patient to rule out delirium
**(E)** Write an order to have rails put on the sides of the patient's bed

**17.** A 19-year-old girl who has been at a party is brought to the emergency room after having a seizure. Her blood is positive for alprazolam, cocaine, and marijuana.

Which of the following is most likely to have caused the seizure in this patient?

**(A)** Overdose of alprazolam
**(B)** Overdose of cocaine
**(C)** Overdose of marijuana
**(D)** Withdrawal of alprazolam
**(E)** Withdrawal of cocaine
**(F)** Withdrawal of marijuana

**18.** The mother of a 15-year-old boy who has asthma tells the doctor that the boy refuses to use his inhaler in school. To increase the boy's adherence, the doctor should most appropriately

**(A)** recommend that the mother and the boy go for counseling together
**(B)** explain to the boy that he can die if he does not use the inhaler
**(C)** shift the boy to oral medication
**(D)** instruct the boy to go to the school nurse whenever he has to use his inhaler
**(E)** put the boy in contact with a support group of teens with asthma

**19.** After a 20-year-old woman ingests red wine and aged cheese at a restaurant, she is brought to the emergency department with elevated blood pressure and a severe occipital headache. The type of drug most likely to have caused this clinical picture is

**(A)** an antidepressant agent
**(B)** an antipsychotic agent
**(C)** an antimanic agent
**(D)** a benzodiazepine
**(E)** a barbiturate

**20.** Which of the following patients is at highest risk for suicide?

**(A)** A 55-year-old divorced woman
**(B)** A 55-year-old divorced man
**(C)** A 55-year-old married woman
**(D)** A 55-year-old married man
**(E)** A 55-year-old widowed woman

**21.** Which of the following is most likely to be seen in healthy 50-year-old women in all cultures?

**(A)** The "empty-nest" syndrome
**(B)** Depression
**(C)** Anxiety
**(D)** Insomnia
**(E)** Hot flashes or flushes

**22.** Patients and physicians commonly prefer selective serotonin reuptake inhibitors (SSRIs) to tricyclic antidepressants because SSRIs are more likely to

**(A)** elevate mood
**(B)** work quickly
**(C)** lower blood pressure
**(D)** enhance sleep
**(E)** be well tolerated

**23.** A 28-year-old man who is afraid to drive a car is taught relaxation techniques and is then shown a photograph of a car. Later in treatment, while relaxed, he is exposed to toy cars, then to real cars. Finally, he drives a car. This treatment technique is best described as

**(A)** implosion
**(B)** biofeedback
**(C)** aversive conditioning
**(D)** token economy
**(E)** flooding
**(F)** systematic desensitization
**(G)** cognitive therapy

**24.** A 59-year-old male patient has just recovered from a myocardial infarction. During a follow-up examination he asks the physician what is the best position for sexual intercourse with his wife. The physician's best recommendation is

**(A)** face to face, lying on their sides
**(B)** face to face, female superior
**(C)** face to face, male superior
**(D)** male behind female, lying on their sides
**(E)** avoid sexual activity for at least 1 year

**25.** A mildly demented 83-year-old man is brought to the emergency department by his daughter, with whom he lives. He smells of urine, is undernourished, and has bruises on both of his arms and abrasions on one wrist. He seems fearful but denies that anyone has harmed him. The most appropriate first action for the physician to take after treating the patient is to

**(A)** speak to the daughter about the possibility that the man has been abused
**(B)** send him home with his daughter as soon as possible
**(C)** contact the appropriate state social service agency
**(D)** order a neurologic evaluation
**(E)** release the patient into the care of another relative

**26.** Of the following, the ethnic group with the longest life expectancy is

**(A)** Hispanic Americans
**(B)** African Americans
**(C)** White Americans
**(D)** Native Americans

**27.** In the United States, which of the following is the most common belief concerning mental illness?

**(A)** It is therapeutic to discuss your internal emotional problems with others.
**(B)** Mental illness signifies personal weakness.
**(C)** Unconscious conflicts can be manifested as physical illness.
**(D)** Mentally ill people have good self-control.
**(E)** Mentally ill people usually seek help.

**28.** A 60-year-old woman presents with chronic headaches. During the interview, she states that the headaches started 3 years ago when her neighbors began to come into her home and harass her at night. The patient has no history of psychiatric illness and physical examination is unremarkable. She has good social and work relationships and, except for her comments about the neighbors, her thoughts seem clear, logical, and appropriate. At this time, the most appropriate diagnosis for this woman is

**(A)** schizophrenia
**(B)** bipolar disorder
**(C)** delusional disorder
**(D)** schizoaffective disorder
**(E)** schizoid personality disorder

**29.** A 26-year-old woman believes that she is pregnant with Ashton Kutcher's child. She has never met the actor and two pregnancy tests are negative. There is no other evidence of a thought disorder. The most appropriate diagnosis for this woman is

**(A)** schizophrenia
**(B)** bipolar disorder
**(C)** delusional disorder
**(D)** somatization disorder
**(E)** schizoid personality disorder

**30.** A 40-year-old woman goes to her gynecologist for a yearly checkup. Which of the following is most likely to cause death in a woman of this age?

(A) Pregnancy and childbirth
(B) An intrauterine device
(C) Oral contraceptives
(D) Barrier contraceptives
(E) A progesterone implant

**31.** A 29-year-old physician with severe psoriasis on his hands and arms asks a colleague how he should deal with the reactions of patients when they notice his condition. The colleague's best response is

(A) "Act like nothing is wrong."
(B) "Wear long-sleeved shirts."
(C) "Reassure patients that the skin condition you have is not contagious."
(D) "See as few patients as possible."
(E) "Tell patient's that it is your problem, not theirs."

**32.** The usual standards of doctor–patient confidentiality are most likely to apply to which of the following patients?

(A) A man who tells his physician that he plans to shoot his partner
(B) A recently bereaved woman who tells her physician that she has had occasional thoughts of suicide
(C) A man who tells his physician that he has been sexually abusing his 10-year-old stepdaughter
(D) An HIV-positive man who is engaging in sexual intercourse with his wife without using condoms
(E) A depressed woman who tells her physician that she has saved up 50 barbiturate tablets and wants to die

**33.** Doctor A is aware that doctor B has made a serious mistake in treating a very ill hospitalized patient. Doctor B refuses to admit that he has made a mistake. Most appropriately, Doctor A should

(A) talk to Doctor B again about his mistake
(B) warn Doctor B that he will be reported if he continues to make mistakes
(C) report Doctor B's action to Doctor B's superior at the hospital
(D) report Doctor B's action to the police
(E) recommend that Doctor B be transferred to another hospital

**34.** To follow improvement or deterioration over time in a 70-year-old patient with suspected neurologic dysfunction, which of the following is the most appropriate test?

(A) Positron emission tomography (PET)
(B) Computed tomography (CT)
(C) Amobarbital sodium (Amytal) interview
(D) Thematic Apperception Test (TAT)
(E) Electroencephalogram (EEG)
(F) Wide Range Achievement Test (WRAT)
(G) Folstein Mini-mental State Examination
(H) Glasgow Coma Scale

**35.** To evaluate unconscious conflicts in a 20-year-old man using drawings depicting ambiguous social situations, which of the following is the most appropriate test?

(A) Positron emission tomography (PET)
(B) Computed tomography (CT)
(C) Amobarbital sodium (Amytal) interview
(D) Thematic Apperception Test (TAT)
(E) Electroencephalogram (EEG)
(F) Wide Range Achievement Test (WRAT)
(G) Folstein Mini-mental State Examination
(H) Glasgow Coma Scale

**36.** An infant's ability to roll over from back to belly and belly to back usually begins at what age?

(A) 0–3 months
(B) 4–6 months
(C) 7–10 months
(D) 12–15 months
(E) 16–30 months

**37.** A patient in the emergency department has just been involved in a car accident. The physician suspects that she has been drinking. In most states the lowest blood alcohol concentration (BAC) to meet the criterion for legal intoxication falls into which of the following ranges?

(A) 0.01%–0.02%
(B) 0.05%–0.15%
(C) 0.40%–0.50%
(D) 1.5%–2.0%
(E) 2.5%–3.0%

**38.** Of the following agents, which is the most appropriate heterocyclic antidepressant for a 45-year-old air traffic controller who must stay alert on the job?

**(A)** Selegilene
**(B)** Tranylcypromine
**(C)** Trazodone
**(D)** Doxepin
**(E)** Amoxapine
**(F)** Fluoxetine
**(G)** Protriptyline
**(H)** Nortriptyline
**(I)** Amitriptyline
**(J)** Imipramine

**39.** A 79-year-old woman reports that she has difficulty sleeping through the night because of persistent muscular contractions in her legs. Which of the following sleep disorders best matches this picture?

**(A)** Kleine–Levin syndrome
**(B)** Nightmare disorder
**(C)** Sleep terror disorder
**(D)** Sleep drunkenness
**(E)** Circadian rhythm sleep disorder
**(F)** Nocturnal myoclonus
**(G)** Restless legs syndrome

**40.** A pilot whose plane is about to crash spends 5 minutes explaining the technical details of the engine malfunction to his copilot. The defense mechanism that the pilot is using is

**(A)** repression
**(B)** sublimation
**(C)** dissociation
**(D)** regression
**(E)** intellectualization

**41.** Most typical children begin to walk without assistance at what age?

**(A)** 0–3 months
**(B)** 4–6 months
**(C)** 7–10 months
**(D)** 12–15 months
**(E)** 16–30 months

**42.** A 40-year-old woman with tension headaches has the tension in the frontalis muscle measured regularly. The readings are projected to her on a computer screen. She is then taught to use mental techniques to decrease tension in this muscle. Which of the following treatment techniques does this example illustrate?

**(A)** Implosion
**(B)** Biofeedback
**(C)** Aversive conditioning
**(D)** Token economy
**(E)** Flooding
**(F)** Systemic desensitization
**(G)** Cognitive therapy

**43.** A patient reports that despite the fact that he goes to sleep at 11:00 PM and wakes up at 7:00 AM, he does not feel fully awake until about noon each day. His wife states that he appears to be sleeping soundly at night. The patient denies substance abuse and physical examination is normal. Which of the following sleep disorders best matches this clinical picture?

**(A)** Kleine–Levin syndrome
**(B)** Nightmare disorder
**(C)** Sleep terror disorder
**(D)** Sleep drunkenness
**(E)** Circadian rhythm sleep disorder
**(F)** Nocturnal myoclonus
**(G)** Restless legs syndrome

**44.** A 33-year-old patient tells the physician that he drinks at least 10 cups of coffee per day. Of the following effects, which is most likely in this patient?

**(A)** Blood pressure reduction
**(B)** Lethargy
**(C)** Tachycardia
**(D)** Decreased gastric acid secretion
**(E)** Depressed mood

**45.** The social smile commonly first appears at what age in typical infants?

**(A)** 0–3 months
**(B)** 4–6 months
**(C)** 7–10 months
**(D)** 12–15 months
**(E)** 16–30 months

**46.** To evaluate reading and arithmetic skills in a 30-year-old hospitalized male patient, which of the following is the most appropriate test?

**(A)** Positron emission tomography (PET)
**(B)** Computed tomography (CT)
**(C)** Amobarbital sodium (Amytal) interview
**(D)** Thematic Apperception Test (TAT)
**(E)** Electroencephalogram (EEG)
**(F)** Wide Range Achievement Test (WRAT)
**(G)** Folstein Mini-mental State Examination
**(H)** Glasgow Coma Scale

**47.** The EEG of a 32-year-old sleeping patient shows mainly slow waves. What stage of sleep is this patient most likely to be in?

**(A)** Stage 1
**(B)** Stage 2
**(C)** Delta
**(D)** REM

**48.** Typical infants begin visually following faces and objects with their eyes (tracking) at what age?

**(A)** 0–3 months
**(B)** 4–6 months
**(C)** 7–10 months
**(D)** 12–15 months
**(E)** 16–30 months

**49.** A 65-year-old physician who has been given a diagnosis of terminal pancreatic cancer repeatedly discusses the technical aspects of his case with other physicians in the hospital. The defense mechanism that this physician is using is

**(A)** acting out
**(B)** sublimation
**(C)** denial
**(D)** regression
**(E)** intellectualization
**(F)** reaction formation

**50.** An anxious, depressed teenager, who has never been in trouble before, steals a car. The defense mechanism that this teenager is using to manage his anxiety and depression is most likely to be

**(A)** acting out
**(B)** sublimation
**(C)** denial
**(D)** regression
**(E)** intellectualization
**(F)** reaction formation

**51.** A 50-year-old hospitalized patient has just received a diagnosis of breast cancer. She states that the biopsy was in error and checks out of the hospital against the advice of her physician. The defense mechanism that this patient is using is

**(A)** acting out
**(B)** sublimation
**(C)** denial
**(D)** regression
**(E)** intellectualization
**(F)** reaction formation

**52.** A patient, although she is unconsciously angry at her physician because he canceled her previous appointment at the last minute, tells him at her next appointment that she really likes his tie. The defense mechanism that this patient is using is

**(A)** acting out
**(B)** sublimation
**(C)** denial
**(D)** regression
**(E)** intellectualization
**(F)** reaction formation

**53.** A 28-year-old woman, who works as an animal caretaker, lives with her elderly aunt and rarely socializes. She reports that, although she would like to have friends, when coworkers ask her to join them for breaks, she refuses because she is afraid that they will not like her. This behavior is most closely associated with which of the following personality disorders?

**(A)** Passive-aggressive personality disorder
**(B)** Schizotypal personality disorder
**(C)** Antisocial personality disorder
**(D)** Paranoid personality disorder
**(E)** Schizoid personality disorder
**(F)** Obsessive-compulsive personality disorder
**(G)** Avoidant personality disorder
**(H)** Histrionic personality disorder

**54.** A 35-year-old man comes to the physician's office dressed all in bright yellow. He reports that he felt like he had "a knife in his ear" and says that he is "burning up" and "must be dying." Physical examination reveals mild otitis externa (inflammation of the ear canal) and temperature of 99.6°F. This patient's behavior is most closely associated with which of the following personality disorders?

**(A)** Passive-aggressive personality disorder
**(B)** Schizotypal personality disorder
**(C)** Antisocial personality disorder
**(D)** Paranoid personality disorder
**(E)** Schizoid personality disorder
**(F)** Obsessive-compulsive personality disorder
**(G)** Avoidant personality disorder
**(H)** Histrionic personality disorder

**55.** A 24-year-old patient is experiencing intense hunger as well as tiredness and headache. This patient is most likely to be withdrawing from which of the following agents?

**(A)** Alcohol
**(B)** Secobarbital
**(C)** Phencyclidine (PCP)
**(D)** Amphetamine
**(E)** Lysergic acid diethylamide (LSD)
**(F)** Diazepam
**(G)** Heroin
**(H)** Marijuana

**56.** A 55-year-old man, who has been taking medications for depression and insomnia, is brought to the emergency department with signs of severe respiratory depression. The agent most likely to be responsible for these symptoms is

**(A)** alcohol
**(B)** secobarbital
**(C)** phencyclidine (PCP)
**(D)** amphetamine
**(E)** lysergic acid diethylamide (LSD)
**(F)** diazepam
**(G)** heroin
**(H)** marijuana

**57.** The police bring a 25-year-old man to the hospital in a coma. His girlfriend tells the physician that prior to having a seizure and fainting, he became combative, showed abnormal eye movements, and said that he felt his body expanding and floating up to the ceiling. Of the following, the drug most likely to be responsible for these symptoms is

**(A)** alcohol
**(B)** secobarbital
**(C)** phencyclidine (PCP)
**(D)** amphetamine
**(E)** lysergic acid diethylamide (LSD)
**(F)** diazepam
**(G)** heroin
**(H)** marijuana

**58.** A patient who has been a heavy coffee drinker is hospitalized and not permitted to take anything except water by mouth. Which of the following is the patient most likely to demonstrate the day after hospitalization?

**(A)** Excitement
**(B)** Euphoria
**(C)** Headache
**(D)** Decreased appetite
**(E)** Pupil dilation

**59.** A 50-year-old female stroke patient opens her eyes in response to a verbal command, speaks but uses inappropriate words, and shows flexion to painful stimulus. For these responses she receives a test score of 9. Which of the following is most likely to be the test that was used?

**(A)** Positron emission tomography (PET)
**(B)** Computed tomography (CT)
**(C)** Amobarbital sodium (Amytal) interview
**(D)** Thematic Apperception Test (TAT)
**(E)** Electroencephalogram (EEG)
**(F)** Wide Range Achievement Test (WRAT)
**(G)** Folstein Mini-mental State Examination
**(H)** Glasgow Coma Scale

**60.** The electroencephalogram of a 28-year-old patient shows mainly alpha waves. This patient is most likely to be

**(A)** awake and concentrating
**(B)** awake, relaxed, with eyes closed
**(C)** in Stage 1 sleep
**(D)** in delta sleep
**(E)** in REM sleep

**61.** A 24-year-old woman experiences pelvic pain when she and her boyfriend attempt to have sexual intercourse. No abnormalities are found during pelvic examination. The most appropriate diagnosis for this patient is

(A) fetishism
(B) functional vaginismus
(C) sexual aversion disorder
(D) orgasmic disorder
(E) functional dyspareunia
(F) female sexual arousal disorder
(G) hypoactive sexual desire

**62.** A 65-year-old woman whose husband died three weeks ago reports that she cries much of the time and sleeps poorly. Also, she states that although she knows her husband is dead, she thought that she saw him walking down the street the day before. The most appropriate first action by her physician is to

(A) recommend that she visit a close relative
(B) provide support and reassurance
(C) prescribe antipsychotic medication
(D) prescribe antidepressant medication
(E) recommend a psychiatric evaluation

**63.** Which of the following individuals has the highest risk for developing schizophrenia?

(A) The dizygotic twin of a person with schizophrenia
(B) The child of two parents with schizophrenia
(C) The monozygotic twin of a person with schizophrenia
(D) The child of one parent with schizophrenia
(E) A child raised in an institutional setting when neither biological parent had schizophrenia

**64.** Which of the following statements is most likely to be evidence of psychotic features in a severely depressed 49-year-old man?

(A) "I am an inadequate person."
(B) "I am a worthless human being."
(C) "I will never get better."
(D) "I am a failure in my profession."
(E) "I am personally responsible for the Tsunami in Japan."

**65.** After a life-threatening bicycle accident, a 9-year-old child requires an immediate blood transfusion. If, for religious reasons, the parents refuse to allow the transfusion, the physician should

(A) tell the parents they will be prosecuted if they do not allow the transfusion
(B) give the child the transfusion
(C) obtain permission from another family member to do the transfusion
(D) have the child moved to another hospital
(E) follow the parents' instructions and do not give the child the transfusion

**66.** A patient states that ever since a long-time lover called to break up their relationship, the patient has had a severe hearing loss. No medical explanation can be found. Which of the following is most likely to be true about this patient?

(A) The patient is old.
(B) The patient is male.
(C) The patient is well educated.
(D) The patient's hearing loss appeared suddenly.
(E) The patient is very upset about the hearing loss.

**67.** Long-term psychiatric hospitals in the United States are owned and operated primarily by

(A) universities
(B) private investors
(C) state governments
(D) municipal governments
(E) the federal government

**68.** A 60-year-old janitor from New York, whose wife died recently, is found in Akron, Ohio, working as a salesman. He does not know how he arrived there and physical examination is unremarkable. Of the following, the most appropriate diagnosis for this man is

(A) dissociative amnesia
(B) dissociative fugue
(C) somatization disorder
(D) conversion disorder
(E) depersonalization disorder

**69.** Which of the following conditions commonly first becomes apparent in the fourth or fifth decade of life?

(A) Dementia of the Alzheimer type
(B) Lesch-Nyhan syndrome
(C) Rett disorder
(D) Tourette disorder
(E) Huntington disease

**70.** During an ophthalmologic examination, a 48-year-old female patient, who has had schizophrenia for more than 30 years, is found to have retinal pigmentation. In the past, this patient is most likely to have taken which one of the following antipsychotic agents?

(A) Chlorpromazine
(B) Haloperidol
(C) Perphenazine
(D) Trifluoperazine
(E) Thioridazine

**71.** A typical 24-year-old woman who is in non-REM sleep is most likely to show which of the following?

(A) Dreaming
(B) Increased pulse
(C) Clitoral erection
(D) Skeletal muscle relaxation
(E) Delta waves on the electroencephalogram

**72.** Of the following disorders, the one most likely to show the largest sex difference in its occurrence is

(A) cyclothymic disorder
(B) major depressive disorder
(C) bipolar disorder
(D) hypochondriasis
(E) schizophrenia

**73.** Negative predictive value is the probability that a person with a

(A) negative test is actually well
(B) positive test is actually well
(C) negative test is actually ill
(D) positive test is actually ill
(E) positive test will eventually show signs of the illness

**74.** In a laboratory study, it is shown that the uterus rises in the pelvic cavity during sexual activity. In which stage of the sexual response cycle does this phenomenon first occur?

(A) Excitement
(B) Plateau
(C) Orgasm
(D) Emission
(E) Resolution

**75.** A married couple tells the physician that their sex life has been poor because the husband ejaculates too quickly. The physician tells them that the "squeeze technique" would be helpful. In this technique, the person who applies the "squeeze" is usually

(A) the husband
(B) the wife
(C) the physician
(D) a sex therapist
(E) a sex surrogate

**76.** Which of the following statistical tests is most appropriately used to evaluate differences among mean body weights of women in three different age groups?

(A) Dependent (paired) $t$-test
(B) Chi-square test
(C) Analysis of variance
(D) Independent (unpaired) $t$-test
(E) Fisher's exact test

**77.** A 39-year-old man (who has never before had problems with erections) begins to have difficulty achieving an erection during sexual activity with his wife. The very first time he had trouble maintaining an erection was after a beach party when he had "too much to drink." This man is showing evidence of which of the following sexual dysfunctions?

(A) Primary erectile dysfunction
(B) Secondary erectile dysfunction
(C) Sexual aversion disorder
(D) Orgasmic disorder
(E) Dyspareunia
(F) Hypoactive sexual desire

**78.** A study was carried out to determine whether exposure to liquid crystal display (LCD) computer screens in the first trimester of pregnancy results in miscarriage. To do this, 50 women who had miscarriages and 90 women who carried to term were questioned the day after miscarriage or delivery, respectively, about their exposure to LCDs during pregnancy. If 10 women who had miscarriages and 10 women who carried to term used LCDs during their pregnancies, the odds–risk ratio associated with LCDs in pregnancy is approximately

(A) 2
(B) 3
(C) 10
(D) 20
(E) 100

**79.** In a cohort study, the ratio of the incidence rate of miscarriage among women who use liquid crystal display (LCD) computer screens to the incidence rate of miscarriage among women who do not use LCD computer screens is the

(A) attributable risk
(B) odds–risk ratio
(C) incidence rate
(D) prevalence ratio
(E) relative risk

**Questions 80 and 81**

In a study, the incidence rate of tuberculosis (TB) in people who have someone with TB living in their home is 5 per 1,000. The incidence rate of TB in people who have no one with TB living in their home is 0.5 per 1,000.

**80.** What is the risk for getting TB attributable to living with someone who has TB (attributable risk)?

(A) 1.5
(B) 4.5
(C) 7.5
(D) 9.5
(E) 10.0

**81.** How many times higher is the risk of getting TB for people who live with a patient with TB than for people who do not live with a TB patient (the relative risk)?

(A) 1.5
(B) 4.5
(C) 7.5
(D) 9.5
(E) 10.0

**82.** To estimate the relative risk in a case-control study, which of the following is calculated?

(A) Attributable risk
(B) Odds–risk ratio
(C) Incidence rate
(D) Prevalence ratio
(E) Sensitivity

**83.** A 50-year-old female high school teacher who had been of normal weight reports that she has been "feeling very low" for the past 3 months. She often misses work because she feels tired and hopeless, has lost 15 pounds without dieting, and has trouble sleeping. When the physician interviews her she says, "Doctor, the Lord calls all his children home." This clinical picture is most closely associated with

(A) cyclothymic disorder
(B) major depressive disorder
(C) bipolar disorder
(D) hypochondriasis
(E) schizophrenia

**84.** A 32-year-old man survives a plane crash in which four passengers died. Two weeks later he reports that he has recurring nightmares about the crash and feels isolated and distant from others. This patient is most likely to have which of the following disorders?

(A) Post-traumatic stress disorder (PTSD)
(B) Generalized anxiety disorder
(C) Obsessive-compulsive disorder (OCD)
(D) Panic disorder
(E) Acute stress disorder

**85.** One year after she was robbed at knife-point in the street, a 28-year-old woman jumps at every loud noise, has recurrent thoughts about the robbery, and is anxious much of the time. Of the following, the best diagnosis for this patient is

(A) post-traumatic stress disorder (PTSD)
(B) generalized anxiety disorder
(C) obsessive-compulsive disorder (OCD)
(D) panic disorder
(E) acute stress disorder

**86.** At the close of a long interview with an elderly male patient, the physician says, "Let's see if I have taken all of the information correctly," and then sums up the information that the patient has given. This interviewing technique is known as

**(A)** confrontation
**(B)** validation
**(C)** recapitulation
**(D)** facilitation
**(E)** reflection
**(F)** direct question
**(G)** support

**87.** "Many people feel the way you do when they first need hospitalization" is an example of the interview technique known as

**(A)** confrontation
**(B)** validation
**(C)** recapitulation
**(D)** facilitation
**(E)** reflection
**(F)** direct question
**(G)** support

**88.** After a patient has described his symptoms and the time of day that they intensify, the interviewer says, "You say that you felt the pain more in the evening?" This question is an example of the interview technique known as

**(A)** confrontation
**(B)** validation
**(C)** recapitulation
**(D)** facilitation
**(E)** reflection
**(F)** direct question
**(G)** support

**89.** "You say that you are not nervous, but you are sweating and shaking and seem very upset to me" is an example of the interviewing technique known as

**(A)** confrontation
**(B)** validation
**(C)** recapitulation
**(D)** facilitation
**(E)** reflection
**(F)** direct question
**(G)** support

**90.** A patient relates to the physician, "If I am seated at a table in the center of a restaurant rather than against the wall, I sud-

denly get dizzy and feel like I cannot breathe." This patient is describing a(n)

**(A)** hallucination
**(B)** delusion
**(C)** illusion
**(D)** panic attack with agoraphobia
**(E)** social phobia

**91.** A patient relates to the physician, "Last week, I thought I saw my father who died last year go around the corner, but I know it wasn't really him." This patient is describing a(n)

**(A)** hallucination
**(B)** delusion
**(C)** illusion
**(D)** panic attack with agoraphobia
**(E)** social phobia

**92.** The most appropriate method to determine the part of the brain used during the translation of a written passage from French to English is

**(A)** computed tomography (CT)
**(B)** dexamethasone suppression test (DST)
**(C)** evoked potentials
**(D)** electroencephalogram (EEG)
**(E)** galvanic skin response
**(F)** positron emission tomography (PET)

**93.** The most appropriate diagnostic technique to evaluate hearing loss in a 3-month-old infant is

**(A)** computed tomography (CT)
**(B)** dexamethasone suppression test (DST)
**(C)** evoked potentials
**(D)** electroencephalogram (EEG)
**(E)** galvanic skin response
**(F)** positron emission tomography (PET)

**94.** A 42-year-old woman pretends that she is paralyzed following an automobile accident in order to collect money from the insurance company. This woman is demonstrating

**(A)** psychogenic fugue
**(B)** derealization
**(C)** factitious disorder
**(D)** malingering
**(E)** conversion disorder
**(F)** multiple personality disorder
**(G)** depersonalization disorder
**(H)** body dysmorphic disorder

**95.** A 42-year-old woman pretends that she is paralyzed following an automobile accident in order to gain attention from her physician. This patient is demonstrating

**(A)** psychogenic fugue
**(B)** derealization
**(C)** factitious disorder
**(D)** malingering
**(E)** conversion disorder
**(F)** multiple personality disorder
**(G)** depersonalization disorder
**(H)** body dysmorphic disorder

**96.** A 54-year-old woman who is depressed awakens at 4:00 AM every morning and cannot fall back asleep. She is then tired all day. This woman is most likely to have which of the following sleep disorders?

**(A)** Narcolepsy
**(B)** Kleine–Levin syndrome
**(C)** Insomnia
**(D)** Obstructive sleep apnea
**(E)** Sleep terror disorder

**97.** A 40-year-old woman who is overweight reports that she feels tired all day despite having 9 hours of sleep each night. The woman's partner reports that she snores loudly. This woman is showing evidence of

**(A)** narcolepsy
**(B)** Kleine–Levin syndrome
**(C)** insomnia
**(D)** obstructive sleep apnea
**(E)** sleep terror disorder

**98.** Following the loss of her job as a cashier, a 23-year-old patient reports, in a dispassionate way, that she has no sensation in her right arm. Physical examination fails to reveal evidence of a physiological problem. This patient is showing evidence of

**(A)** hypochondriasis
**(B)** body dysmorphic disorder
**(C)** conversion disorder
**(D)** somatization disorder
**(E)** somatoform pain disorder

**99.** Despite the physician's reassurances and negative biopsies of five different moles, a 45-year-old patient appears very worried and tells the physician that he believes that his remaining moles should be biopsied because they are "probably melanomas." This patient is showing evidence of

**(A)** hypochondriasis
**(B)** body dysmorphic disorder
**(C)** conversion disorder
**(D)** somatization disorder
**(E)** somatoform pain disorder

**100.** A dog learns to turn a doorknob with its teeth because this behavior has been rewarded with a treat. This is an example of the type of learning best described as

**(A)** operant conditioning
**(B)** aversive conditioning
**(C)** spontaneous recovery
**(D)** modeling
**(E)** stimulus generalization

**101.** Each time a 35-year-old man receives physical therapy for a shoulder injury, his pain lessens. Because of this improvement in pain, the patient returns for more physical therapy sessions. This patient's increase in physical therapy sessions is an example of which of the following?

**(A)** Implosion
**(B)** Stimulus generalization
**(C)** Systematic desensitization
**(D)** Flooding
**(E)** Positive reinforcement
**(F)** Fixed ratio reinforcement
**(G)** Negative reinforcement

**102.** A 75-year-old woman who lives alone develops a high fever and is brought to the hospital by a neighbor. Although the woman can state her name, she is not oriented to place or time and mistakes the nursing assistant for her nephew. This clinical picture is most consistent with

**(A)** depression (pseudodementia)
**(B)** Tourette disorder
**(C)** dementia of the Alzheimer type
**(D)** delirium
**(E)** amnestic disorder (Korsakoff syndrome)

**103.** A 19-year-old man is brought to the hospital by the police. The policeman states that when stopped for a minor traffic violation, the man cursed at him and showed bizarre grimacing and twitching movements. This young man is showing evidence of

(A) depression (pseudodementia)
(B) Tourette disorder
(C) dementia of the Alzheimer type
(D) delirium
(E) amnestic disorder (Korsakoff syndrome)

**104.** A 63-year-old female patient, who has been having memory problems for the past year, now cannot identify the man sitting next to her (her husband). Physical examination is unremarkable and there is no history of drug or alcohol abuse. The patient is alert and seems to be paying attention to the physician. This patient is most likely to have

(A) depression (pseudodementia)
(B) Tourette disorder
(C) dementia of the Alzheimer type
(D) delirium
(E) amnestic disorder (Korsakoff syndrome)

**105.** A dying patient tells his physician, "I will go to church every day if only I can get rid of this illness." This statement indicates that the patient is in which of the following stages of dying?

(A) Denial
(B) Anger
(C) Bargaining
(D) Depression
(E) Acceptance

**106.** A mother puts a bitter substance on her 9-year-old son's fingernails in order to break his nail-biting habit. This is an example of the type of learning best described as

(A) operant conditioning
(B) aversive conditioning
(C) spontaneous recovery
(D) modeling
(E) stimulus generalization

**107.** A 29-year-old woman comes to the physician with symptoms of anxiety which have been present for over 2 years and have no obvious precipitating event. The patient has never previously taken an antianxiety agent. Of the following psychoactive agents, the best choice for this woman is

(A) diazepam (Valium)
(B) haloperidol (Haldol)
(C) fluoxetine (Prozac)
(D) buspirone (BuSpar)
(E) lithium

**108.** "Head Start," an early-intervention enrichment program for disadvantaged preschoolers, is aimed at reducing the likelihood of failure in grade school. "Head Start" is an example of

(A) primary prevention
(B) secondary prevention
(C) tertiary prevention
(D) systematic desensitization
(E) behavior modification

**109.** The basic defense mechanism on which all others are based, and which is used to prevent unacceptable emotions from reaching awareness, is known as

(A) repression
(B) sublimation
(C) dissociation
(D) regression
(E) intellectualization

**110.** In telling a physician about her younger sister's death in a car accident, a 33-year-old woman tries to speak but keeps breaking into tears. The most appropriate statement for the physician to make at this point is

(A) "It is sad but everybody loses a loved one at some time."
(B) "Don't cry, you will feel better in a few months."
(C) "You must feel terrible about her death."
(D) "She was too young to die."
(E) "Please take your time."

**111.** The parents of a 17-year-old young woman with Down syndrome and an intelligence quotient (IQ) of 70 bring her in for a school physical. The physical is required for admission to a highly recommended special education co-ed boarding school. The parents are worried about sending their daughter to the school because she is sexually active and they are afraid that she will get pregnant. Although she has been on oral contraceptives for the past year, her mother must often remind her to take them. The parents ask for the physician's advice. The physician's most appropriate recommendation is to

**(A)** do a tubal ligation
**(B)** do an oophorectomy
**(C)** enroll her in a local day school so that she can live at home
**(D)** prescribe a long-acting contraceptive
**(E)** send her to the boarding school and take no further action

**112.** A 6-year-old child with an intelligence quotient (IQ) of 50 is most likely to be able to do which of the following?

**(A)** Read a sentence
**(B)** Identify colors
**(C)** Copy a triangle
**(D)** Ride a two-wheeled bicycle
**(E)** Understand the moral difference between right and wrong

**113.** A physician diagnoses genital herpes in a 16-year-old male high school student. Prior to treating him, the physician should

**(A)** notify his parents
**(B)** get permission from his parents
**(C)** notify his sexual partner(s)
**(D)** recommend that he tell his sexual partner(s)
**(E)** notify the appropriate state agency

**114.** A 9-month-old infant is brought to a pediatrician by his mother. The child can sit unassisted and pull himself up to stand. He babbles and makes noises when his mother speaks to him but he cannot say any words. The mother tells the physician that when the child sees his baby-sitter on Saturday nights, he cries and refuses to go to her. With respect to physical, social, and cognitive/verbal development, respectively, this child is best described as

**(A)** normal, normal, needs evaluation
**(B)** normal, needs evaluation, normal

**(C)** needs evaluation, normal, normal
**(D)** needs evaluation, needs evaluation, normal
**(E)** normal, normal, normal
**(F)** needs evaluation, needs evaluation, needs evaluation
**(G)** normal, needs evaluation, needs evaluation

**115.** A typical boy can walk up stairs 1 foot at a time, but when told to copy a circle, he just scribbles on paper. At the playground, he often moves away from his mother to watch the other children, but then comes right back to her. With respect to verbal skills, this child is most likely to be able to

**(A)** speak in complete sentences
**(B)** use about 900 words
**(C)** use prepositions
**(D)** understand about 3,500 words
**(E)** use about 10 words

**116.** As a 60-year-old male patient is leaving the hospital after surgery for prostate cancer, he turns to the physician and says, "You know doctor, I have a gun in my house." The most appropriate action for the physician to take at this time is to

**(A)** call the patient's wife and tell her to find the gun and remove it
**(B)** suggest that the patient remain in the hospital for further evaluation
**(C)** give the patient a prescription for an antidepressant
**(D)** warn the patient about taking medications that are dangerous in overdose
**(E)** release the patient from the hospital as planned

**117.** A bond trader states that sometimes he makes money and sometimes he loses money. The trader complains that he is so preoccupied with trading bonds that he cannot seem to stop following the bond markets, even on weekends when the markets are closed. Which of the following is most likely to have influenced this trader's preoccupation with trading bonds?

**(A)** Continuous reinforcement
**(B)** Fixed ratio reinforcement
**(C)** Fixed interval reinforcement
**(D)** Variable ratio reinforcement
**(E)** Stimulus generalization

**118.** A mother brings her 3-year-old son to the pediatrician for a well-child checkup. The physician observes that the child relates well to his mother and is able to speak in complete sentences. In speaking to the mother, the physician determines that the child has a tricycle but cannot pedal it, and he does not play cooperatively with other children. Select the best description of this child's development in language, motor, and social skills, respectively.

**(A)** Typical, typical, needs evaluation
**(B)** Typical, needs evaluation, typical
**(C)** Needs evaluation, typical, typical
**(D)** Needs evaluation, needs evaluation, typical
**(E)** Typical, typical, typical
**(F)** Needs evaluation, needs evaluation, needs evaluation
**(G)** Typical, needs evaluation, needs evaluation

**119.** A 14-year-old boy tells his physician that he is concerned because he masturbates everyday. He is doing well in school and is the captain of the school debating team. The physician's next move should be to

**(A)** notify his parents
**(B)** refer him to an adolescent psychologist
**(C)** reassure him that his behavior is normal
**(D)** tell him to become more involved in school sports
**(E)** measure his level of circulating testosterone

**120.** A 49-year-old sexually active woman tells her physician that she is experiencing hot flashes and has not menstruated in four months. She asks the physician when she can discontinue the use of birth control. The physician's most correct response is

**(A)** 6 months after the last menstrual period
**(B)** 1 year after the last menstrual period
**(C)** after age 55
**(D)** immediately
**(E)** when the hot flashes subside

**121.** Whenever a new child is admitted to the pediatrics floor, an 8-year-old girl, who has been hospitalized for more than 2 months, calms the fearful child by drawing pictures with him or her. This behavior by the 8-year-old is an example of her use of which of the following defense mechanisms?

**(A)** Repression
**(B)** Sublimation
**(C)** Dissociation
**(D)** Regression
**(E)** Intellectualization

**122.** Of the following people, which one is likely to use the most Medicare services and funds during his or her lifetime?

**(A)** African-American male smoker
**(B)** African-American female smoker
**(C)** African-American male nonsmoker
**(D)** African-American female nonsmoker
**(E)** White male smoker
**(F)** White female smoker
**(G)** White male nonsmoker
**(H)** White female nonsmoker

**123.** A child uses about 900 individual words, can stack nine blocks, and does well in a preschool program each day. This child's age is most likely to be

**(A)** 8 months
**(B)** 12 months
**(C)** 18 months
**(D)** 36 months
**(E)** 48 months

**124.** Of the following, the most likely reason for a physician to be sued for malpractice is that the physician

**(A)** prescribed a medication incorrectly
**(B)** had poor rapport with a patient
**(C)** did an unsuccessful surgical procedure
**(D)** cancelled an appointment with a patient
**(E)** made a poor medical decision

**125.** A 65-year-old woman signs a document that gives her neighbor durable power of attorney. Five days later she has a stroke, enters a vegetative state from which she will never recover, and requires life support. The most appropriate action for the physician to take at this time with respect to life support is to

**(A)** get a court order to continue life support
**(B)** follow the wishes of the neighbor
**(C)** not provide life support
**(D)** follow the wishes of the woman's adult children
**(E)** turn the case over to the ethics committee of the hospital

**126.** An elderly American woman is most likely to spend most of the last 5 years of her life

(A) in a nursing home
(B) with family
(C) on her own
(D) in a hospice
(E) in a hospital

**127.** The husband of an 85-year-old patient with Alzheimer disease tells the physician that he wants to keep his wife at home but is worried because the patient keeps wandering out the front door of the house. Of the following, the most appropriate recommendation for the physician to make at this time is to

(A) place the patient in restraints
(B) label all the doors as to their function
(C) prescribe diazepam (Valium)
(D) prescribe donepezil (Aricept)
(E) place the patient in a nursing home

**128.** An 8-year-old child with normal intelligence reads, communicates well, and gets along well with the other children in school. However, he often argues with the teacher and gets bad marks for his behavior. His parents tell the physician that he often also seems angry toward them and rarely follows their rules. The best description for this child's behavior is

(A) typical
(B) attention deficit hyperactivity disorder (ADHD)
(C) autistic disorder
(D) oppositional defiant disorder
(E) conduct disorder

**129.** Which of the following agents is most useful in the management of a 28-year-old male patient who experiences cataplexy, hypnagogic hallucinations, and a very short rapid eye movement (REM) latency?

(A) A benzodiazepine
(B) A barbiturate
(C) An amphetamine
(D) An antipsychotic
(E) An opioid

**130.** A woman who had a normal delivery of a normal child 2 days ago tells her physician that she feels sad and cries for no reason. She appears well groomed and is taking congratulatory calls and visits from friends and family. Her physician should

(A) tell her to stop worrying
(B) have her call him daily over the next 2 weeks to report how she is feeling
(C) recommend a consultation with a psychiatrist
(D) prescribe an antidepressant
(E) prescribe a benzodiazepine

**131.** Although transplants can save many lives, there are fewer transplants done than are needed. Of the following, the primary reason for this is that

(A) there are not enough donors
(B) patients are usually too ill to withstand surgery
(C) transplants are too expensive
(D) transplants have a high chance of rejection
(E) the drugs used to prevent rejection are too toxic

**132.** A 22-year-old medical student has a parotid gland abscess and an excessive number of dental caries. She is of normal weight for her height, but seems distressed when the physician questions her about her eating habits. This young woman is most likely to have

(A) bulimia nervosa
(B) anorexia nervosa
(C) conversion disorder
(D) avoidant personality disorder
(E) passive-aggressive personality disorder

**133.** The adoptive parents of a newborn ask their physician when they should tell the child that she is adopted. The pediatrician correctly suggests that they tell her

(A) when she questions them about her background
(B) when she enters school
(C) as soon as possible
(D) at 4 years of age
(E) if she develops an illness that has a known genetic basis

**134.** An internist observes that one of her colleagues at the hospital, a surgeon, has been getting very intoxicated at social gatherings. The nurses, residents, and fellow physicians complain that the surgeon's notes are always late, illegible, or nonsensical. One of the internist's patients told her that he smelled alcohol on the breath of the surgeon. After ceasing to refer patients to him, the internist's next best course of action is to

(A) suggest to her colleagues that they also stop referring patients to the surgeon
(B) do nothing. She has done enough by ceasing to refer patients to the surgeon
(C) notify the police
(D) notify the state impaired physicians' program
(E) talk to the surgeon and tell him about her concerns

**135.** The autopsy of a 65-year-old man who was killed when he walked across the street without looking at the traffic light shows degeneration of cholinergic neurons in the hippocampus. In life, this man is most likely to have had which of the following disorders?

(A) Mania
(B) Depression
(C) Alzheimer disease
(D) Anxiety
(E) Schizophrenia

**136.** A woman, who gave birth to a healthy child 3 weeks ago, tells her doctor that since the birth, she has felt emotional and frightened and has had repeated thoughts that the baby would be better off without her as its mother. The patient is poorly groomed but the medical examination is unremarkable. The best explanation for this woman's feelings is:

(A) Normal postpartum reaction
(B) Adjustment disorder with depressed mood
(C) Major depressive disorder
(D) Adjustment disorder with conduct disturbance
(E) Generalized anxiety disorder

**137.** A 27-year-old woman who shows evidence of major depressive disorder reports that during the night she often wakes up, goes into the kitchen, and eats large amounts of chocolate candy or multiple bags of chips. After binging on these treats she puts her fingers down her throat to induce vomiting. Her body weight is normal and physical examination is unremarkable. Of the following antidepressants which would be the best initial choice for treating this patient?

(A) Fluoxetine
(B) Sertraline
(C) Bupropion
(D) Phenelzine
(E) Clomipramine

**138.** A 2-year-old girl who has reached all of her developmental milestones at the typical ages cannot seem to pay attention to a task for more than 15 minutes at a time in nursery school. She often gets out of her seat to walk around the room or to play on the floor. The girl plays with the other children but refuses to share her toys with them. Physical examination is unremarkable. The best explanation for this child's behavior is

(A) age-typical behavior
(B) attention deficit-hyperactivity disorder (ADHD)
(C) autism spectrum disorder (ASD)
(D) oppositional defiant disorder
(E) Rett's disorder

**139.** Parents of a typical 8-month-old girl ask their pediatrician what skills they can expect that their daughter will develop over the next 2 months. The physician's best response is

(A) speaking in two-word sentences
(B) crawling on hands and knees
(C) sitting unassisted
(D) climbing stairs
(E) walking unassisted

**140.** The Federal EMTALA act is most closely associated with which of the following?

(A) Control of emergent pathogens
(B) Reporting of impaired medical personnel
(E) Reporting of contagious illnesses
(D) Treatment of patients in hospital emergency rooms
(E) Confidentiality of medical information

**141.** Which of the following agents used to treat patients with Alzheimer disease is *not* an acetylcholinesterase inhibitor?

(A) Galantamine
(B) Rivastigmine
(C) Memantine
(D) Tacrine
(E) Donepezil

**142.** A 28-year-old woman with a family history of lupus visits the physician. Her symptoms include weakness and muscle aches. After physical examination and negative test results, the doctor tells the patient that she does not have lupus and in fact shows no signs of rheumatologic illness. That afternoon the patient calls another rheumatologist to make an appointment to be evaluated for lupus. The best explanation for this clinical picture is

(A) conversion disorder
(B) hypochondriasis
(C) PTSD
(D) malingering
(E) factitious disorder

**143.** Which of the following neurotransmitters is most likely to be metabolized to MHPG (3-methoxy-4-hydroxyphenylglycol)?

(A) Serotonin
(B) Norepinephrine
(C) Dopamine
(D) g-aminobutyric acid (GABA)
(E) Acetylcholine (Ach)
(F) Glutamate

**144.** A 76-year-old man whose wife died 1 month ago tells his physician that since her death he sometimes feels that he "does not want to go on." The patient denies suicidal plans and shows no evidence of psychotic thinking. He also reports that he sleeps well most nights and that his appetite is essentially normal. Physical examination and laboratory testing are unremarkable. Of the following, the most appropriate description of the patient's behavior at this time is

(A) adjustment disorder with depression
(B) adjustment disorder with anxiety
(C) major depressive disorder
(D) normal bereavement
(E) dysthymic disorder

**145.** Parents bring their 12-year-old daughter to the doctor. They are worried because the girl refuses to eat breakfast or lunch and has been losing weight over the past 3 months. The girl is 65 inches tall and weighs 110 pounds. Physical examination reveals that the girl is in Tanner Stage 3 and both this examination and laboratory test results are unremarkable. The next step in management is for the physician to

(A) speak to the parents alone
(B) speak to the girl alone
(C) speak to the girl and the parents together
(D) recommend a consultation with a specialist in adolescent eating disorders
(E) reassure the parents that the girl's behavior is normal

**146.** A 45-year-old man is admitted to the ICU for trauma-related injuries sustained in a car accident. Thirty-six hours after admission he becomes agitated. He is pulling at his IV access lines and is disoriented to place and time. His blood pressure is 190/110 mm Hg, and his pulse is 114/min. A reliable history from the patient's son reveals that the patient is dependent on alcohol. Which of the following is the most appropriate next step in management?

(A) Give haloperidol
(B) Give lithium
(C) Give lorazepam
(D) Give propranolol
(E) Refer to Alcoholics Anonymous

**147.** A 59-year-old woman tells her physician that she has been taking estrogen and progesterone replacement therapy since she stopped menstruating, 5 years ago. Compared with women of her age who have not taken hormone replacement therapy, this patient is likely to be at decreased risk for

(A) breast cancer
(B) uterine cancer
(C) cardiovascular disease
(D) osteoporosis
(E) depression

**148.** A 21-year-old student reports that he becomes very anxious when he must use a public restroom but otherwise does not report episodes of anxiety. Because he becomes so uncomfortable about using public restrooms, he refuses when his classmates ask him to join them when they go out. Of the following, the pharmacologic agent that has been approved for the long-term management of this student's symptoms is

(A) imipramine (Tofranil)
(B) chlordiazepoxide (Librium)
(C) clomipramine (Anafranil)
(D) venlafaxine (Effexor)
(E) clonazepam (Klonopin)

**149.** A 17-year-old college student comes to the physician complaining of facial swelling and pain. The student has a BMI of 17 and physical examination reveals a parotid gland abscess. The patient notes that she only eats healthy "diet" foods and then tells the doctor that sometimes she feels like her eating is "out of control." This clinical picture most closely suggests

**(A)** anorexia nervosa restricting type
**(B)** anorexia nervosa binge-eating/purging type
**(C)** bulimia nervosa binge-eating/purging type
**(D)** hypochondriasis
**(E)** acute stress disorder

**150.** Parents of a 45-year-old, mildly mentally retarded patient tell the doctor that the patient has recently started to experience memory loss. The doctor notes that the patient has odd facial features. The genetic abnormality most likely to be responsible for this clinical picture is most likely to be on chromosome

**(A)** 1
**(B)** 14
**(C)** 19
**(D)** 21
**(E)** 22

**151.** Since being started on a new antipsychotic medication, a 25-year-old female patient has begun to experience abnormal motor movements. She also reports that she has started to have a discharge from the nipples. Which of the following agents is most likely to be the new medication?

**(A)** Aripiprazole (Abilify)
**(B)** Olanzapine (Zyprexa)
**(C)** Ziprasidone (Geodon)
**(D)** Iloperidone (Fanapt)
**(E)** Lurasidone (Latuda)

**152.** A 43-year-old woman reports that since being put on an antidepressant, she has started to have difficulty having an orgasm. The medication that this patient is most likely to be taking is

**(A)** sertraline
**(B)** vilazodone
**(C)** mirtazapine
**(D)** duloxetine
**(E)** bupropion
**(F)** venlafaxine

**153.** A 36-year-old patient tells the physician that she is having difficult falling asleep. While the physical examination is essentially unremarkable, it reveals that the patient is about 8 weeks pregnant. If the doctor decides to prescribe something to help the patient fall asleep, which of the following agents should be avoided?

**(A)** Temazepam
**(B)** Buspirone
**(C)** Zolpidem
**(D)** Bupropion
**(E)** Zaleplon

**154.** Five hours after birth, a male infant begins to show excessive salivation and lacrimation. The doctor notes that the child, who has a rapid heart rate and appears restless and agitated, is sweating, although the room is cool. Prior to delivery, the mother of this infant is most likely to have used which of the following substances?

**(A)** PCP
**(B)** Cocaine
**(C)** Marijuana
**(D)** Alcohol
**(E)** Heroin

**155.** A 70-year old man, who, over the past year, has developed memory loss, spatial impairment, and language difficulties, has recently started to show a fine tremor and gait disturbances. The patient tells the doctor that he is also disturbed by vivid visual hallucinations. The patient's wife reports that at night the patient is very restless during sleep and often hits and punches her. Two days after being started on risperidone to control the hallucinations, the patient begins to show severe muscular rigidity. Aside from these symptoms, physical findings and laboratory studies are unremarkable. This clinical picture is most consistent with

**(A)** delirium
**(B)** Huntington disease
**(C)** Lewy body dementia
**(D)** Alzheimer disease
**(E)** acquired immunodeficiency syndrome

# Answers and Explanations

1. **The answer is B.** While smoking, red meat and alcohol, and working as a police officer are related to long-term mortality, the leading cause of death in people under age 35 is motor vehicle accidents, particularly when passengers fail to wear seat belts (and see Chapter 24). So, as in children (and see Chapter 24, Question 1), the most important recommendation for decreasing mortality in the short- or long-term for this patient is for her to consistently wear a seat belt in the car.

2. **The answer is B.** The most likely explanation for this student's behavior which began with a stressful life event (going away to college) is adjustment disorder (with depressive symptoms). This student's behavior is not normal homesickness because her symptoms are affecting her ability to function (e.g., she is in danger of failing her courses). The absence of a previous psychiatric history or suicidal thinking and the fact that she can enjoy time with friends indicates that her symptoms would probably not fulfill criteria for an anxiety or mood disorder. The fact that the stressor provoking the symptoms was not life-threatening rules out acute stress disorder (see also Chapter 13).

3. **The answer is C.** This 48-year-old man who believes that his fellow employees are conspiring to get him fired is most likely to have delusional disorder, paranoid type. This disorder is characterized by one chronic and fixed non-bizarre delusional system such as this patient's belief in a non-existent conspiracy. Because there is no other evidence of a thought disorder, schizophrenia is ruled out. Personality disorders are not characterized by frank delusions such as the one this patient exhibits.

4. **The answer is E.** This patient with sinus tachycardia, flattening of T waves, and prolonged QT interval is most likely to be taking a tricyclic antidepressant such as imipramine. Fluoxetine, bupropion, lorazepam, and sertraline are less likely than imipramine to cause these cardiac symptoms.

5. **The answer is A.** The physician's most appropriate response to this patient's comment is "Tell me about the problems." The physician should first get all of the information about the problem before reassuring the patient or suggesting a course of action.

6. **The answer is C.** Most correctly the physician should follow the current wishes of the patient and not put him on life support. The current preference of the patient was expressed directly to the doctor, so the prior written instructions no longer apply. The hospital chaplain, ethics committee, or court order are not involved in this decision since the patient's wishes have been directly expressed to and documented by the doctor.

7. **The answer is D.** This man is showing normal bereavement. In the first 2 months after the death of a close relative, many patients have occasional thoughts that life is no longer worth living. Because this patient does not show frank suicidality, sleep problems, or eating problems, it is unlikely that he has major depressive disorder. Dysthymic disorder involves at least 2 years of mild depressive symptoms. Adjustment disorder cannot be diagnosed when bereavement is a more appropriate description.

8. **The answer is B.** The most appropriate diagnosis for this manic patient is bipolar I disorder. While a single episode of mania defines this illness, this patient also has a history of depression. The grandiose religious belief that this patient exhibits is a delusion and delusions are not seen in hypomania (hypomania and depression characterize bipolar II disorder). Brief psychotic disorder and schizophrenia both involve psychotic symptoms such as delusions, but, in contrast to this patient, the delusions must occur independent of elevation or depression of mood.

9. **The answer is D**. Chromosome 16 is associated with tuberous sclerosis (TSC) (see Table 4.1), a rare genetic disorder that causes benign tumors to grow in the brain and in other organs leading to seizures, mental retardation, and autistic behavior. Skin abnormalities such as forehead plaques are also seen in TSC. TSC is caused by a mutation on one of two genes, TSC1 on chromosome 9 or TSC2 on chromosome 16.

10. **The answer is D**. Because he engages in behavior that is dangerous and would be considered illegal in an adult, the most likely cause of this child's difficulties is conduct disorder. While children with oppositional defiant disorder, attention deficit hyperactivity disorder, or adjustment disorder also may show behavioral problems they are unlikely to harm pets or set fires.

11. **The answer is A**. Most appropriately, the doctor should talk to the patient alone. While the mother and brother obviously want to help, the doctor must first elicit the teen's perspective on the issue privately and then address it. The patient can indicate whether or not he wants his mother and brother to be involved. Patients must recognize that there is a problem and indicate that they are willing to change their behavior before change can begin.

12. **The answer is E**. The most likely reason that this patient would not hit the other patients in the day care center is that he would not want them to hit him back. Like a 2-year-old child (the patient's mental age), this patient's main interest is in getting pleasure and avoiding pain. He has not yet developed a superego (typically developed after age 6 in children with normal intelligence) and so will not feel badly later. Like any 2-year-old, he is also unlikely to care about hurting the other patients, whether or not they like him, or invoking anger in the teacher.

13. **The answer is D**. This woman is now at the highest risk for osteoporosis, a sequela of anorexia nervosa. Dermatitis and osteoarthritis are not associated with a history of anorexia nervosa. In biliary atresia, ducts to transport bile from the liver to the duodenum fail to develop in a fetus. Amenorrhea usually resolves when a patient with anorexia nervosa recovers from the illness.

14. **The answer is C**. Memantine (Namenda), an N-Methyl-D-aspartate (NMDA) receptor antagonist, is approved to slow deterioration in patients with moderate to severe Alzheimer disease. While also used to treat Alzheimer disease, tacrine (Cognex), donepezil (Aricept), rivastigmine (Exelon), and galantamine (Remiryl) are all acetylcholinesterase inhibitors.

15. **The answer is C**. Of the listed agents, the most appropriate one to treat sleep apnea in this patient is medroxyprogesterone acetate (Provera). Progesterone raises resting ventilation in patients with decreased respiratory drive, and overweight post-menopausal women with sleep apnea such as this patient can benefit. While they may be used to treat sleep apnea in some patients, protriptyline and other tricyclic antidepressants are less effective for patients such as this than hormone treatment. Benzodiazepines such as diazepam and alprazolam can promote sleep but are not useful in sleep apnea.

16. **The answer is A**. The physician's next step is to ask the patient about his relationship with his caretakers. Elder abuse is a real possibility in this case, particularly since the patient seems to be avoiding eye contact. Assessing the patient for a cognitive disorder or ordering measures to protect the patient (if necessary) can wait until the patient is questioned about his caretakers.

17. **The answer is B**. Overdose of cocaine is most likely to have caused the seizure in this patient. Withdrawal from benzodiazepines such as alprazolam also can cause seizures, but this patient had alprazolam in her system and so is unlikely to be in withdrawal. Marijuana overdose, marijuana withdrawal, and cocaine withdrawal are not associated with seizures.

18. **The answer is E**. As children with chronic illnesses such as asthma reach their teen years, they are less likely to adhere to treatment that sets them apart from other teens.

The most effective way to increase adherence in such teenagers is to encourage inter-action with other teens who have the same condition. Frightening the boy, or recom-mending counseling or going to the school nurse will not be effective in increasing his adherence. Oral medication for asthma may not be medically appropriate for this patient.

19. **The answer is A.** The type of drug most likely to have caused this problem is an anti-depressant agent, namely a monoamine oxidase inhibitor. These agents block the breakdown of tyramine (a pressor) in the gastrointestinal tract as well as in the brain, resulting in elevated blood pressure, occipital headache, and other serious symptoms following ingestion of tyramine-rich foods (e.g., cheese and red wine).

20. **The answer is B.** Being divorced and being male are high-risk factors for suicide.

21. **The answer is E.** Because their cause is completely physiological, hot flashes or flushes are the symptom of menopause most likely to be seen in 50-year-old women in all cultures. The "empty-nest" syndrome, depression, anxiety, and insomnia are more closely associated with societal factors and so are more likely to differ across cultures.

22. **The answer is E.** Patients and physicians commonly prefer selective serotonin reuptake inhibitors (SSRIs) to tricyclic antidepressants because SSRIs have fewer side effects and thus are more likely to be well tolerated. Both groups of antidepressants have similar action on mood and sleep. All take 3–4 weeks to work and neither group is particularly effective at lowering blood pressure.

23. **The answer is F.** This treatment technique in which a phobic patient is taught relaxa-tion techniques and is then exposed to increased "doses" of the feared object is best described as systematic desensitization (see Chapter 7).

24. **The answer is B.** Because it is likely to cause the least exertion for the patient, the physician's best recommendation is face to face, female superior (woman on the top). To enhance the patient's recovery, the couple should be encouraged to return to their normal activities (including sex) as soon as it is safe to do so. Avoiding sexual activity can delay the patient's recovery.

25. **The answer is C.** Poor physical care, bruises, and abrasions in this demented elderly patient indicate that he has been neglected and abused. Even though he denies that anyone has harmed him, the most likely abuser is his daughter. Therefore, the most appropriate action for the physician to take after treating this patient is to contact the appropriate state social service agency. As in cases of child abuse, speaking to the likely abuser about the physician's concerns is not necessary. The physician also can-not send the patient home with the likely abuser or with another relative. The social service agency will deal with the patient's ultimate placement. If necessary, a neuro-logic evaluation can be done at a later date.

26. **The answer is A.** Hispanic Americans have longer life expectancies than African Americans, white Americans, or Native Americans.

27. **The answer is B.** While some Americans may understand that it is therapeutic to dis-cuss your internal emotional problems with others or that unconscious conflicts can be manifested as physical illness, a significant number of Americans believe that men-tal illness is a sign of personal weakness or failure. Many also believe that mentally ill people have poor self-control. For these and other reasons, many mentally ill people do not seek help.

28. **The answer is C.** In persons with delusional disorder (paranoid type), paranoid delu-sions (i.e., neighbors entering one's home at night) are present without abnormal thought processes. Absence of affective symptoms makes the diagnosis of bipolar disorder and schizoaffective disorder unlikely. Social withdrawal but no frank delu-sions characterize schizoid personality disorder (see also answers to Questions 3 and 29).

29. **The answer is C.** This woman who believes that she is pregnant with the child of a celebrity probably has another type of delusional disorder, the erotomanic type (see also answers to Questions 3 and 28).

30. **The answer is A.** Pregnancy and childbirth are more likely to cause death in this 40-year-old woman than any contraceptive technique.

31. **The answer is C.** The colleague's best response is "Reassure patients that the skin condition you have is not contagious." It is better to face the problem than to act like nothing is wrong or to put patients off by telling them it is not their problem. The physician should be encouraged to see patients and deal with the problem openly rather than to avoid questions by wearing long-sleeved shirts or avoiding social interaction.

32. **The answer is B.** The usual standards of doctor–patient confidentiality apply to the recently bereaved woman who has not expressed a plan and is currently not at high risk to kill herself. In contrast, the depressed woman who tells her physician that she has saved up 50 Nembutal tablets (has a suicidal plan) and wants to die is at high risk to kill herself. Other exceptions to confidentiality include patients who commit child abuse, put their sexual partners at risk for HIV infection, or indicate that they plan to harm someone (see also answer to Question 7).

33. **The answer is C.** The most appropriate action for Doctor A to take is to report Doctor B to his superior at the hospital. Reporting of a lapse by a colleague is required ethically because patients must be protected. Talking to Doctor B about his lapse again, warning him, reporting to the police, or recommending a transfer is not likely to accomplish the immediate goal of protecting patients.

34. **The answer is G.** The Folstein Mini-mental State Examination is used to follow improvement or deterioration in patients with suspected neurologic dysfunction. Positron emission tomography (PET) localizes physiologically active brain areas by measuring glucose metabolism. Computed tomography (CT) identifies organically based brain changes, such as enlarged ventricles. The Thematic Apperception Test (TAT) utilizes drawings depicting ambiguous social situations to evaluate unconscious conflicts. The sodium amobarbital (Amytal) interview is used to determine whether psychological factors are responsible for behavioral symptoms. The electroencephalogram (EEG), which measures electrical activity in the cortex, is useful in diagnosing epilepsy and in differentiating delirium from dementia. The Wide Range Achievement Test (WRAT) is used clinically to evaluate reading, arithmetic, and other school-related skills in patients. The Glasgow Coma Scale quantifies level of consciousness on a scale of 3 to 15.

35. **The answer is D.** The Thematic Apperception Test (TAT) utilizes drawings depicting ambiguous social situations to evaluate unconscious conflicts in patients (see answer to Question 34).

36. **The answer is B.** Typically, infants begin to roll over from back to belly and belly to back at about 5 months of age.

37. **The answer is B.** Legal intoxication is defined by blood alcohol concentrations of 0.05%–0.15%, depending on individual state law.

38. **The answer is G.** Protriptyline is less sedating than doxepin, nortriptyline, amitriptyline and imipramine and thus is the most appropriate heterocyclic antidepressant for someone who must stay alert on the job. While fluoxetine is also unlikely to be sedating, it is a selective serotonin reuptake inhibitor (SSRI), not a heterocyclic agent.

39. **The answer is F.** This elderly woman who reports that she has difficulty sleeping through the night because of muscular contractions in her legs is showing evidence of nocturnal myoclonus.

40. **The answer is E.** Intellectualization, using the mind's higher functions to avoid experiencing emotion associated with the likelihood of crashing, is the defense mechanism being used by this pilot.

41. **The answer is D.** Typically, children begin to walk unassisted between 12 and 15 months of age.

42. **The answer is B.** The treatment technique described here is biofeedback. In this treatment, the patient is given ongoing physiologic information about the tension in the frontalis muscle and learns to use mental techniques to control this tension.

43. **The answer is D.** This patient who has a full night's sleep but does not feel fully awake until hours after he first wakes up is showing evidence of a sleep disorder known as sleep drunkenness. This condition is rare and the diagnosis can only be made in the absence of other more common problems during sleep (e.g., sleep apnea) or substance abuse.

44. **The answer is C.** Tachycardia (increased heart rate) is seen with the use of all of the stimulant drugs, including caffeine. Stimulant drugs also tend to increase energy, blood pressure, and gastric acid secretion, and improve mood.

45. **The answer is A.** The social smile commonly first appears at about 2 months of age in typical infants.

46. **The answer is F.** The Wide Range Achievement Test (WRAT) is clinically used to evaluate reading, arithmetic, and other school-related skills in patients (see also answer 34).

47. **The answer is C.** Slow waves are characteristic of delta sleep (stages 3 and 4).

48. **The answer is A.** Infants can visually track a human face and objects starting at birth.

49. **The answer is E.** Like the pilot in Question 40, this physician, who has been given a diagnosis of terminal pancreatic cancer, is using the defense mechanism of intellectualization (i.e., he is using his intellect and knowledge to avoid experiencing the frightening emotions associated with his illness).

50. **The answer is A.** By acting out, the teenager's unacceptable anxious and depressed feelings are expressed in actions (stealing a car).

51. **The answer is C.** By using denial, this woman unconsciously refuses to believe, what to her is the intolerable fact, that she has breast cancer.

52. **The answer is F.** This patient is using the defense mechanism of reaction formation, which involves adopting behavior (i.e., complimenting the physician) that is the opposite of the way she really feels (i.e., anger toward the physician).

53. **The answer is G.** This woman is showing evidence of the avoidant personality disorder. Because she is overly sensitive to rejection, she has become socially withdrawn. In contrast to the schizoid patient who prefers to be alone, this patient is interested in meeting people but is unable to do so because of her shyness, feelings of inferiority, and timidity.

54. **The answer is H.** This behavior is most closely associated with the histrionic personality disorder. Persons with this disorder are dramatic when reporting their symptoms to physicians, and call attention to themselves with their dress and behavior.

55. **The answer is D.** Intense hunger, tiredness, and headache are all signs of withdrawal from an amphetamine.

56. **The answer is B.** The history of insomnia indicates that this patient may have been given a prescription for a barbiturate such as secobarbital (Seconal). His history of depression further suggests that he has taken an overdose of the drug in a suicide attempt.

57. **The answer is C.** Use of both phencyclidine (PCP) and lysergic acid diethylamide (LSD) results in feelings of altered body state such as this patient describes. However, in contrast to LSD, increased aggressivity and nystagmus (i.e., abnormal horizontal or vertical eye movements) are seen particularly with PCP use.

58. **The answer is C.** Withdrawal from caffeine and other stimulant drugs is associated with headache, lethargy, depression, and increased appetite. Pupil dilation is associated with the use of, rather than withdrawal from, stimulants.

59. **The answer is H.** The Glasgow Coma Scale (scores range from 3–15) is used to evaluate the level of consciousness in patients (see also answer to Question 34).

60. **The answer is B.** Alpha waves are associated with the awake relaxed state with eyes closed.

61. **The answer is E.** This woman has symptoms of functional dyspareunia (i.e., physically unexplained pain with sexual intercourse).

62. **The answer is B.** Within the first 2 months of an important loss, people may respond intensely. They may even have the illusion that they see the dead person. The physician should provide support and reassurance since this patient probably is experiencing a normal grief reaction. While limited use of medications for sleep is appropriate, antipsychotic or antidepressant medications are not indicated in the management of normal grief.

63. **The answer is C.** The monozygotic twin of a person with schizophrenia has about a 50% chance of developing the disorder. The child of one parent with schizophrenia or the dizygotic twin of a patient with schizophrenia has about a 10% chance, and the child of two parents with schizophrenia has about a 40% chance. Environmental events such as being raised in an institutional setting are not risk factors for schizophrenia.

64. **The answer is E.** Feeling that one is personally responsible for a major disaster when one had nothing to do with it is a delusion in this depressed 49-year-old man. His other statements, while indicating feelings of inadequacy and hopelessness, are commonly seen in depression but do not suggest psychotic thinking.

65. **The answer is B.** Parents cannot refuse life-saving treatment for their child for any reason. Because there is no time before the child must have the transfusion, treatment can proceed on an emergency basis. There is no reason to threaten the parents with legal action.

66. **The answer is D.** This patient shows evidence of conversion disorder. This disorder involves neurological symptoms with no physical cause occurring after a stressful life event. Sensory loss in patients with conversion disorder appears suddenly. Patients with this disorder are more likely to be young and female. They frequently show "la belle indifférence," a curious lack of concern about the dramatic symptom.

67. **The answer is C.** Long-term psychiatric hospitals are owned and operated primarily by state governments.

68. **The answer is B.** Patients with dissociative fugue, a dissociative disorder, wander away from their homes and do not know how they got to another destination. This memory loss and wandering often occur following a stressful life event, in this case the patient's loss of his wife.

69. **The answer is E.** Huntington disease commonly first appears between the ages of 35 and 45 years. Lesch-Nyhan syndrome and Rett Disorder are apparent during childhood; schizophrenia usually appears in adolescence or early adulthood; Alzheimer disease most commonly appears in old age.

70. **The answer is E.** Retinal pigmentation is primarily associated with use of the low-potency antipsychotic agent thioridazine.

71. **The answer is E.** Delta waves are seen in non-REM sleep stages 3 and 4. Penile and clitoral erection, increased pulse, increased respiration, elevated blood pressure, dreaming, and complete relaxation of skeletal muscles are all seen in REM sleep.

72. **The answer is B**. Of the disorders listed, the largest sex difference in the occurrence of a disorder is seen in major depressive disorder. Two times more women than men are diagnosed with this disorder. There is no significant sex difference in the occurrence of schizophrenia, cyclothymic disorder, hypochondriasis, or bipolar disorder.

73. **The answer is A**. Negative predictive value is the probability that a person with a negative test is actually well.

74. **The answer is A**. Rising of the uterus in the pelvic cavity with sexual activity (i.e., "the tenting effect") first occurs during the excitement phase of the sexual response cycle.

75. **The answer is B**. The sexual partner, e.g., the wife, applies the squeeze in the squeeze technique, a method used to delay ejaculation in men who ejaculate prematurely. In this technique, the man identifies a point at which ejaculation can still be prevented. He then instructs his partner to apply gentle pressure to the corona of the penis. The erection then subsides and ejaculation is delayed.

76. **The answer is C**. Analysis of variance is used to examine differences among means of more than two samples or groups. In this example there are three samples (i.e., age groups).

77. **The answer is B**. This man has secondary erectile dysfunction, problems with erection occurring after a period of normal functioning. Alcohol use is commonly associated with secondary erectile dysfunction.

78. **The answer is A**. The odds–risk ratio (odds ratio) of 2 in this case-control study is calculated as follows

|  | Liquid Crystal Display (LCD) Exposure | No LCD Exposure |
| --- | --- | --- |
| Women who miscarried | A = 10 | B = 40 |
| Women who carried to term | C = 10 | D = 80 |

**Odds ratio** = $(A)(D)/(B)(C) = (10)(80)/(40)(10) = 2$.

79. **The answer is E**. In a cohort study, the ratio of the incidence rate of a condition (e.g., miscarriage) in exposed people to the incidence rate in unexposed people is the relative risk.

80. **The answer is B. 81. The answer is E**. The attributable risk is the incidence rate in exposed people (5.0) minus the incidence rate in unexposed people (0.5) = 4.5. Therefore, 4.5 is the additional risk of getting TB associated with living with someone with TB. The relative risk is the incidence rate in exposed people (5.0) divided by the incidence rate in unexposed people (0.5) = 10.0. Therefore, the chances of getting TB are 10 times greater when living with someone who has TB than when living in a household in which no one has TB.

82. **The answer is B**. The odds–risk ratio is used to estimate the relative risk (i.e., estimated relative risk) in a case-control study.

83. **The answer is B**. This patient is most likely to have major depressive disorder. Evidence for this is missing work, feeling hopeless and tired, losing >5% of body weight, and having trouble sleeping. Suicidal ideation is shown by her reference to death (i.e., "Doctor, the Lord calls all his children home").

84. **The answer is E**. As it is only 2 weeks since the traumatic event occurred, this patient is most likely to have acute stress disorder. Post-traumatic stress disorder (PTSD) cannot be diagnosed until at least 1 month has passed after the traumatic event. Obsessive-compulsive disorder (OCD) is an anxiety disorder characterized by obsessions and compulsions, and panic disorder is characterized by sudden attacks of intense anxiety and a feeling that one is about to die. In OCD, generalized anxiety disorder, and panic disorder, there is no obvious precipitating event.

85. **The answer is A.** After a life-threatening event, hypervigilance (e.g., jumping at every loud noise), flashbacks (re-experiencing of the event), and persistent anxiety suggest PTSD. Acute stress disorder can only be diagnosed within 1 month of the traumatic event (see also answer 84).

86. **The answer is C.** Using recapitulation, the interviewer sums up all of the information given by the patient to ensure that it has been correctly documented.

87. **The answer is B.** "Many people feel the way you do when they first need hospitalization" is an example of the interview technique known as validation. In validation, the interviewer gives credence to the patient's feelings and fears.

88. **The answer is E.** "You say that you felt the pain more in the evening?" is an example of the interview technique known as reflection.

89. **The answer is A.** Commenting on body language indicating anxiety and noting inconsistencies between verbal responses and body language demonstrate the interviewing technique known as confrontation.

90. **The answer is D.** Suddenly feeling anxious, becoming dizzy, and feeling like one cannot breathe when exposed to an open area are manifestations of a panic attack with agoraphobia.

91. **The answer is C.** In an illusion, an individual misperceives a real external stimulus. In this case, the individual has seen someone but has interpreted the person as being her father. Illusions are not uncommon in a normal grief reaction (and see also answer to Chapter 3, Question 14)

92. **The answer is F.** Positron emission tomography (PET) scans, which are used mainly as research tools, can localize metabolically active brain areas in persons who are performing specific tasks.

93. **The answer is C.** Auditory evoked potentials, the responses of the brain to sound as measured by electrical activity, are used to evaluate loss of hearing in infants.

94. **The answer is D.** In malingering, the patient pretends that she is ill in order to realize an obvious (e.g., financial) gain.

95. **The answer is C.** In factitious disorder (formerly Munchausen syndrome), the patient simulates illness for medical attention. The gain to this patient, attention from a physician, is not obvious as it is in the malingering patient (see also answer to Question 94).

96. **The answer is C.** Early morning awakening is a type of insomnia that is commonly seen in people with major depressive disorder.

97. **The answer is D.** Patients with obstructive sleep apnea are frequently unaware that they have awakened often during the night because they cannot breathe. They snore loudly and often become chronically tired.

98. **The answer is C.** Conversion disorder involves a dramatic loss of motor or sensory function with no medical cause. There is often a curious lack of concern ("la belle indifférence") about the symptoms. Hypochondriasis is an exaggerated concern with illness or normal bodily functions. People with body dysmorphic disorder feel that there is something seriously wrong with their appearance. In somatization disorder, patients have many different physical symptoms over many years that have no biological cause. In somatoform pain disorder, a patient has long-lasting unexplainable pain (and see also answer to Question 66).

99. **The answer is A.** This patient is showing evidence of hypochondriasis, an exaggerated concern with illness (see also answer to Question 98).

100. **The answer is A.** In operant conditioning, a non-reflexive behavior, such as a dog turning a doorknob, is learned by using reinforcement, such as a treat.

101. **The answer is G.** In this example of negative reinforcement, a patient increases his behavior (e.g., going to physical therapy sessions) in order to reduce an aversive stimulus (e.g., his shoulder pain).

102. **The answer is D.** This woman is most likely to have delirium caused by the high fever.

103. **The answer is B.** Facial tics, cursing, and grimacing seen in this young man are symptoms of Tourette disorder.

104. **The answer is C.** This patient is most likely to have Alzheimer disease. Because her level of attention is normal, this is not delirium. There is no evidence of depression (pseudodementia) and this patient has no history of alcohol abuse to suggest amnestic disorder.

105. **The answer is C.** This statement is an example of the Kübler-Ross stage of dying known as bargaining.

106. **The answer is B.** In aversive conditioning, an unwanted behavior (nail biting) is paired with an unpleasant stimulus (noxious-tasting substance) and the behavior ceases.

107. **The answer is D.** Because it is less likely than the benzodiazepines (e.g., diazepam) to cause dependence, the best choice of medication for this patient with generalized anxiety disorder (i.e., chronic anxiety) is buspirone. Lithium is used to treat bipolar disorder, and while it can be helpful, fluoxetine is more likely to be used to treat other anxiety disorders, such as obsessive-compulsive disorder.

108. **The answer is A.** Head Start and educational programs like it are examples of primary prevention, mechanisms to reduce the incidence of a problem (e.g., school failure) by reducing its associated risk factors (e.g., lack of educational enrichment).

109. **The answer is A.** Repression, the defense mechanism in use when unacceptable emotions are prevented from reaching awareness, is the defense mechanism on which all others are based.

110. **The answer is E.** Most appropriately, the physician should tell the patient that she can take her time and not try to speak while she is crying.

111. **The answer is D.** The parent's concerns are real. Therefore, to take no further action is not an acceptable choice for the physician. The physician's most appropriate recommendation is to recommend a long-acting contraceptive for this young woman. Permanent forms of birth control, such as tubal ligation or oophorectomy, are not appropriate. Preventing her from going to the school for fear of pregnancy could limit the social, academic, and employment potential of this young woman.

112. **The answer is B.** Using the intelligence quotient (IQ) formula (i.e., mental age [MA]/chronological age [CA] $\times$ 100 = IQ), the MA of this child is 3 years (MA/6 $\times$ 100 = 50). Like a typical 3-year-old child, someone with a mental age of 3 years can identify colors but cannot read, copy a triangle, ride a two-wheeled bicycle, or understand the moral difference between right and wrong.

113. **The answer is D.** Prior to treating the 16-year-old patient, the physician should recommend that he tell his sexual partner(s). There is no need to break doctor–patient confidentiality by telling the sexual partner(s) since the illness is not life-threatening. Parents do not have to be told or give permission to treat sexually transmitted diseases in teenagers. Genital herpes is not generally reportable to state or federal health authorities.

114. **The answer is E.** With respect to physical, social, and cognitive/verbal development, respectively, this 9-month-old child is best described as normal, normal, normal. Children can sit unassisted and pull themselves up to stand by about age 10 months. At about age 7 months, children begin to show stranger anxiety (the baby-sitter is

essentially a stranger because the child sees her only once a week). Children commonly do not speak using understandable words until they are about 1-year old.

115. **The answer is E.** This child's motor skills (e.g., walking up stairs 1 foot at a time, scribbling when told to copy a circle) and social skills (e.g., moving away from and then toward his mother) indicate that this child is about $1^1/_2$ years old. With respect to verbal skills, children of this age are able to use about 10 individual words. Children 3 years of age use about 900 words, understand about 3,500 words, and speak in complete sentences. At about 4 years of age, children use prepositions (e.g., below, under) in speech.

116. **The answer is B.** A statement such as "I have a gun in my house" made to a physician is a warning sign suggesting that this patient is planning to harm himself or someone else. Therefore, the most appropriate action for the physician to take at this time is to suggest that the patient remain in the hospital for further evaluation. If the patient refuses, he can be held against his will for a limited period of time. Informing the wife of the threat, removing the gun, or avoiding dangerous medications are useful strategies, but will not prevent the dangerous act from occurring.

117. **The answer is D.** The mechanism that is likely to underlie this man's preoccupation with bond trading is that he makes money on a variable ratio reinforcement schedule. Since he never knows how many trades he has to make to get reinforcement (i.e., money), his preoccupation persists (i.e., is resistant to extinction) on weekends even though he cannot receive reinforcement because the markets are closed.

118. **The answer is B.** Most typical 3-year-old children can ride a tricycle, speak in complete sentences, and play in parallel with (next to) other children. They generally do not play cooperatively with other children until about 4 years of age. Thus, this child may need evaluation in motor skills (e.g., he should be able to pedal a tricycle), but is typical in language and social skills.

119. **The answer is C.** The physician should reassure this 14-year-old boy that masturbation is normal. Any amount of masturbation is normal, provided it does not prevent a person from having an active, successful life. There is no dysfunction in this boy and it is not appropriate to notify his parents, refer him to a psychologist, measure his testosterone level, or tell him to become involved in school sports.

120. **The answer is B.** One year after the last menstrual period usually signals the end of menopause, and the use of birth control can be discontinued. The age of menopause and the occurrence of hot flashes vary considerably among women and thus cannot be used to predict the end of fertility.

121. **The answer is B.** Helping other children to adjust to the hospital is an example of this 8-year-old girl's use of the defense mechanism of sublimation. In sublimation, the child reroutes her own unconscious, anxious feelings about her hospitalization into socially acceptable behavior (e.g., helping other frightened children).

122. **The answer is H.** Because Medicare coverage lasts for life and because she has the longest life expectancy, a white female nonsmoker is likely to use more Medicare services and funds than men, African Americans, and smokers during her lifetime.

123. **The answer is D.** This child is most likely to be 36 months of age. At age 3 years, children can use about 900 words and stack nine blocks. They are also able to spend a few hours away from their primary caregiver each day.

124. **The answer is B.** The most likely reason for a physician to be sued for malpractice is that the physician had poor rapport with a patient. The doctor–patient relationship is the most important factor in whether or not a patient will sue a physician. The physician's medical or surgical skills have less to do with whether or not the physician will be sued by a patient.

**125. The answer is B.** The most appropriate action for the physician is to follow the wishes of the neighbor. In this example, the neighbor can decide whether or not to continue life support since she has assumed the power to speak for the patient by virtue of the document giving her durable power of attorney.

**126. The answer is C.** Most elderly Americans spend the last 5 years of their lives living on their own in their own residences. Approximately 5% end up in nursing homes and 20% live with family members. Hospice care is aimed at people expected to die within 6 months. Hospital stays currently average only 4.8 days.

**127. The answer is B.** The most effective intervention for this 85-year-old patient with Alzheimer disease, who wanders out of the house, is to label all the doors. She may wander out because she no longer knows where each door leads. Medications can be helpful for associated symptoms (e.g., diazepam for anxiety) and to delay further decline (e.g., donepezil, an acetylcholinesterase inhibitor), but cannot replace lost function. Nursing home placement should be considered if the caregiver wishes it. Long-term use of restraints is never appropriate.

**128. The answer is D.** Since this child's problem is with authority figures like his parents and teachers, the best description for his behavior is oppositional defiant disorder. He reads and communicates well and there is no evidence of attention deficit hyperactivity disorder (ADHD) or autistic disorder. Because this child relates well to the other children in school, he is unlikely to have conduct disorder.

**129. The answer is C.** Cataplexy, hypnagogic hallucinations, and a very short rapid eye movement (REM) latency indicate that this patient has narcolepsy. Amphetamines are more likely than benzodiazepines, barbiturates, antipsychotics, or opioids to be used in the management of narcolepsy.

**130. The answer is B.** The physician's most appropriate action is to have this patient call him over the next few weeks to report how she is feeling. This woman has the "baby blues" (i.e., sadness for no obvious reason after a normal delivery). There is no specific treatment for baby blues and the symptoms usually disappear within 2 weeks. However, because some women with the baby blues go on to develop a major depressive episode requiring treatment, the physician should speak to this patient daily until her symptoms remit.

**131. The answer is A.** Fewer transplants are done than are needed primarily because there are not enough people willing to donate their organs at death.

**132. The answer is A.** This young woman is most likely to have bulimia nervosa, an eating disorder characterized by binge eating and purging, but normal body weight. Parotid gland enlargement and abscesses and dental caries are seen in bulimia as a result of the forced vomiting.

**133. The answer is C.** The best time to tell a child she is adopted is as soon as possible, usually when the child can first understand language. Waiting any longer than this will increase the probability that someone else will tell the child before the parents are able to.

**134. The answer is D.** Reporting of an impaired colleague is required ethically because patients must be protected. If, as in this case, the colleague is a licensed physician, it is appropriate to notify the state impaired physicians' program. If the internist talks to the surgeon about her concerns, there is no guarantee that the surgeon will listen and that the patients will be protected. Reporting the surgeon to the police is not appropriate (and see Chapter 23).

**135. The answer is C.** Degeneration of cholinergic neurons in the hippocampus indicates that this man is most likely to have had Alzheimer disease. Mania, depression, anxiety, and schizophrenia are not specifically associated with degeneration of cholinergic neurons.

136. **The answer is C.** Tearfulness and over-emotionality are normal postpartum reactions, i.e., the "baby blues." However, because this patient has had symptoms including suicidality for 3 weeks, the best diagnosis is major depressive disorder (see also answer to Question 130).

137. **The answer is A.** Fluoxetine is the only listed agent that is indicated in the management of both major depressive disorder and bulimia. Bupropion should be avoided in patients with eating disorders because it lowers the seizure threshold.

138. **The answer is A.** This 2-year-old child is showing typical behavior for her age. A typical 2-year-old child cannot be expected to pay attention for more than a few minutes at a time. Typical 2-year-old children also do not yet play cooperatively with other children and commonly are reluctant to share their toys (see Chapter 1).

139. **The answer is B.** Typical infants begin to crawl on hands and knees between 9 and 11 months of age. In typical infants, sitting unassisted is seen at about 6 months, walking unassisted at about 12 months, climbing stairs at about 18 months, and speaking in two-word sentences at about 24 months (and see Chapter 1).

140. **The answer is D.** Hospitals are legally required to provide care to anyone needing emergency management whether they have the means to pay or not via the Emergency Medical Treatment and Active Labor Act (EMTALA).

141. **The answer is C.** Memantine is an NMDA receptor antagonist. Galantamine, rivastigmine, tacrine, and donepezil are acetylcholinesterase inhibitors.

142. **The answer is B.** The best explanation for this clinical picture is hypochondriasis. Despite negative findings, this patient continues to believe she has lupus and goes "doctor shopping," that is, she makes an appointment with another rheumatologist. There is no indication that this patient is malingering (there is no obvious gain from the symptoms) or factitious disorder (there is no evidence of a desire to be considered a sick person) and there is no evidence of a precipitating life-threatening stressor as in PTSD. Conversion disorder is not likely because the symptoms are chronic and not neurological and the patient is worried rather than indifferent.

143. **The answer is B.** The neurotransmitter most likely to be metabolized to MHPG (3-methoxy-4-hydroxyphenylglycol) is norepinephrine.

144. **The answer is D.** The most appropriate description of this patient's behavior is normal bereavement. Occasionally thinking that one does not want "to go on" is common in normal bereavement and this patient does not have suicidal plans. Because he sleeps and eats normally, major depressive disorder is not likely and his symptoms have not lasted long enough to diagnose dysthymic disorder. Adjustment disorder (see Chapter 13, Table 13-1.) cannot be diagnosed if death of a loved one was the life stressor that preceded the symptoms.

145. **The answer is B.** Because this girl is well into puberty (Tanner Stage 3 is the middle stage in adolescent sexual development, see Chapter 2), the next step in management is to speak to the girl alone. Whenever the problem (here a possible eating disorder) involves privacy issues in a post-pubescent patient, the doctor should first speak only to the patient (see Chapter 21 and Comprehensive Examination, Question 11). It is best for the physician to take the first step in management, referral to a specialist is not appropriate at this time.

146. **The answer is C.** This 45-year-old man is showing evidence of alcohol withdrawal. The most appropriate next step in the acute management of alcohol withdrawal is a benzodiazepine such as lorazepam. His history of drinking alcohol (as provided by his son), the delayed (36 hours) onset of agitation and disorientation, and elevated blood pressure and pulse indicate that he has become dependent on alcohol. Haloperidol, lithium, and propranolol are less likely to be useful for immediate management.

Referral to Alcoholics Anonymous typically is a long-term, not an immediate strategy in management.

147. **The answer is D.** In menopausal women, estrogen replacement therapy (ERT) is most closely associated with decreased risk for osteoporosis. ERT has also been associated with increased risk of breast cancer (when administered in combination with progesterone [P]) and uterine cancer (when administered without P), but not with prevention of cardiovascular disease or psychiatric illnesses such as depression.

148. **The answer is D.** This student's symptoms of anxiety in a public situation (e.g., using public restrooms) but not in other situations suggest that he has social phobia. This phobia has limited the patient's ability to socialize freely. While heterocyclic antidepressants such as imipramine and clomipramine, and benzodiazepines such as chlordiazepoxide and clonazepam may be helpful, venlafaxine (as well as paroxetine, sertraline and some MAOIs) is the only one of the listed agents that is approved to manage social phobia (see Table 16.3).

149. **The answer is B.** This clinical picture most closely suggests anorexia nervosa, binge-eating/purging type. Calluses on the knuckles (Russell sign) and the parotid gland abscess are evidence of self-induced vomiting. Because her BMI is only 17 she does not have bulimia nervosa, binge-eating/purging type. This patient neither worries excessively about her health, as would a person with hypochondriasis, nor does she report exposure to a life-threatening stressor, as would someone with acute stress disorder (and see also answer to Question 132).

150. **The answer is D.** Mild mental retardation and unusual facial features suggest that this patient has Down syndrome. Down syndrome patients who live to middle age commonly develop Alzheimer disease. Chromosome 21 is associated with both Down's syndrome and Alzheimer disease.

151. **The answer is E.** Abnormal motor movements and galactorrhea (fluid discharge from the nipples) are side effects of lurasidone. Aripiprazole, olanzapine, ziprasidone, and iloperidone are less likely to be associated with these adverse effects (see Table 16.2).

152. **The answer is A.** Like other SSRIs, sertraline is likely to cause sexual side effects such as delayed orgasm. Vilazodone, mirtazapine, duloxetine, bupropion, and venlafaxine have low rates of sexual side effects (see Table 16.3).

153. **The answer is A.** Temazepam, a hypnotic benzodiazepine, is in FDA pregnancy category X and so should be avoided in pregnant patients. In contrast, buspirone, zolpidem, and bupropion are in category A and zaleplon is in category B (see Table 16.5).

154. **The answer is E.** Salivation, lacrimation, rapid heart rate, sweating, restlessness, and agitation are signs of heroin withdrawal. Thus, the mother of this infant is most likely to have been using heroin and the infant is in withdrawal. Withdrawal from PCP, cocaine, marijuana, and alcohol are unlikely to produce this symptom picture.

155. **The answer is C.** This patient is showing evidence of Lewy body dementia. Patients with this disorder show signs of dementia similar to those of Alzheimer disease (e.g., memory loss and language difficulties), but they also show Parkinsonian symptoms (e.g., fine tremor and gait disturbances), psychotic symptoms (e.g., visual hallucinations), motor activity during REM sleep (REM sleep behavior disorder [see Chapter 10]), and hypersensitivity reactions to antipsychotic medications (e.g., muscular rigidity). Delirium is unlikely because the symptoms have been present over a long period and there are no significant medical findings. Huntington disease and acquired immunodeficiency syndrome do not fit this clinical picture.

# Index

Note: Page number followed by f and t indicates figure and table respectively.